Skeletal Radiology

Skeletal Radiology

Editor

Majid Chalian

MDPI • Basel • Beijing • Wuhan • Barcelona • Belgrade • Manchester • Tokyo • Cluj • Tianjin

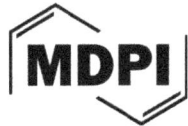

Editor
Majid Chalian
Department of Radiology
University of Washington
Seattle
United States

Editorial Office
MDPI
St. Alban-Anlage 66
4052 Basel, Switzerland

This is a reprint of articles from the Special Issue published online in the open access journal *Diagnostics* (ISSN 2075-4418) (available at: www.mdpi.com/journal/diagnostics/special_issues/ Skeletal_Radiology).

For citation purposes, cite each article independently as indicated on the article page online and as indicated below:

LastName, A.A.; LastName, B.B.; LastName, C.C. Article Title. *Journal Name* **Year**, *Volume Number*, Page Range.

ISBN 978-3-0365-8435-5 (Hbk)
ISBN 978-3-0365-8434-8 (PDF)

Cover image courtesy of Majid Chalian

© 2023 by the authors. Articles in this book are Open Access and distributed under the Creative Commons Attribution (CC BY) license, which allows users to download, copy and build upon published articles, as long as the author and publisher are properly credited, which ensures maximum dissemination and a wider impact of our publications.
The book as a whole is distributed by MDPI under the terms and conditions of the Creative Commons license CC BY-NC-ND.

Contents

About the Editor vii

Atefe Pooyan, Ehsan Alipour, Arash Azhideh and Majid Chalian
Editorial on Special Issue "Skeletal Radiology"
Reprinted from: *Diagnostics* **2023**, *13*, 2396, doi:10.3390/diagnostics13142396 1

Pooya Torkian, Javid Azadbakht, Pietro Andrea Bonaffini, Behrang Amini and Majid Chalian
Advanced Imaging in Multiple Myeloma: New Frontiers for MRI
Reprinted from: *Diagnostics* **2022**, *12*, 2182, doi:10.3390/diagnostics12092182 5

Mehrzad Shafiei, Firoozeh Shomal Zadeh, Bahar Mansoori, Hunter Pyle, Nnenna Agim and Jorge Hinojosa et al.
Imaging More than Skin-Deep: Radiologic and Dermatologic Presentations of Systemic Disorders
Reprinted from: *Diagnostics* **2022**, *12*, 2011, doi:10.3390/diagnostics12082011 17

Reza Talaie, Pooya Torkian, Alexander Clayton, Stephanie Wallace, Hoiwan Cheung and Majid Chalian et al.
Emerging Targets for the Treatment of Osteoarthritis: New Investigational Methods to Identify Neo-Vessels as Possible Targets for Embolization
Reprinted from: *Diagnostics* **2022**, *12*, 1403, doi:10.3390/diagnostics12061403 49

Sara Haseli, Bahar Mansoori, Mehrzad Shafiei, Firoozeh Shomal Zadeh, Hamid Chalian and Parisa Khoshpouri et al.
A Review of Posteromedial Lesions of the Chest Wall: What Should a Chest Radiologist Know?
Reprinted from: *Diagnostics* **2022**, *12*, 301, doi:10.3390/diagnostics12020301 61

Fatemeh Ezzati and Parham Pezeshk
Radiographic Findings of Inflammatory Arthritis and Mimics in the Hands
Reprinted from: *Diagnostics* **2022**, *12*, 2134, doi:10.3390/diagnostics12092134 93

Maryam Soltanolkotabi, Chris Mallory, Hailey Allen, Brian Y. Chan, Megan K. Mills and Richard L. Leake
Postoperative Findings of Common Foot and Ankle Surgeries: An Imaging Review
Reprinted from: *Diagnostics* **2022**, *12*, 1090, doi:10.3390/diagnostics12051090 109

Pietro Venezia, Ludovica Nucci, Serena Moschitto, Alessia Malgioglio, Gaetano Isola and Vincenzo Ronsivalle et al.
Short-Term and Long-Term Changes of Nasal Soft Tissue after Rapid Maxillary Expansion (RME) with Tooth-Borne and Bone-Borne Devices. A CBCT Retrospective Study.
Reprinted from: *Diagnostics* **2022**, *12*, 875, doi:10.3390/diagnostics12040875 125

Filippo Del Grande, Shivani Ahlawat, Edward McCarthy and Laura M. Fayad
Grade 1 and 2 Chondrosarcomas of the Chest Wall: CT Imaging Features and Review of the Literature
Reprinted from: *Diagnostics* **2022**, *12*, 292, doi:10.3390/diagnostics12020292 139

Fayaz Khan, Mohamed Faisal Chevidikunnan, Mashael Ghazi Alsobhi, Israa Anees Ibrahim Ahmed, Nada Saleh Al-Lehidan and Mohd Rehan et al.
Diagnostic Accuracy of Various Radiological Measurements in the Evaluation and Differentiation of Flatfoot: A Cross-Sectional Study
Reprinted from: *Diagnostics* **2022**, *12*, 2288, doi:10.3390/diagnostics12102288 149

Alberto Stefano Tagliafico, Clarissa Valle, Pietro Andrea Bonaffini, Ali Attieh, Matteo Bauckneht and Liliana Belgioia et al.
Myeloma Spine and Bone Damage Score (MSBDS) on Whole-Body Computed Tomography (WBCT): Multiple Reader Agreement in a Multicenter Reliability Study
Reprinted from: *Diagnostics* **2022**, *12*, 1894, doi:10.3390/diagnostics12081894 161

Adrián Cardín-Pereda, Daniel García-Sánchez, Nuria Terán-Villagrá, Ana Alfonso-Fernández, Michel Fakkas and Carlos Garcés-Zarzalejo et al.
Osteonecrosis of the Femoral Head: A Multidisciplinary Approach in Diagnostic Accuracy
Reprinted from: *Diagnostics* **2022**, *12*, 1731, doi:10.3390/diagnostics12071731 173

Andrea S. Klauser, Sylvia Strobl, Christoph Schwabl, Werner Klotz, Gudrun Feuchtner and Bernhard Moriggl et al.
Prevalence of Monosodium Urate (MSU) Deposits in Cadavers Detected by Dual-Energy Computed Tomography (DECT)
Reprinted from: *Diagnostics* **2022**, *12*, 1240, doi:10.3390/diagnostics12051240 183

Seyed Mohammad Gharavi, Yujie Qiao, Armaghan Faghihimehr and Josephina Vossen
Imaging of the Temporomandibular Joint
Reprinted from: *Diagnostics* **2022**, *12*, 1006, doi:10.3390/diagnostics12041006 195

Ki-Taek Hong, Yongwon Cho, Chang Ho Kang, Kyung-Sik Ahn, Heegon Lee and Joohui Kim et al.
Lumbar Spine Computed Tomography to Magnetic Resonance Imaging Synthesis Using Generative Adversarial Network: Visual Turing Test
Reprinted from: *Diagnostics* **2022**, *12*, 530, doi:10.3390/diagnostics12020530 211

Tzu-Herng Hsu, Che-Li Lin, Chin-Wen Wu, Yi-Wen Chen, Timporn Vitoonpong and Lien-Chieh Lin et al.
Accuracy of Critical Shoulder Angle and Acromial Index for Predicting Supraspinatus Tendinopathy
Reprinted from: *Diagnostics* **2022**, *12*, 283, doi:10.3390/diagnostics12020283 227

Miju Cheon and Jang Yoo
Visualization of Dialysis-Related Amyloid Arthropathy on ^{18}F-FDG PET-CT Scan
Reprinted from: *Diagnostics* **2022**, *12*, 113, doi:10.3390/diagnostics12010113 237

Hyo Jin Kim, Joon Woo Lee, Eugene Lee, Yusuhn Kang and Joong Mo Ahn
Incidence of Spinal CSF Leakage on CT Myelography in Patients with Nontraumatic Intracranial Subdural Hematoma
Reprinted from: *Diagnostics* **2021**, *11*, 2278, doi:10.3390/diagnostics11122278 241

About the Editor

Majid Chalian

Dr. Chalian is a Musculoskeletal Radiologist and an Associate Professor of Radiology at the University of Washington. He grew up in Tehran, Iran and received his M.D. from Iran University of Medical Sciences followed by Postdoctoral Research Fellowship in Musculoskeletal Imaging at the Johns Hopkins University. Dr. Chalian completed his Diagnostic Radiology Residency at Case Western Reserve University and his fellowship in Musculoskeletal Imaging and Intervention at University of Virginia. Dr. Chalian is a certified diplomate of the American Board of Radiology.

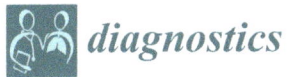

Editorial

Editorial on Special Issue "Skeletal Radiology"

Atefe Pooyan, Ehsan Alipour, Arash Azhideh and Majid Chalian *

Division of Musculoskeletal Imaging and Intervention, Department of Radiology, University of Washington, Seattle, WA 98105, USA; atefe@uw.edu (A.P.)
* Correspondence: mchalian@uw.edu; Tel.: +1-206-598-6868; Fax: +1-206-598-2847

Citation: Pooyan, A.; Alipour, E.; Azhideh, A.; Chalian, M. Editorial on Special Issue "Skeletal Radiology". *Diagnostics* 2023, 13, 2396. https://doi.org/10.3390/diagnostics13142396

Received: 11 July 2023
Accepted: 14 July 2023
Published: 18 July 2023

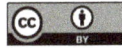

Copyright: © 2023 by the authors. Licensee MDPI, Basel, Switzerland. This article is an open access article distributed under the terms and conditions of the Creative Commons Attribution (CC BY) license (https://creativecommons.org/licenses/by/4.0/).

1. Introduction

Musculoskeletal (MSK) disorders are among the top five contributors to disability-adjusted life years (DALYs) worldwide [1]. These disorders include a wide range of conditions, spanning from fractures, sports injuries, rheumatoid arthritis, and musculoskeletal pain syndromes to those mostly affecting older age groups like osteoarthritis and osteoporosis. MSK conditions often present diagnostic challenges due to overlapping symptoms, complex anatomical aspects, and the variety of potential causes [2]. Imaging plays a pivotal role in diagnosing and guiding treatment for these disorders. In the past decade, the MSK radiology field has witnessed significant progress driven by breakthroughs in artificial intelligence (AI), the development of high-resolution equipment and novel imaging sequences, and the adoption of innovative multidisciplinary approaches. This Special Issue on skeletal radiology brings together a diverse collection of articles that showcase the latest advancements in this field. From evaluating flatfoot to exploring emerging targets for osteoarthritis treatment, the included studies provide valuable insights into diagnostic accuracy and the expanding applications of skeletal radiology techniques. This editorial aims to highlight the significance of these articles and their contributions to the field of skeletal radiology.

1.1. Diagnostic Accuracy in Musculoskeletal Radiology

Several articles in this Special Issue delve into the diagnostic accuracy of radiological measurements in different musculoskeletal conditions. Tagliafico et al. investigated the reliability of the Myeloma Spine and Bone Damage Score (MSBDS) in assessing myeloma-related spine and bone damage using whole-body computed tomography (WBCT) [3]. This multicenter study emphasizes the need for standardized scoring systems to accurately evaluate myeloma-related skeletal complications. The researchers propose a consensus-based, semiquantitative scoring system based on CT data on multiple myeloma, which demonstrated a substantial level of agreement among readers of varying experience levels, highlighting its potential for widespread use. Another noteworthy study focuses on the diagnostic challenges of the osteonecrosis of the femoral head [4]. This disorder afflicts at least 30,000 Americans each year and can be undetectable in radiographs during the early stages [5]. Cardin-Pereda et.al. highlight the significance of a multidisciplinary approach in enhancing diagnostic accuracy. By considering various radiological modalities and incorporating clinical expertise, this study provides valuable insights into optimizing the diagnostic pathway for patients with osteonecrosis. Various radiologic measures are available for evaluating flatfoot; however, the accuracy of these measures is still unknown [6]. Thus, one of our studies provided a cross-sectional evaluation and differentiation of flatfoot that explores the sensitivity and specificity of six different measures, namely, arch angle, calcaneal pitch, talar-first metatarsal angle, lateral talar angle, talar inclination angle, and navicular index, in diagnosing flatfoot deformity [6]. This study will help to improve the accuracy of diagnosing flatfoot, leading to more appropriate treatment strategies. In another study, the accuracy of critical shoulder angle (CSA) and the acromial index in predicting supraspinatus tendinopathy was explored, emphasizing the significance of radiological measurements in assessing shoulder pathologies [7]. Critical shoulder angle, defined as the angle between the plane of the glenoid and the most lateral border of the acromion process, has been reported to be a predictor of several shoulder pathologies [8]. However, its association with supraspinatus tendinopathy had not yet been investigated. This retrospective case-control study shows that CSA can also predict supraspinatus tendinopathy.

1.2. Novel Applications and Techniques in Skeletal Radiology

This Special Issue also explores the application of novel techniques to skeletal radiology. New sequences are expanding diagnostic capabilities, and AI-based techniques are revolutionizing the field via enhancing image interpretation and improving image acquisition protocols. Despite being introduced some time ago, the utilization of relatively new MRI sequences like DWI in skeletal radiology has been limited due to their susceptibility to artifacts and inhomogeneity [9]. However, with the advancement of rapid acquisition techniques, researchers are now actively investigating the effectiveness of DWI in detecting and evaluating musculoskeletal pathologies. In their review study on advanced imaging techniques for assessing multiple myeloma, Torkian et al. explored the emerging role of MRI sequences such as DWI, intravoxel incoherent motion (IVIM), and positron emission tomography–magnetic resonance imaging (PET-MRI) in the evaluation of multiple myeloma [10]. The growing role of AI in medical imaging is exemplified in the study by Hong et al. [11]. In their study on lumbar spine computed tomography to magnetic resonance imaging (CT to MRI) synthesis, the researchers employed a generative adversarial network (GAN) model to generate synthesized images. They assessed the accuracy of these synthesized images through a visual Turing test, demonstrating the potential of GANs in bridging the gap between CT and MRI. Significant progress has also been achieved in the discovery of potential therapeutic approaches. For example, Talaie et. al. reviewed the emerging targets for osteoarthritis treatment [12]. They focused on exploring new investigational methods, such as genicular artery embolization (GAE), to identify neo-vessels as potential targets for the treatment of osteoarthritis, emphasizing the importance of understanding the mechanisms of inflammation, neovascularization, and joint remodeling in the pathogenesis of osteoarthritis.

1.3. Clinical Applications and Reviews

In addition to diagnostic accuracy and advancements in skeletal radiology, this Special Issue features studies focusing on specific clinical applications. The diagnosis of systemic disorders, characterized by their wide-ranging impact on different organs, significantly relies on the field of skeletal radiology. Due to the non-specific nature of their clinical presentations and the presence of overlapping features, familiarity with the radiologic findings of these disorders is crucial. Radiologic and dermatologic presentations of systemic disorders, the visualization of dialysis-related amyloid arthropathy via 18F-FDG PET-CT scans, and radiographic findings of inflammatory arthritis and mimics in the hands are the topics of the studies focusing on systemic disorders in this issue [13–15]. The other included reviews focus on pathologies presenting in specific anatomic locations. The imaging of the temporomandibular joint and postoperative findings of common foot and ankle surgeries are the topics of two of the included image-rich reviews that discuss common skeletal findings [16,17]. Notably, one article delves into posteromedial lesions of the chest wall, while the other focuses on reviewing grade 1 and 2 chondrosarcomas of the chest wall, providing crucial insights into accurate diagnosis and treatment planning for these complex cases [18,19].

2. Conclusions

This Special Issue on skeletal radiology encompasses a comprehensive array of articles that contribute to the advancement of this dynamic field. From studies on diagnostic accuracy to emerging applications and clinical reviews, the included articles show the progress and potential of skeletal radiology in improving patient care. The field of skeletal radiology offers promising prospects. Ongoing discussions focus on leveraging emerging technologies to enhance diagnostic capabilities and treatment planning. However, challenges persist, such as the need for standardized protocols, the addressal of data quality and privacy concerns, and the optimization of the integration of artificial intelligence. Further research is required to explore the potential of novel imaging techniques, including advanced MRI sequences and functional imaging modalities, in providing valuable insights into skeletal pathologies. The corresponding evolving technology and imaging techniques have the potential to revolutionize the practice of skeletal radiology, enabling more accurate diagnoses, personalized treatment approaches, and improved patient outcomes.

Author Contributions: Conceptualization and writing—original draft preparation, A.P.; writing—review and editing, E.A. and A.A.; supervision, M.C. All authors have read and agreed to the published version of the manuscript.

Funding: Disclosures: Majid Chalian, RSNA R&E Scholar Grant, Boeing Technology Development Grant.

Conflicts of Interest: The authors declare no conflict of interest.

References

1. Cooper, C. Global, regional, and national disability-adjusted life-years (DALYs) for 359 diseases and injuries and healthy life expectancy (HALE) for 195 countries and territories, 1990–2017: A systematic analysis for the Global Burden of Disease Study 2017. *Lancet* **2018**, *392*, 1859–1922.
2. Botchu, R.; Gupta, H. Updates of the imaging of musculoskeletal problems. *J. Clin. Orthop. Trauma* **2021**, *22*, 101612. [CrossRef] [PubMed]
3. Tagliafico, A.S.; Valle, C.; Bonaffini, P.A.; Attieh, A.; Bauckneht, M.; Belgioia, L.; Bignotti, B.; Brunetti, N.; Bonsignore, A.; Capaccio, E.; et al. Myeloma Spine and Bone Damage Score (MSBDS) on Whole-Body Computed Tomography (WBCT): Multiple Reader Agreement in a Multicenter Reliability Study. *Diagnostics* **2022**, *12*, 1894. [CrossRef]
4. Cardín-Pereda, A.; García-Sánchez, D.; Terán-Villagrá, N.; Alfonso-Fernández, A.; Fakkas, M.; Garcés-Zarzalejo, C.; Pérez-Campo, F.M. Osteonecrosis of the Femoral Head: A Multidisciplinary Approach in Diagnostic Accuracy. *Diagnostics* **2022**, *12*, 1731. [CrossRef]
5. Lavernia, C.J.; Villa, J.M. Total hip arthroplasty in the treatment of osteonecrosis of the femoral head: Then and now. *Curr. Rev. Musculoskelet. Med.* **2015**, *8*, 260–264. [CrossRef] [PubMed]
6. Khan, F.; Chevidikunnan, M.F.; Alsobhi, M.G.; Ahmed, I.A.I.; Al-Lehidan, N.S.; Rehan, M.; Alalawi, H.A.; Abduljabbar, A.H. Diagnostic Accuracy of Various Radiological Measurements in the Evaluation and Differentiation of Flatfoot: A Cross-Sectional Study. *Diagnostics* **2022**, *12*, 2288. [CrossRef]
7. Hsu, T.H.; Lin, C.L.; Wu, C.W.; Chen, Y.W.; Vitoonpong, T.; Lin, L.C.; Huang, S.W. Accuracy of Critical Shoulder Angle and Acromial Index for Predicting Supraspinatus Tendinopathy. *Diagnostics* **2022**, *12*, 283. [CrossRef]
8. Rose-Reneau, Z.; Moorefield, A.K.; Schirmer, D.; Ismailov, E.; Downing, R.; Wright, B.W. The Critical Shoulder Angle as a Diagnostic Measure for Osteoarthritis and Rotator Cuff Pathology. *Cureus* **2020**, *12*, e11447. [CrossRef] [PubMed]
9. Hillengass, J.; Bäuerle, T.; Bartl, R.; Andrulis, M.; McClanahan, F.; Laun, F.B.; Zechmann, C.M.; Shah, R.; Wagner-Gund, B.; Simon, D.; et al. Diffusion-weighted imaging for non-invasive and quantitative monitoring of bone marrow infiltration in patients with monoclonal plasma cell disease: A comparative study with histology. *Br. J. Haematol.* **2011**, *153*, 721–728. [CrossRef] [PubMed]
10. Torkian, P.; Azadbakht, J.; Andrea Bonaffini, P.; Amini, B.; Chalian, M. Advanced Imaging in Multiple Myeloma: New Frontiers for MRI. *Diagnostics* **2022**, *12*, 2182. [CrossRef]
11. Hong, K.T.; Cho, Y.; Kang, C.H.; Ahn, K.S.; Lee, H.; Kim, J.; Hong, S.J.; Kim, B.H.; Shim, E. Lumbar Spine Computed Tomography to Magnetic Resonance Imaging Synthesis Using Generative Adversarial Network: Visual Turing Test. *Diagnostics* **2022**, *12*, 530. [CrossRef]
12. Talaie, R.; Torkian, P.; Clayton, A.; Wallace, S.; Cheung, H.; Chalian, M.; Golzarian, J. Emerging Targets for the Treatment of Osteoarthritis: New Investigational Methods to Identify Neo-Vessels as Possible Targets for Embolization. *Diagnostics* **2022**, *12*, 1403. [CrossRef]
13. Shafiei, M.; Shomal Zadeh, F.; Mansoori, B.; Pyle, H.; Agim, N.; Hinojosa, J.; Dominguez, A.; Thomas, C.; Chalian, M. Imaging More than Skin-Deep: Radiologic and Dermatologic Presentations of Systemic Disorders. *Diagnostics* **2022**, *12*, 2011. [CrossRef]
14. Ezzati, F.; Pezeshk, P. Radiographic Findings of Inflammatory Arthritis and Mimics in the Hands. *Diagnostics* **2022**, *12*, 2134. [CrossRef]
15. Cheon, M.; Yoo, J. Visualization of Dialysis-Related Amyloid Arthropathy on 18F-FDG PET-CT Scan. *Diagnostics* **2022**, *12*, 113. [CrossRef]
16. Gharavi, S.M.; Qiao, Y.; Faghihimehr, A.; Vossen, J. Imaging of the Temporomandibular Joint. *Diagnostics* **2022**, *12*, 1006. [CrossRef]

17. Soltanolkotabi, M.; Mallory, C.; Allen, H.; Chan, B.Y.; Mills, M.K.; Leake, R.L. Postoperative Findings of Common Foot and Ankle Surgeries: An Imaging Review. *Diagnostics* **2022**, *12*, 1090. [CrossRef]
18. Haseli, S.; Mansoori, B.; Shafiei, M.; Shomal Zadeh, F.; Chalian, H.; Khoshpouri, P.; Yousem, D.; Chalian, M. A Review of Posteromedial Lesions of the Chest Wall: What Should a Chest Radiologist Know? *Diagnostics* **2022**, *12*, 301. [CrossRef]
19. Del Grande, F.; Ahlawat, S.; McCarthy, E.; Fayad, L.M. Grade 1 and 2 Chondrosarcomas of the Chest Wall: CT Imaging Features and Review of the Literature. *Diagnostics* **2022**, *12*, 292. [CrossRef]

Disclaimer/Publisher's Note: The statements, opinions and data contained in all publications are solely those of the individual author(s) and contributor(s) and not of MDPI and/or the editor(s). MDPI and/or the editor(s) disclaim responsibility for any injury to people or property resulting from any ideas, methods, instructions or products referred to in the content.

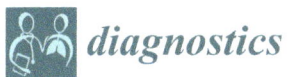

Review

Advanced Imaging in Multiple Myeloma: New Frontiers for MRI

Pooya Torkian [1], Javid Azadbakht [2], Pietro Andrea Bonaffini [3], Behrang Amini [4] and Majid Chalian [5,*]

1. Vascular and Interventional Radiology, Department of Radiology, University of Minnesota, Minneapolis, MN 55455, USA
2. Department of Radiology, Kashan University of Medical Sciences, Kashan 8715988141, Iran
3. Department of Radiology, Papa Giovanni XXIII Hospital, Piazza OMS, 1, 24127 Bergamo, Italy
4. Department of Musculoskeletal Imaging, The University of Texas MD Anderson Cancer Center, Huoston, TX 77030, USA
5. Musculoskeletal Imaging and Intervention, Department of Radiology, University of Washington, Seattle, WA 98105, USA
* Correspondence: mchalian@uw.edu

Abstract: Plasma cell dyscrasias are estimated to newly affect almost 40,000 people in 2022. They fall on a spectrum of diseases ranging from relatively benign to malignant, the malignant end of the spectrum being multiple myeloma (MM). The International Myeloma Working Group (IMWG) has traditionally outlined the diagnostic criteria and therapeutic management of MM. In the last two decades, novel imaging techniques have been employed for MM to provide more information that can guide not only diagnosis and staging, but also treatment efficacy. These imaging techniques, due to their low invasiveness and high reliability, have gained significant clinical attention and have already changed the clinical practice. The development of functional MRI sequences such as diffusion weighted imaging (DWI) or intravoxel incoherent motion (IVIM) has made the functional assessment of lesions feasible. Moreover, the growing availability of positron emission tomography (PET)–magnetic resonance imaging (MRI) scanners is leading to the potential combination of sensitive anatomical and functional information in a single step. This paper provides an organized framework for evaluating the benefits and challenges of novel and more functional imaging techniques used for the management of patients with plasma cell dyscrasias, notably MM.

Keywords: multiple myeloma; plasma cell dyscrasia; diffusion weighted imaging; whole body MRI

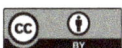

1. Introduction

Multiple myeloma (MM), the second most prevalent hematopoietic malignancy, is a plasma cell dyscrasia where monoclonal plasma cells infiltrate bone marrow, resulting in marrow failure and/or bone destruction, mainly in the axial skeleton and proximal appendicular bones [1,2]. MM exists on the end of a spectrum of disease progression, from an asymptomatic premalignant state, namely monoclonal gammopathy of undetermined significance (MGUS), to smoldering multiple myeloma (SMM), and finally to symptomatic MM, commonly with MM-associated end-organ damage, also known as CRAB (hyperCalcemia, Renal failure, Anemia, and Bone disease) [3,4].

Currently, MM is identified and staged according to the International Myeloma Working Group (IMWG) criteria. IMWG criteria outlines the MM diagnosis as clonal bone marrow plasma cells > 10%, or biopsy-proven bony or extramedullary plasmacytoma, in addition to one or more of the following: evidence of end organ damage (hypercalcemia, renal insufficiency, anemia and/or osteolytic bone lesions) and/or biomarkers positive for malignancy (serum-free light chain ratio, and clonal plasma cell proportion), and the presence of more than one focal marrow lesions on MRI [5]. There are several limitations to some of the tests involved in these criteria. The biomarkers outlined above are of limited value in non-secretory or extramedullary MM cases [3–5]. While bone marrow biopsy is the gold standard diagnostic test and is required for the assessment of treatment response, it is invasive, with a risk of local hemorrhage and infection, and it is not representative of the whole spectrum of the marrow [6].

Earlier in 2009, the consensus statement of the IMWG recommended conventional radiography (CR) as the standard imaging modality to stage MM, both in new cases and for relapsed patients, being widely available and inexpensive [5]. However, radiographs lack sensitivity and specificity, and they poorly detect extra-osseous lesions and diffuse medullary invasion. Therefore, skeletal surveys have been replaced with more sophisticated imaging techniques (computed tomography (CT), magnetic resonance imaging (MRI), and positron emission tomography (PET)) in many tertiary centers [7,8]. Newer staging systems incorporate more sensitive imaging modalities, such as whole-body MRI (WB-MRI) or ^{18}F-fluorodeoxyglucose (FDG) PET/CT into the staging system [9]. The need for whole-body imaging in MM is related to the fact that myelomatous lesions can potentially affect any bony segment in the body.

Once it has been diagnosed and staged, as with most other malignancies, MM treatment management is also dependent on bone imaging to determine the extent of tumor cell burden, both for prognostic stratification and to assess post-therapy changes [10,11].

This paper describes available advanced imaging techniques in an assessment of MM, with a greater focus on whole-body diffusion weighted imaging (WB-DWI).

2. MRI

2.1. Conventional Whole-Body MRI (WB-MRI)

According to IMWG guidelines, MRI should be considered as the complementary adequate imaging modality for the diagnosis of MM, as it is more sensitive than FDG-PET/CT [12,13]. As opposed to computed tomography (CT) or positron emission tomography (PET), an advantage of MRI is that it causes no radiation exposure. In contrast to ^{18}F-FDG PET/CT, MRI is widely available, relatively faster, has no pre-scan diet requirement, and is not reliant on the metabolic activity of tumor cells. This is specifically important in the case of MM, as frequent follow-up imaging is necessary, and survival time is increasing in light of recent therapeutic advancements. Conventional MRI can relatively accurately measure the size and extension of MM pathology, but it takes longer to interpret and requires more training to read than other imaging modalities [14–17].

Nearly half of MM lesions may be missed when imaging only covers the spine [14]. Thus, for a more sensitive assessment, MRI should cover the entire axial skeleton and the proximal appendicular skeleton, defining the idea of the "whole body" MRI technique. WB-MRI has gained popularity since the last decade. for diagnosing and assessing the treatment response in MM by providing morphological information on tumor spread. Around one-third to a half of MM patients show diffuse infiltration or focal deposits on WB-MRI [18,19].

The Myeloma Response Assessment and Diagnosis System (MY-RADS) comprehensively characterizes the myeloma state at diagnosis, initiation of treatment, and during follow-up, as the disease course changes in response to therapy. MY-RADS recommendations will help to improve response assessments by increasing standardization, and by decreasing the variations seen in the acquisition, interpretation, and reporting of whole-body MRI. For response assessments, the classified response assessment category (RAC) is according to anatomical regions. For each region, the RAC should use a five-point scale as follows: (1) highly likely to be responding; (2) likely to be responding; (3) stable; (4) likely to be progressing; and (5) highly likely to be progressing. MY-RADS functions to categorize patients with regard to specific disease patterns to aid in clinical trial stratification [20].

Different MRI sequences are being used based on imaging protocols of the radiology department [21–24]. Fat-suppressed T2-weighted (FS T2W), Short Tau Inversion recovery (STIR), and T1-weighted (T1W) MRI sequences are most commonly utilized for MM [23–27]. The signal intensity on FS T2W and STIR images correlates with the plasma cell concentration in the bone marrow. However, it lacks enough accuracy to differentiate between hyperplastic/red marrow and myeloma marrow. Changes on T1W images occur relatively late in the course of disease, and might differentiate MM from MGUS and SMM, although to a lesser extent compared to FS T2-WI, but they offer increased specificity [28]. While the T1W, STIR, and T2W sequences are more frequently used, diffusion weighted imaging (DWI) is the most promising MRI sequence for distinguishing MM from MGUS and SMM through visual assessment, and for the qualitative evaluation of lesion activity and treatment response [28].

2.2. Whole-Body Diffusion Weighted Imaging (WB-DWI)

DWI is a functional MRI sequence that can quantitatively evaluate tissue cellularity by measuring the random thermal movements of water molecules (Brownian motion) using the apparent diffusion coefficient (ADC) map [29]. Although DWI MRI was limited to brain imaging for many years due to its sensitivity to motion, its use has been recently expanded to include other anatomic locations, due to the introduction of echoplanar imaging and the use of fast acquisition techniques capable of capturing images during breath holds [30]. Thus, DWI MRI, including WB-DWI, have revolutionized the assessment of myeloma lesions from simple evaluations based on size to quantitative data based on free water molecule movement and tissue cellularity [29,31].

From 2010 on, the utilization of WB-DWI in MM has steadily increased [30–33]. WB-DWI can be performed relatively rapidly with low technical and operational efforts when added to the standard WB-MRI protocol. WB-DWI keeps the aforementioned advantages of WB-MRI, and adds further details to morphological imaging, as compared to the conventional sequences of WB-MRI during the assessment of treatment response and extramedullary disease, which are critical for MM management [21].

ADC mapping, which is derived from DW images, can distinguish bone marrow changes in active myeloma from those in remission, providing clinically relevant data on tumor viability [34]. ADC values above 600–700 $\mu m^2/s$ in a non-treated and newly diagnosed patient with multiple myeloma could be used to increase confidence for the diagnosis of diffuse marrow involvement, while normal marrow ADC value mostly falls below 600 $\mu m^2/s$, with even lower values in elderly patients with prominent fatty marrow [32,35–37]. Koutoulidis et al. reported a higher ADC value for diffuse MM patterns in imaging comparing to focal lesions, and they found that an ADC value of >548 $\mu mm^2/s$ shows 100% sensitivity and 98% specificity for comparing a diffuse pattern of myeloma infiltration, than normal marrow [36]. Messiou et al. reported a significant decrease in the ADC values of MM patients who were responders from 4 weeks to 20 weeks after treatment, while patients with stable or progressive disease did not show a significant decrease in ADC value within the same time period [35].

If cellularity was the dominant factor in determining the ADC value in myeloma marrow, there should be a negative correlation between the ADC value and marrow cellularity. However, this is not the case. For this reason, cellularity is not the main factor affecting the DWI-ADC image signal in MM. Recent studies on liver fibrosis and pancreatic cancer have suggested that the perfusion effect on the measured ADC value dominates over hypercellularity [30,38,39]. This has been suggested for MM as well [40], as the ADC number decreases with hypercellularity and increases with hypervascularity, which parallels hypercellularity in the myeloma marrow [30]: the net effect is an increase of the ADC value in MM relative to the normal reference. This explains the Intravoxel Incoherent Motion (IVIM) MRI advantage for MM diagnosis/monitoring, which will be discussed in the following section. Employing lower b-values offer a better Signal to Noise Ratio (SNR), whereas higher b-values are more accurate for detecting MM lesions (Figures 1 and 2) [41]. Most of the studies on DWI in MM have been conducted with a high b-value of 600–800, which offers a good MM lesion detection rate at a reasonable SNR [42–44].

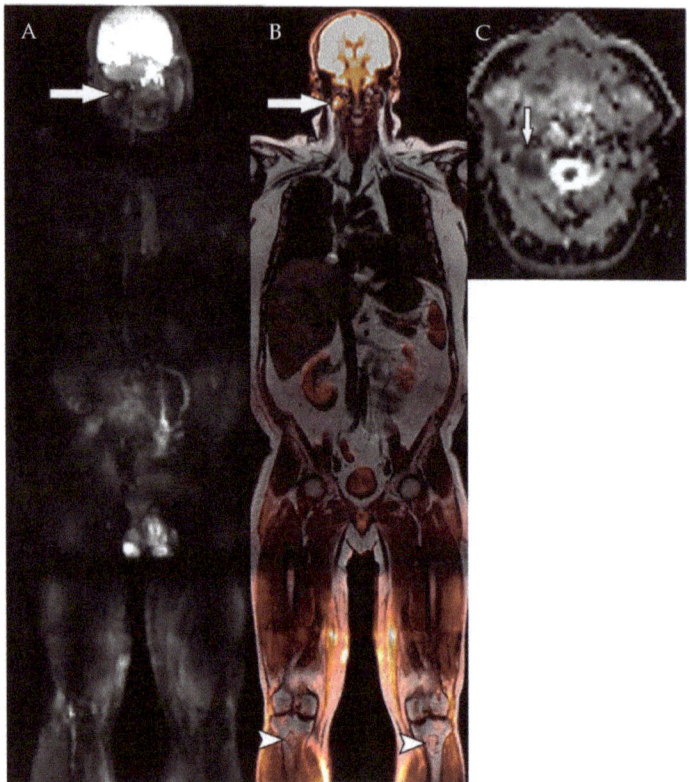

Figure 1. A 45-year-old man with hyposecretory IgG kappa multiple myeloma (MM) and a history of autologous stem cell transplantation 3 years before imaging. Patient had received radiation therapy to L1 vertebral body 2 years ago, and has been on maintenance therapy (carfilzomob, pomalidomide, and dexamethasone) for 6 months. WB-MRI images failed to demonstrate any osseous lesion, but showed a 12 mm extramedullary lesion deep to right parotid gland (arrow) on coronal high b-value (b = 800) DWI MIP image (**A**). Fused coronal DWI MIP and T1-weighted Dixon image (**B**) confirms the finding (arrow). Axial ADC map (**C**) confirms diffusion restriction (mean value of 0.8 ($\times 10^{-3}$ mm^2/s). Note areas of marrow infarction at bilateral proximal tibial metaphysis (arrowheads, (**B**)).

One of the main advantages to WB-DWI is that it provides an excellent visual contrast between the normal marrow and bone marrow lesions, differentiating them with a higher sensitivity than the conventional MRI sequence, radiologic skeletal survey, or PET/CT scan [45–47]. For example, lesion conspicuity is greater in DWI as compared to the conventional T1-MRI and STIR sequences, and has a higher lesion detection rate compared to PET/CT [48,49].

DWI was able to identify 11% more patients than PET/CT in a cohort of 227 patients, and had a sensitivity of 77% versus 47% in PET/CT compared to a conventional MRI and CT in a smaller study of 24 patients [50]. WB-DWI also offers an excellent interobserver agreement for quantifying the disease burden in MM, both for the whole-body assessment and regional evaluation for any location across the body [48,51]. This superiority offers a substantial impact on treatment planning and patient classification, and it allows clinicians to make better decisions [35,52]. Importantly, WB-DWI has also been found to be useful in differentiating the stages of monoclonal gammopathies [35,52]. In addition, WB-DWI provides more reliable differentiation between benign tumors and pathological vertebral compression fractures [49]. DWI differentiates benign vertebral body collapse from malignant fractures with a reported sensitivity and specificity of 95.6% and 90%, respectively [36,48].

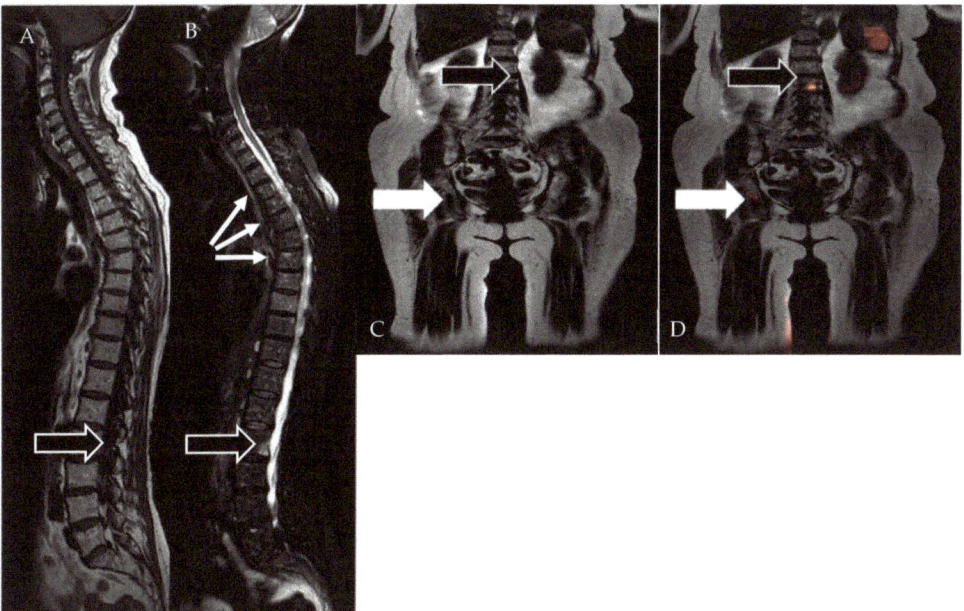

Figure 2. WB-MRI in a 75-year-old woman with mixed active and treated disease. (**A**) Sagittal T1-WI shows a lesion (black arrow) in the posterior and inferior L2 vertebral body. (**B**) Sagittal STIR image shows the L2 lesion (black arrow), as well as at several other sites of disease (thin white arrows) that were not obvious on the T1-WI. (**C**) Coronal T1 Dixon Fat image shows the L2 lesion (black arrow) and another lesion in the right ischium (white arrow). (**D**) Fused b800-Dixon image shows increased signal at L2 (black arrow) and to a lesser extent at the ischial lesion (white arrow).

DWI-MRI is also useful in evaluating treatment efficacy, remission, and prognostication. ADC images, similar to other functional imaging modalities, account for the heterogeneous pathologic distribution and patchy marrow infiltration in MM (which is accentuated after relapse) [53], and thus can help to monitor the treatment response in MM patients.

With effective treatment, responders show an increased ADC value at 4–6 weeks post-treatment: hemorrhage, edema, vascular congestion, and liquefaction necrosis from tumor cell death contribute to an increased diffusivity [35,46]. ADC then decreases at 20 weeks after therapy, due to a reappearance of normal fatty marrow. Conversely, patients who are resistant to therapy show a persistent marrow hyperintensity on DWI, and hypointensity on ADC images [35,37,54,55].

DWI images have also been proven to detect prognostically relevant residual focal lesions with a higher sensitivity than PET and PET/CT [56,57]. For a diffuse pattern of myeloma infiltration, there are controversies regarding the correlation between the ADC signal and therapy response, as some studies support its use [47] while others do not [47,58]. A previous study has related this issue to the slower transition from replaced to recovered fatty marrow in focal MM lesions that make it possible to be captured when imaged post-treatment [36]. WB-MRI with DWI also offers a quantitative analysis of the entire bone marrow after treatment, which is invaluable for clinicians directing further need for therapies and remission.

The limitations of WB-DWI include some issues with a definitive identification of lesions, and with resolution. The ADC value of MM lesions increases early after effective treatment, and for an interpreter who is blind to previous exams, this might resemble a hemangioma. However, when previous images are not available, corresponding T1 and T2-weighted imaging solves this issue. Additionally, DWI suffers from some limitations in resolution, rendering, and field of view (FOV). Therefore, when interpreted with the available anatomical data, DWI is an important support for MM, and should be added to morphologic imaging sequences in WB protocols; and it currently cannot be relied on as a stand-alone imaging modality [49].

2.3. IVIM MRI

IVIM theory was first introduced by Le Bihan et al. more than two decades ago, describing the role of the perfusion effects on the significant signal decay at b-values of less than 300 s/mm^2 [59]. The recorded ADC value is influenced by a combination of tissue microarchitecture/cellularity and perfusion. Given that the routine clinical implementation of DWI does not include a complete set of b-values (low, intermediate, and high), it does not provide information on the perfusion component of the signal derived from the imaged tissues [59].

As previously mentioned, in MM, the impact of the perfusion component on the ADC value seems to be larger than the effect of hypercellularity; hence, IVIM may be even more promising than DWI for MM patients [59]. IVIM decontaminates the ADC maps from the so-called "pseudo-diffusion" (D*), and marks out a part of the ADC signal that arises from any process other than diffusion, which is predominantly microperfusion at the capillary level. By taking three or more DWI images that are set at low, intermediate, and high b-values, two or more ADC maps could be generated, where ADC maps of low to moderate b-values reflect a combination of perfusion (D*: pseudo or enhanced diffusivity) and true diffusion (D). Subtracting these ADC maps will achieve tissue vascularity, which would be of added value to predict prognosis and assess treatment response in MM.

IVIM parameter D, the molecular diffusion coefficient, has been reported to be significantly higher in a diffuse pattern of myeloma marrow infiltration [60]. IVIM parameters are also associated with serum levels of biomarkers, showing that IVIM could be another useful tool for the prognostication of disease activity in MM [61].

2.4. Marrow Fat Quantification Techniques

Recently, gradient echo-based Dixon MRI as a fat quantification method approach has been evolved to include the generation of four separate image types: in-phase (IP), out-of-phase (OP), water-only (WO), and fat-only (FO) [62–64]. This method has been used for anatomical WB-MRI in MM, and it has several benefits over conventional T1- or T2-weighted imaging. The fat fraction is obtained using OP and IP images, and it can be efficient for both the lesion detection and the response assessment of bone lesions in MM patients [62]. It also has been shown that T2 Dixon fat-only Dixon images are more efficient by providing higher lesion detection rates compared to in-phase images alone in multiple myeloma [65].

2.5. Whole-Body Dynamic Contrast-Enhanced MRI (WB-DCE MRI)

WB-DCE MRI refers to the acquisition of serial images pre- and post-contrast administration, which can provide functional data on marrow infiltration in MM. WB-DCE MRI data can be computed into time-signal intensity curves providing a quantitative assessment of myeloma marrow infiltration, which could be valuable for diagnosis, prognosis, and monitoring treatment response. With regard to diagnosis, higher peaks and steeper slopes of WB-DCE MRI curves are associated with a higher percentage of plasma cell infiltration [66–68]. Prior studies have also found WB-DCE MRI curves to be well-correlated with MM disease activity and serum biomarkers [67]. In terms of prognosis, the relative signal enhancement of marrow in SMM predicts its rapid progression into symptomatic disease, and more severe enhancement in progressive MM predicting a shorter progression-free survival [69,70]. After treatment, persistent abnormally elevated peaks of marrow enhancement and the foci of early enhancement portend disease progression or relapse (poor treatment response) [71]. Due to the paucity of research on standard acquisition protocols and reporting systems, WB-DCE MRI is not presently recommended for daily practice [72].

3. ^{18}F-Fluorodeoxyglucose Positron Emission Tomography (18FDG PET)

3.1. ^{18}FDG PET

^{18}F-fluorodeoxyglucose (FDG) is the most commonly used radiotracer in PET imaging for MM [73]. FDG uptake, which is widely semi-quantitatively assessed via the maximum standardized uptake value (SUVmax), is known to be correlated with biological tumor aggressiveness [74]. ^{18}FDG PET may over- or underestimate MM disease activity; for example, over-calling pathologic fractures or under-identifying small sized lesions. Moreover, SUVmax measures ^{18}FDG uptake in a single-voxel region of interest, which might emit a distorted signal due to noise, reconstruction protocols, and post-processing (if applicable). Additionally, a single-voxel measurement may not be representative of marrow disease in its entirety [75]. Reporting SUVmean and SUVpeak instead of SUVmax addresses these setbacks, but is rarely performed in clinical practice [76]. Additionally, recent studies have suggested that measuring total lesion glycolysis (TLG) and metabolic tumor volume (MTV) may represent the tumor burden/activity and the patient's prognosis more accurately [77,78]. However, these measurements can be time-consuming and not routinely performed in clinical practice. Hybrid imaging and adding the morphological data from CT or MRI into the functional data from PET imaging resolves these issues to a considerable extent.

3.2. ^{18}FDG PET/CT

^{18}FDG PET/CT is a sensitive diagnostic modality for both medullary and extramedullary plasma cell dyscrasias, and can accurately detect MM lesions, assess treatment response, and predict prognosis and progression in MM [77,79–81]. The wider employment of ^{18}FDG PET/CT has also resulted in a significantly increased detection rate for extramedullary MM at diagnosis compared to older imaging techniques [82].

The International Myeloma Working Group (IMWG) recently introduced the evaluation of minimal residual disease (MRD) within the multiple myeloma (MM) response criteria. Currently the most powerful predictor of favorable outcomes over long-term follow-up, MRD negativity can be assessed both inside and outside of the bone marrow. Functional imaging techniques such as PET/CT and magnetic resonance imaging (MRI) serve in sensitive response assessment, and have been shown to be promising in terms of evaluating the response to treatment. Not only have they helped to assess MRD status in MM patients, but they also provide a global representation of the tumor burden by including several prognostic markers in addition to lesion type [83].

The sensitivity of ^{18}FDG PET/CT for focal MM lesions has been reported to be more than WB-MRI, roughly estimated at 75% [84]; however, a diffuse pattern of marrow infiltration is better detected using WB-MRI. Additionally, ^{18}FDG PET/CT was shown to have more promising results in having a higher impact on clinical decisions than WB-MRI in MM patients in terms of prognosis and management [85]. In a recent meta-analysis, a high ^{18}FDG uptake significantly and independently predicted a shorter overall and progression-free survival in MM patients [81] when considering whole-body burden disease [81].

WB-MRI with DWI provides a non-invasive and quantitative assessment of the entire bone marrow after treatment. Based on a study by Torkian et al., DWI had a pooled sensitivity of 78% (95% CI: 72–83) and a specificity of 73% (95% CI: 61–83) in distinguishing responders from non-responders, emphasizing the prominent role of DWI for treatment response assessment in patients with MM [86]. In a cohort of 49 cases, WB DWI has been shown to be more sensitive than ^{18}FDG PET/CT for detecting intramedullary lesions in all regions except the skull, both in patients with a new diagnosis and previously treated patients. Additionally, WB DWI has been shown to have a sensitivity equivalent to that of ^{18}FDG PET/CT for detecting extramedullary lesions [87].

3.3. ^{18}FDG PET/MRI

Finally, hybrid ^{18}FDG PET/MRI techniques combine the morphological information provided by MRI and the metabolic and functional data furnished via ^{18}FDG PET imaging, which allows for both the ability to detect the marrow foci of myeloma infiltration and to assess prognosis and treatment response. ^{18}FDG PET/MRI increases the visibility of focal MM lesions at diagnosis and initial staging, and localizes residual disease activity after treatment [12]. ^{18}FDG PET/MRI has been reported to have a higher lesion detectability rate than ^{18}FDG PET/CT in evaluating skeletal lesions [88]. However, Sachpekidis et al. concluded that these two techniques are equally sensitive in detecting MM lesions [89]. As with WB-DCE MRI, there are few studies on a standard acquisition protocol and reporting system in ^{18}FDG PET/MRI for MM; thus, further studies are warranted to test repeatability and validity before ^{18}FDG PET/MRI can be considered as a viable tool in a routine imaging work-up of MM.

4. Conclusions

In the last two decades, novel imaging techniques have been developed or employed for MM to provide more information that can guide not only diagnosis and staging, but also treatment efficacy. These imaging techniques, due to their low invasiveness and high reliability, have gained significant clinical attention and have changed the clinical practice. The development of functional MRI sequences such as diffusion weighted imaging (DWI) and Intravoxel Incoherent Motion (IVIM) has made the functional assessment of lesions feasible.

DWI-MRI provides a high utility tool for not only the diagnosis and initial staging of plasma cell dyscrasias such as MM, but also for the evaluation of treatment efficacy and for re-staging. It can reliably detect tissue hypercellularity with high sensitivity, challenging the use of other procedures or imaging modalities for the management of MM. Therefore, DWI-MRI presents a promising option for clinicians engaged in the management of plasma cell dyscrasias like MM.

Author Contributions: Conceptualization, P.T., J.A. and M.C.; methodology, P.T. and M.C.; investigation, P.T. and J.A.; data curation, P.T. and J.A.; writing—original draft preparation, P.T., J.A. and M.C.; writing—review and editing, M.C., P.A.B. and B.A.; visualization, P.T., J.A. and B.A.; supervision, M.C., B.A., P.A.B. and B.A. All authors have read and agreed to the published version of the manuscript.

Funding: This research received no external funding.

Institutional Review Board Statement: Not applicable.

Informed Consent Statement: Not applicable.

Data Availability Statement: Not applicable.

Conflicts of Interest: The authors declare no competing interest.

References

1. Dimopoulos, M.; Terpos, E.; Comenzo, R.L.; Tosi, P.; Beksac, M.; Sezer, O.; Siegel, D.; Lokhorst, H.; Kumar, S.; Rajkumar, S.V.; et al. International myeloma working group consensus statement and guidelines regarding the current role of imaging techniques in the diagnosis and monitoring of multiple Myeloma. *Leukemia* **2009**, *23*, 1545–1556. [CrossRef] [PubMed]
2. Bataille, R.; Harousseau, J.-L. Multiple Myeloma. *N. Engl. J. Med.* **1997**, *336*, 1657–1664. [CrossRef] [PubMed]
3. Kyle, R.A.; Durie, B.G.M.; Rajkumar, S.V.; Landgren, O.; Blade, J.; Merlini, G.; Kröger, N.; Einsele, H.; Vesole, D.H.; Dimopoulos, M.; et al. Monoclonal gammopathy of undetermined signif-icance (MGUS) and smoldering (asymptomatic) multiple myeloma: IMWG consensus perspectives risk factors for progression and guidelines for monitoring and management. *Leukemia* **2010**, *24*, 1121–1127. [CrossRef] [PubMed]
4. Smith, D.; Yong, K. Multiple myeloma. *BMJ* **2013**, *346*, f3863. [CrossRef] [PubMed]

5. Rajkumar, S.V.; Dimopoulos, M.A.; Palumbo, A.; Blade, J.; Merlini, G.; Mateos, M.V.; Kumar, S.; Hillengass, J.; Kastritis, E.; Richardson, P.; et al. International Myeloma Working Group updated criteria for the diagnosis of multiple myeloma. *Lancet Oncol.* **2014**, *15*, e538–e548. [CrossRef]
6. Durie, B.G.; Harousseau, J.L.; Miguel, J.S.; Bladé, J.; Barlogie, B.; Anderson, K.; Gertz, M.; Dimopoulos, M.; Westin, J.; Sonneveld, P.; et al. International uniform response criteria for multiple myeloma. *Leukemia* **2006**, *20*, 1467–1473. [CrossRef] [PubMed]
7. Ormond Filho, A.G.; Carneiro, B.C.; Pastore, D.; Silva, I.P.; Yamashita, S.R.; Consolo, F.D.; Hungria, V.T.M.; Sandes, A.F.; Rizzatti, E.G.; Nico, M.A.C. Whole-Body Imaging of Multiple Myeloma: Diagnostic Criteria. *Radiographics* **2019**, *39*, 1077–1097. [CrossRef] [PubMed]
8. Hotta, T. Classification, staging and prognostic indices for multiple myeloma. *Nihon Rinsho Jpn. J. Clin. Med.* **2007**, *65*, 2161–2166.
9. Durie, B.G. The role of anatomic and functional staging in myeloma: Description of Durie/Salmon plus staging system. *Eur. J. Cancer* **2006**, *42*, 1539–1543. [CrossRef]
10. Hillengass, J.; Fechtner, K.; Weber, M.A.; Bäuerle, T.; Ayyaz, S.; Heiss, C.; Hielscher, T.; Moehler, T.M.; Egerer, G.; Neben, K.; et al. Prognostic significance of focal lesions in whole-body magnetic resonance imaging in patients with asymptomatic multiple myeloma. *J. Clin. Oncol. Off. J. Am. Soc. Clin. Oncol.* **2010**, *28*, 1606–1610. [CrossRef]
11. Walker, R.; Barlogie, B.; Haessler, J.; Tricot, G.; Anaissie, E.; Shaughnessy, J.D., Jr.; Epstein, J.; van Hemert, R.; Erdem, E.; Hoering, A.; et al. Magnetic resonance imaging in multiple myeloma: Diagnostic and clinical implications. *J. Clin. Oncol. Off. J. Am. Soc. Clin. Oncol.* **2007**, *25*, 1121–1128. [CrossRef] [PubMed]
12. Dimopoulos, M.A.; Hillengass, J.; Usmani, S.; Zamagni, E.; Lentzsch, S.; Davies, F.E.; Raje, N.; Sezer, O.; Zweegman, S.; Shah, J.; et al. Role of magnetic resonance imaging in the management of patients with multiple myeloma: A consensus statement. *J. Clin. Oncol. Off. J. Am. Soc. Clin. Oncol.* **2015**, *33*, 657–664. [CrossRef] [PubMed]
13. Pawlyn, C.; Fowkes, L.; Otero, S.; Jones, J.R.; Boyd, K.D.; Davies, F.E.; Morgan, G.J.; Collins, D.J.; Sharma, B.; Riddell, A.; et al. Whole-body diffusion-weighted MRI: A new gold standard for assessing disease burden in patients with multiple myeloma? *Leukemia* **2016**, *30*, 1446–1448. [CrossRef] [PubMed]
14. Bäuerle, T.; Hillengass, J.; Fechtner, K.; Zechmann, C.M.; Grenacher, L.; Moehler, T.M.; Christiane, H.; Wagner-Gund, B.; Neben, K.; Kauczor, H.U.; et al. Multiple myeloma and monoclonal gammopathy of undetermined significance: Importance of whole-body versus spinal MR imaging. *Radiology* **2009**, *252*, 477–485. [CrossRef] [PubMed]
15. Baur, A.; Stäbler, A.; Nagel, D.; Lamerz, R.; Bartl, R.; Hiller, E.; Wendtner, C.; Bachner, F.; Reiser, M. Magnetic resonance imaging as a supplement for the clinical staging system of Durie and Salmon? *Cancer* **2002**, *95*, 1334–1345. [CrossRef]
16. Kusumoto, S.; Jinnai, I.; Itoh, K.; Kawai, N.; Sakata, T.; Matsuda, A.; Tominaga, K.; Murohashi, I.; Bessho, M.; Harashima, K.; et al. Magnetic resonance imaging patterns in patients with multiple myeloma. *Br. J. Haematol.* **1997**, *99*, 649–655. [CrossRef] [PubMed]
17. Moulopoulos, L.A.; Gika, D.; Anagnostopoulos, A.; Delasalle, K.; Weber, D.; Alexanian, R.; Dimopoulos, M.A. Prognostic significance of magnetic resonance imaging of bone marrow in previously untreated patients with multiple myeloma. *Ann. Oncol. Off. J. Eur. Soc. Med. Oncol.* **2005**, *16*, 1824–1828. [CrossRef]
18. Hillengass, J.; Ayyaz, S.; Kilk, K.; Weber, M.-A.; Hielscher, T.; Shah, R.; Hose, D.; Delorme, S.; Goldschmidt, H.; Neben, K. Changes in magnetic resonance imaging before and after autologous stem cell transplantation correlate with response and survival in multiple myeloma. *Haematologica* **2012**, *97*, 1757–1760. [CrossRef]
19. Moulopoulos, L.A.; Dimopoulos, M.A.; Alexanian, R.; Leeds, N.E.; Libshitz, H.I. Multiple myeloma: MR patterns of response to treatment. *Radiology* **1994**, *193*, 441–446. [CrossRef]
20. Messiou, C.; Hillengass, J.; Delorme, S.; Lecouvet, F.E.; Moulopoulos, L.A.; Collins, D.J.; Blackledge, M.D.; Abildgaard, N.; Østergaard, B.; Schlemmer, H.P.; et al. Guidelines for Acquisition, Interpretation, and Reporting of Whole-Body MRI in Myeloma: Myeloma Response Assessment and Diagnosis System (MY-RADS). *Radiology* **2019**, *291*, 5–13. [CrossRef]
21. Schmidt, G.P.; Reiser, M.F.; Baur-Melnyk, A. Whole-body MRI for the staging and follow-up of patients with metastasis. *Eur. J. Radiol.* **2009**, *70*, 393–400. [CrossRef] [PubMed]
22. Weininger, M.; Lauterbach, B.; Knop, S.; Pabst, T.; Kenn, W.; Hahn, D.; Beissert, M. Whole-body MRI of multiple myeloma: Comparison of different MRI sequences in assessment of different growth patterns. *Eur. J. Radiol.* **2009**, *69*, 339–345. [CrossRef] [PubMed]
23. Albano, D.; Stecco, A.; Micci, G.; Sconfienza, L.M.; Colagrande, S.; Reginelli, A.; Grassi, R.; Carriero, A.; Midiri, M.; Lagalla, R.; et al. Whole-body magnetic resonance imaging (WB-MRI) in oncology: An Italian survey. *La Radiol. Med.* **2021**, *126*, 299–305. [CrossRef] [PubMed]
24. Feldhaus, J.M.; Garner, H.W.; Wessell, D.E. Society of skeletal radiology member utilization and performance of whole-body MRI in adults. *Skelet. Radiol.* **2020**, *49*, 1731–1736. [CrossRef]
25. Dinter, D.J.; Neff, W.K.; Klaus, J.; Böhm, C.; Hastka, J.; Weiss, C.; Schoenberg, S.O.; Metzgeroth, G. Comparison of whole-body MR imaging and conventional X-ray examination in patients with multiple myeloma and implications for therapy. *Ann. Hematol.* **2009**, *88*, 457–464. [CrossRef] [PubMed]
26. Engelhardt, M.; Kleber, M.; Frydrychowicz, A.; Pache, G.; Schmitt-Gräff, A.; Wäsch, R.; Durie, B.G. Superiority of magnetic resonance imaging over conventional radiographs in multiple myeloma. *Anticancer. Res.* **2009**, *29*, 4745–4750. [PubMed]

27. Ghanem, N.; Lohrmann, C.; Engelhardt, M.; Pache, G.; Uhl, M.; Saueressig, U.; Kotter, E.; Langer, M. Whole-body MRI in the detection of bone marrow infiltration in patients with plasma cell neoplasms in comparison to the radiological skeletal survey. *Eur. Radiol.* **2006**, *16*, 1005–1014. [CrossRef]
28. Dutoit, J.C.; Vanderkerken, M.A.; Anthonissen, J.; Dochy, F.; Verstraete, K.L. The diagnostic value of SE MRI and DWI of the spine in patients with monoclonal gammopathy of undetermined significance, smouldering myeloma and multiple myeloma. *Eur. Radiol.* **2014**, *24*, 2754–2765. [CrossRef]
29. Jacobs, M.A.; Pan, L.; Macura, K.J. Whole-body diffusion-weighted and proton imaging: A review of this emerging technology for monitoring metastatic cancer. *Semin. Roentgenol.* **2009**, *44*, 111–122. [CrossRef]
30. Hillengass, J.; Bäuerle, T.; Bartl, R.; Andrulis, M.; McClanahan, F.; Laun, F.B.; Zechmann, C.M.; Shah, R.; Wagner-Gund, B.; Simon, D.; et al. Diffusion-weighted imaging for non-invasive and quantitative monitoring of bone marrow infiltration in patients with monoclonal plasma cell disease: A comparative study with histology. *Br. J. Haematol.* **2011**, *153*, 721–728. [CrossRef]
31. Horger, M.; Weisel, K.; Horger, W.; Mroue, A.; Fenchel, M.; Lichy, M. Whole-body diffusion-weighted MRI with apparent diffusion coefficient mapping for early response monitoring in multiple myeloma: Preliminary results. *AJR Am. J. Roentgenol.* **2011**, *196*, 6. [CrossRef]
32. Messiou, C.; Collins, D.J.; Morgan, V.A.; Desouza, N.M. Optimising diffusion weighted MRI for imaging metastatic and myeloma bone disease and assessing reproducibility. *Eur. Radiol.* **2011**, *21*, 1713–1718. [CrossRef] [PubMed]
33. Sommer, G.; Klarhöfer, M.; Lenz, C.; Scheffler, K.; Bongartz, G.; Winter, L. Signal characteristics of focal bone marrow lesions in patients with multiple myeloma using whole body T1w-TSE, T2w-STIR and diffusion-weighted imaging with background suppression. *Eur. Radiol.* **2011**, *21*, 857–862. [CrossRef]
34. Fenchel, M.; Konaktchieva, M.; Weisel, K.; Kraus, S.; Claussen, C.D.; Horger, M. Response assessment in patients with multiple myeloma during antiangiogenic therapy using arterial spin labeling and diffusion-weighted imaging: A feasibility study. *Acad. Radiol.* **2010**, *17*, 1326–1333. [CrossRef]
35. Messiou, C.; Giles, S.; Collins, D.J.; West, S.; Davies, F.E.; Morgan, G.J.; Desouza, N.M. Assessing response of myeloma bone disease with diffusion-weighted MRI. *Br. J. Radiol.* **2012**, *85*, 1020. [CrossRef]
36. Koutoulidis, V.; Fontara, S.; Terpos, E.; Zagouri, F.; Matsaridis, D.; Christoulas, D.; Panourgias, E.; Kastritis, E.; Dimopoulos, M.A.; Moulopoulos, L.A. Quantitative Diffusion-weighted Imaging of the Bone Marrow: An Adjunct Tool for the Diagnosis of a Diffuse MR Imaging Pattern in Patients with Multiple Myeloma. *Radiology* **2017**, *282*, 484–493. [CrossRef]
37. Giles, S.L.; Messiou, C.; Collins, D.J.; Morgan, V.A.; Simpkin, C.J.; West, S.; Davies, F.E.; Morgan, G.J.; deSouza, N.M. Whole-Body Diffusion-weighted MR Imaging for Assessment of Treatment Response in Myeloma. *Radiology* **2014**, *271*, 785–794. [CrossRef]
38. Lemke, A.; Laun, F.B.; Klauss, M.; Re, T.J.; Simon, D.; Delorme, S.; Schad, L.R.; Stieltjes, B. Differentiation of pancreas carcinoma from healthy pancreatic tissue using multiple b-values: Comparison of apparent diffusion coefficient and intravoxel incoherent motion derived parameters. *Investig. Radiol.* **2009**, *44*, 769–775. [CrossRef]
39. Luciani, A.; Vignaud, A.; Cavet, M.; Nhieu, J.T.; Mallat, A.; Ruel, L.; Laurent, A.; Deux, J.F.; Brugieres, P.; Rahmouni, A. Liver cirrhosis: Intravoxel incoherent motion MR imaging—Pilot study. *Radiology* **2008**, *249*, 891–899. [CrossRef]
40. Sezer, O.; Niemöller, K.; Jakob, C.; Zavrski, I.; Heider, U.; Eucker, J.; Kaufmann, O.; Possinger, K. Relationship between bone marrow angiogenesis and plasma cell infiltration and serum beta2-microglobulin levels in patients with multiple myeloma. *Ann. Hematol.* **2001**, *80*, 598–601.
41. Chu, H.H.; Choi, S.H.; Ryoo, I.; Kim, S.C.; Yeom, J.A.; Shin, H.; Jung, S.C.; Lee, A.L.; Yoon, T.J.; Kim, T.M.; et al. Differentiation of true progression from pseudoprogression in glioblastoma treated with radiation therapy and concomitant temozolomide: Comparison study of standard and high-b-value diffusion-weighted imaging. *Radiology* **2013**, *269*, 831–840. [CrossRef]
42. Ajit, M.; Maruvaneni, S.; Kumar, A.; Ullal, S.; Fernandes, M. Role of Diffusion Weighted Imaging in Differentiating Benign from Pathological Vertebral Collapse using ADC Values. *J. Clin. Diagn. Res.* **2019**, *13*, 1–5.
43. Biffar, A.; Baur-Melnyk, A.; Schmidt, G.P.; Reiser, M.F.; Dietrich, O. Multiparameter MRI assessment of normal-appearing and diseased vertebral bone marrow. *Eur. Radiol.* **2010**, *20*, 2679–2689. [CrossRef]
44. Plank, C.; Koller, A.; Mueller-Mang, C.; Bammer, R.; Thurnher, M.M. Diffusion-weighted MR imaging (DWI) in the evaluation of epidural spinal lesions. *Neuroradiology* **2007**, *49*, 977–985. [CrossRef] [PubMed]
45. Pearce, T.; Philip, S.; Brown, J.; Koh, D.M.; Burn, P.R. Bone metastases from prostate, breast and multiple myeloma: Differences in lesion conspicuity at short-tau inversion recovery and diffusion-weighted MRI. *Br. J. Radiol.* **2012**, *85*, 1102–1106. [CrossRef] [PubMed]
46. Padhani, A.R.; Koh, D.M.; Collins, D.J. Whole-body diffusion-weighted MR imaging in cancer: Current status and research directions. *Radiology* **2011**, *261*, 700–718. [CrossRef]
47. Lacognata, C.; Crimì, F.; Guolo, A.; Varin, C.; De March, E.; Vio, S.; Ponzoni, A.; Barilà, G.; Lico, A.; Branca, A.; et al. Diffusion-weighted whole-body MRI for evaluation of early response in multiple myeloma. *Clin. Radiol.* **2017**, *72*, 850–857. [CrossRef] [PubMed]
48. Giles, S.L.; deSouza, N.M.; Collins, D.J.; Morgan, V.A.; West, S.; Davies, F.E.; Morgan, G.J.; Messiou, C. Assessing myeloma bone disease with whole-body diffusion-weighted imaging: Comparison with x-ray skeletal survey by region and relationship with laboratory estimates of disease burden. *Clin. Radiol.* **2015**, *70*, 614–621. [CrossRef]

49. Sachpekidis, C.; Mosebach, J.; Freitag, M.T.; Wilhelm, T.; Mai, E.K.; Goldschmidt, H.; Haberkorn, U.; Schlemmer, H.-P.; Delorme, S.; Dimitrakopoulou-Strauss, A. Application of (18)F-FDG PET and diffusion weighted imaging (DWI) in multiple myeloma: Comparison of functional imaging modalities. *Am. J. Nucl. Med. Mol. Imaging* **2015**, *5*, 479–492.
50. Rasche, L.; Angtuaco, E.; McDonald, J.E.; Buros, A.; Stein, C.; Pawlyn, C.; Thanendrarajan, S.; Schinke, C.; Samant, R.; Yaccoby, S.; et al. Low expression of hexokinase-2 is associated with false-negative FDG-positron emission tomography in multiple myeloma. *Blood* **2017**, *130*, 30–34. [CrossRef]
51. Lai, A.Y.T.; Riddell, A.; Barwick, T.; Boyd, K.; Rockall, A.; Kaiser, M.; Koh, D.M.; Saffar, H.; Yusuf, S.; Messiou, C. Interobserver agreement of whole-body magnetic resonance imaging is superior to whole-body computed tomography for assessing disease burden in patients with multiple myeloma. *Eur. Radiol.* **2020**, *30*, 320–327. [CrossRef] [PubMed]
52. Hernandez, J.; Montesinos, O.; Mateo, A.G.; Queizán, J.A.; Peral, G.S.d.; Olivier, C.; Fisac, R.M.; Coca, A.G.d.; López, R.; Ocio, E.M.; et al. Usefulness of Whole-Body Diffusion-Weighted MRI (WB-MRI) With Apparent Diffusion Coefficient (ADC) In The Differentiation of Monoclonal Gammopathies. *Clin. Lymphoma Myeloma Leuk.* **2015**, *15*, e90–e91. [CrossRef]
53. Rasche, L.; Schinke, C.D.; Alapat, D.; Gershner, G.; Johnson, S.K.; Thanendrarajan, S.; Epstein, J.; van Rhee, F.; Zangari, M.; McDonald, J.E.; et al. Functional Imaging Detects Residual Disease in MRD-Negative Multiple Myeloma Patients Who Subsequently Relapse. *Blood* **2017**, *130*, 4510.
54. Lecouvet, F.E.; Larbi, A.; Pasoglou, V.; Omoumi, P.; Tombal, B.; Michoux, N.; Malghem, J.; Lhommel, R.; Vande Berg, B.C. MRI for response assessment in metastatic bone disease. *Eur. Radiol.* **2013**, *23*, 1986–1997. [CrossRef] [PubMed]
55. Khoo, M.M.; Tyler, P.A.; Saifuddin, A.; Padhani, A.R. Diffusion-weighted imaging (DWI) in musculoskeletal MRI: A critical review. *Skelet. Radiol.* **2011**, *40*, 665–681. [CrossRef]
56. Rasche, L.; Alapat, D.; Kumar, M.; Gershner, G.; McDonald, J.; Wardell, C.P.; Samant, R.; Van Hemert, R.; Epstein, J.; Williams, A.F.; et al. Combination of flow cytometry and functional imaging for monitoring of residual disease in myeloma. *Leukemia* **2019**, *33*, 1713–1722. [CrossRef]
57. Fernández-Poveda, E.; Cabañas, V.; Moreno, M.J.; Blanquer Blanquer, M.; Moraleda, J.M. Prognostic Value of Diffusion-Weighted Magnetic Resonance Imaging in Newly Diagnosed Multiple Myeloma Patients Treated with up-Front Autologous Transplantation. *Blood* **2019**, *134*, 3146. [CrossRef]
58. Zhang, Y.; Xiong, X.; Fu, Z.; Dai, H.; Yao, F.; Liu, D.; Deng, S.; Hu, C. Whole-body diffusion-weighted MRI for evaluation of response in multiple myeloma patients following bortezomib-based therapy: A large single-center cohort study. *Eur. J. Radiol.* **2019**, *120*, 108695. [CrossRef]
59. Le Bihan, D.; Breton, E.; Lallemand, D.; Aubin, M.L.; Vignaud, J.; Laval-Jeantet, M. Separation of diffusion and perfusion in intravoxel incoherent motion MR imaging. *Radiology* **1988**, *168*, 497–505. [CrossRef]
60. Bourillon, C.; Rahmouni, A.; Lin, C.; Belhadj, K.; Beaussart, P.; Vignaud, A.; Zerbib, P.; Pigneur, F.; Cuenod, C.A.; Bessalem, H.; et al. Intravoxel Incoherent Motion Diffusion-weighted Imaging of Multiple Myeloma Lesions: Correlation with Whole-Body Dynamic Contrast Agent-enhanced MR Imaging. *Radiology* **2015**, *277*, 773–783. [CrossRef]
61. Shah, R.; Stieltjes, B.; Andrulis, M.; Pfeiffer, R.; Sumkauskaite, M.; Delorme, S.; Schlemmer, H.P.; Goldschmidt, H.; Landgren, O.; Hillengass, J. Intravoxel incoherent motion imaging for assessment of bone marrow infiltration of monoclonal plasma cell diseases. *Ann. Hematol.* **2013**, *92*, 1553–1557. [CrossRef]
62. Bray, T.J.P.; Singh, S.; Latifoltojar, A.; Rajesparan, K.; Rahman, F.; Narayanan, P.; Naaseri, S.; Lopes, A.; Bainbridge, A.; Punwani, S.; et al. Diagnostic utility of whole body Dixon MRI in multiple myeloma: A multi-reader study. *PLoS ONE* **2017**, *12*, e0180562. [CrossRef] [PubMed]
63. Koutoulidis, V.; Terpos, E.; Papanikolaou, N.; Fontara, S.; Seimenis, I.; Gavriatopoulou, M.; Ntanasis-Stathopoulos, I.; Bourgioti, C.; Santinha, J.; Moreira, J.M.; et al. Comparison of MRI Features of Fat Fraction and ADC for Early Treatment Response Assessment in Participants with Multiple Myeloma. *Radiology* **2022**, *304*, 211388. [CrossRef] [PubMed]
64. Berardo, S.; Sukhovei, L.; Andorno, S.; Carriero, A.; Stecco, A. Quantitative bone marrow magnetic resonance imaging through apparent diffusion coefficient and fat fraction in multiple myeloma patients. *La Radiol. Med.* **2021**, *126*, 445–452. [CrossRef]
65. Danner, A.; Brumpt, E.; Alilet, M.; Tio, G.; Omoumi, P.; Aubry, S. Improved contrast for myeloma focal lesions with T2-weighted Dixon images compared to T1-weighted images. *Diagn. Interv. Imaging* **2019**, *100*, 513–519. [CrossRef]
66. Lin, C.; Luciani, A.; Belhadj, K.; Maison, P.; Vignaud, A.; Deux, J.F.; Zerbib, P.; Pigneur, F.; Itti, E.; Kobeiter, H.; et al. Patients with plasma cell disorders examined at whole-body dynamic contrast-enhanced MR imaging: Initial experience. *Radiology* **2009**, *250*, 905–915. [CrossRef] [PubMed]
67. Nosàs-Garcia, S.; Moehler, T.; Wasser, K.; Kiessling, F.; Bartl, R.; Zuna, I.; Hillengass, J.; Goldschmidt, H.; Kauczor, H.U.; Delorme, S. Dynamic contrast-enhanced MRI for assessing the disease activity of multiple myeloma: A comparative study with histology and clinical markers. *J. Magn. Reson. Imaging JMRI* **2005**, *22*, 154–162. [CrossRef]
68. Rahmouni, A.; Montazel, J.L.; Divine, M.; Lepage, E.; Belhadj, K.; Gaulard, P.; Bouanane, M.; Golli, M.; Kobeiter, H. Bone marrow with diffuse tumor infiltration in patients with lymphoproliferative diseases: Dynamic gadolinium-enhanced MR imaging. *Radiology* **2003**, *229*, 710–717. [CrossRef]
69. Hillengass, J.; Ritsch, J.; Merz, M.; Wagner, B.; Kunz, C.; Hielscher, T.; Laue, H.; Bäuerle, T.; Zechmann, C.M.; Ho, A.D.; et al. Increased microcirculation detected by dynamic contrast-enhanced magnetic resonance imaging is of prognostic significance in asymptomatic myeloma. *Br. J. Haematol.* **2016**, *174*, 127–135. [CrossRef]

70. Hillengass, J.; Wasser, K.; Delorme, S.; Kiessling, F.; Zechmann, C.; Benner, A.; Kauczor, H.U.; Ho, A.D.; Goldschmidt, H.; Moehler, T.M. Lumbar bone marrow microcirculation measurements from dynamic contrast-enhanced magnetic resonance imaging is a predictor of event-free survival in progressive multiple myeloma. *Clin. Cancer Res. Off. J. Am. Assoc. Cancer Res.* **2007**, *13*, 475–481. [CrossRef]
71. Lin, C.; Luciani, A.; Belhadj, K.; Deux, J.F.; Kuhnowski, F.; Maatouk, M.; Beaussart, P.; Cuenod, C.A.; Haioun, C.; Rahmouni, A. Multiple myeloma treatment response assessment with whole-body dynamic contrast-enhanced MR imaging. *Radiology* **2010**, *254*, 521–531. [CrossRef] [PubMed]
72. Mulé, S.; Reizine, E.; Blanc-Durand, P.; Baranes, L.; Zerbib, P.; Burns, R.; Nouri, R.; Itti, E.; Luciani, A. Whole-Body Functional MRI and PET/MRI in Multiple Myeloma. *Cancers* **2020**, *12*, 3155. [CrossRef]
73. Matteucci, F.; Paganelli, G.; Martinelli, G.; Cerchione, C. PET/CT in Multiple Myeloma: Beyond FDG. *Front. Oncol.* **2021**, *10*, 622501. [CrossRef]
74. Bartel, T.B.; Haessler, J.; Brown, T.L.; Shaughnessy, J.D., Jr.; van Rhee, F.; Anaissie, E.; Alpe, T.; Angtuaco, E.; Walker, R.; Epstein, J.; et al. F18-fluorodeoxyglucose positron emission tomography in the context of other imaging techniques and prognostic factors in multiple myeloma. *Blood* **2009**, *114*, 2068–2076. [CrossRef] [PubMed]
75. Soret, M.; Bacharach, S.L.; Buvat, I. Partial-volume effect in PET tumor imaging. Journal of nuclear medicine: Official publication. *Soc. Nucl. Med.* **2007**, *48*, 932–945. [CrossRef] [PubMed]
76. Wahl, R.L.; Jacene, H.; Kasamon, Y.; Lodge, M.A. From RECIST to PERCIST: Evolving Considerations for PET response criteria in solid tumors. *J. Nucl. Med. Off. Publ. Soc. Nucl. Med.* **2009**, *50*, 122s–150s. [CrossRef]
77. Fonti, R.; Larobina, M.; Del Vecchio, S.; De Luca, S.; Fabbricini, R.; Catalano, L.; Pane, F.; Salvatore, M.; Pace, L. Metabolic tumor volume assessed by 18F-FDG PET/CT for the prediction of outcome in patients with multiple myeloma. *J. Nucl. Med. Off. Publ. Soc. Nucl. Med.* **2012**, *53*, 1829–1835. [CrossRef]
78. McDonald, J.E.; Kessler, M.M.; Gardner, M.W.; Buros, A.F.; Ntambi, J.A.; Waheed, S.; van Rhee, F.; Zangari, M.; Heuck, C.J.; Petty, N.; et al. Assessment of Total Lesion Glycolysis by (18)F FDG PET/CT Significantly Improves Prognostic Value of GEP and ISS in Myeloma. *Clin. Cancer Res. Off. J. Am. Assoc. Cancer Res.* **2017**, *23*, 1981–1987. [CrossRef]
79. Derlin, T.; Bannas, P. Imaging of multiple myeloma: Current concepts. *World J. Orthop.* **2014**, *5*, 272–282. [CrossRef]
80. Dimitrakopoulou-Strauss, A.; Hoffmann, M.; Bergner, R.; Uppenkamp, M.; Haberkorn, U.; Strauss, L.G. Prediction of progression-free survival in patients with multiple myeloma following anthracycline-based chemotherapy based on dynamic FDG-PET. *Clin. Nucl. Med.* **2009**, *34*, 576–584. [CrossRef]
81. Han, S.; Woo, S.; Kim, Y.I.; Yoon, D.H.; Ryu, J.S. Prognostic value of (18)F-fluorodeoxyglucose positron emission tomography/computed tomography in newly diagnosed multiple myeloma: A systematic review and meta-analysis. *Eur. Radiol.* **2021**, *31*, 152–162. [CrossRef]
82. Varettoni, M.; Corso, A.; Pica, G.; Mangiacavalli, S.; Pascutto, C.; Lazzarino, M. Incidence, presenting features and outcome of extramedullary disease in multiple myeloma: A longitudinal study on 1003 consecutive patients. *Ann. Oncol. Off. J. Eur. Soc. Med. Oncol.* **2010**, *21*, 325–330. [CrossRef] [PubMed]
83. Zamagni, E.; Tacchetti, P.; Barbato, S.; Cavo, M. Role of Imaging in the Evaluation of Minimal Residual Disease in Multiple Myeloma Patients. *J. Clin. Med.* **2020**, *9*, 3519. [CrossRef] [PubMed]
84. Hillengass, J.; Usmani, S.; Rajkumar, S.V.; Durie, B.G.M.; Mateos, M.V.; Lonial, S.; Joao, C.; Anderson, K.C.; García-Sanz, R.; Riva, P.; et al. International myeloma working group consensus recommendations on imaging in monoclonal plasma cell disorders. *Lancet Oncol.* **2019**, *20*, e302–e312. [CrossRef]
85. Lecouvet, F.E.; Boyadzhiev, D.; Collette, L.; Berckmans, M.; Michoux, N.; Triqueneaux, P.; Pasoglou, V.; Jamar, F.; Vekemans, M.C. MRI versus (18)F-FDG-PET/CT for detecting bone marrow involvement in multiple myeloma: Diagnostic performance and clinical relevance. *Eur. Radiol.* **2020**, *30*, 1927–1937. [CrossRef] [PubMed]
86. Torkian, P.; Mansoori, B.; Hillengass, J.; Azadbakht, J.; Rashedi, S.; Lee, S.S.; Amini, B.; Bonaffini, P.A.; Chalian, M. Diffusion-weighted imaging (DWI) in diagnosis, staging, and treatment response assessment of multiple myeloma: A systematic review and meta-analysis. *Skelet. Radiol.* **2022**. [CrossRef]
87. Chen, J.; Li, C.; Tian, Y.; Xiao, Q.; Deng, M.; Hu, H.; Wen, B.; He, Y. Comparison of Whole-Body DWI and ^{18}F-FDG PET/CT for Detecting Intramedullary and Extramedullary Lesions in Multiple Myeloma. *Am. J. Roentgenol.* **2019**, *213*, 514–523. [CrossRef]
88. Beiderwellen, K.; Huebner, M.; Heusch, P.; Grueneisen, J.; Ruhlmann, V.; Nensa, F.; Kuehl, H.; Umutlu, L.; Rosenbaum-Krumme, S.; Lauenstein, T.C. Whole-body [^{18}F]FDG PET/MRI vs. PET/CT in the assessment of bone lesions in oncological patients: Initial results. *Eur. Radiol.* **2014**, *24*, 2023–2030. [CrossRef]
89. Sachpekidis, C.; Hillengass, J.; Goldschmidt, H.; Mosebach, J.; Pan, L.; Schlemmer, H.-P.; Haberkorn, U.; Dimitrakopoulou-Strauss, A. Comparison of (18)F-FDG PET/CT and PET/MRI in patients with multiple myeloma. *Am. J. Nucl. Med. Mol. Imaging* **2015**, *5*, 469–478.

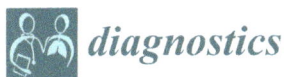

Review

Imaging More than Skin-Deep: Radiologic and Dermatologic Presentations of Systemic Disorders

Mehrzad Shafiei [1], Firoozeh Shomal Zadeh [1], Bahar Mansoori [2], Hunter Pyle [3], Nnenna Agim [4], Jorge Hinojosa [4], Arturo Dominguez [4,5], Cristina Thomas [4,5] and Majid Chalian [1,*]

1. Division of Musculoskeletal Imaging and Intervention, Department of Radiology, University of Washington, Seattle, WA 98195, USA
2. Division of Abdominal Imaging, Department of Radiology, University of Washington, Seattle, WA 98195, USA
3. University of Texas Southwestern Medical School, University of Texas Southwestern Medical Center, Dallas, TX 75390, USA
4. Department of Dermatology, University of Texas Southwestern Medical Center, Dallas, TX 75390, USA
5. Department of Internal Medicine, University of Texas Southwestern Medical Center, Dallas, TX 75390, USA
* Correspondence: mchalian@uw.edu; Tel.: +1-(206)598-2405

Abstract: Background: Cutaneous manifestations of systemic diseases are diverse and sometimes precede more serious diseases and symptomatology. Similarly, radiologic imaging plays a key role in early diagnosis and determination of the extent of systemic involvement. Simultaneous awareness of skin and imaging manifestations can help the radiologist to narrow down differential diagnosis even if imaging findings are nonspecific. Aims: To improve diagnostic accuracy and patient care, it is important that clinicians and radiologists be familiar with both cutaneous and radiologic features of various systemic disorders. This article reviews cutaneous manifestations and imaging findings of commonly encountered systemic diseases. Conclusions: Familiarity with the most disease-specific skin lesions help the radiologist pinpoint a specific diagnosis and consequently, in preventing unnecessary invasive workups and contributing to improved patient care.

Keywords: dermatology; systemic; cutaneous; radiologic features; congenital; genetic; autoimmune; vasculitis; neoplasms; multidisciplinary

Citation: Shafiei, M.; Shomal Zadeh, F.; Mansoori, B.; Pyle, H.; Agim, N.; Hinojosa, J.; Dominguez, A.; Thomas, C.; Chalian, M. Imaging More than Skin-Deep: Radiologic and Dermatologic Presentations of Systemic Disorders. *Diagnostics* **2022**, *12*, 2011. https://doi.org/10.3390/diagnostics12082011

Academic Editor: Ernesto Di Cesare

Received: 27 July 2022
Accepted: 17 August 2022
Published: 19 August 2022

Publisher's Note: MDPI stays neutral with regard to jurisdictional claims in published maps and institutional affiliations.

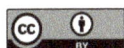

Copyright: © 2022 by the authors. Licensee MDPI, Basel, Switzerland. This article is an open access article distributed under the terms and conditions of the Creative Commons Attribution (CC BY) license (https://creativecommons.org/licenses/by/4.0/).

1. Introduction

Systemic disorders often present with both cutaneous and radiologic findings. Some presenting skin lesions are disease-specific (e.g., shagreen patch in tuberous sclerosis); others signify internal organ involvement (e.g., erythema nodosum in sarcoidosis, tuberculosis, or inflammatory bowel disease). These cutaneous manifestations sometimes precede more serious findings and should prompt clinicians to investigate further systemic involvement by radiologic examinations. Familiarity with dermatologic signs of these disorders can help radiologists interpret imaging findings more precisely. This may result in early diagnosis of the disease entity and obviate further, often invasive, diagnostic testing, ultimately improving patient management [1–3].

This article aims to provide a review of both dermatologic and radiologic manifestations of various systemic diseases, emphasizing findings that are disease-specific. We describe characteristic radiologic findings of common systemic disorders through a multimodality approach after a brief overview of clinical and dermatologic manifestations. Disease entities are broadly categorized into three areas: (1) autoimmune/inflammatory disorders and vasculitides, (2) genetic/congenital disorders, and (3) neoplasms (Table 1).

Table 1. Clinical, Dermatologic, and Imaging Findings in Systemic Diseases.

Disorder	Clinical and Dermatologic Findings	Imaging Findings
Autoimmune/Inflammatory Disorders and Vasculitides		
Dermatomyositis	Atrophic dermal papules of dermatomyositis (Gottron papules), Gottron sign, heliotrope rash, V sign, shawl sign, calcinosis cutis Proximal nailfold erythema, capillary loop dilation and dropout, ragged cuticles Esophageal dysmotility Myositis ILD Malignancy	Calcinosis cutis Feathery edema-like SI of the muscles NSIP, OP, UIP
Sarcoidosis	Lupus pernio Erythema nodosum Lung nodules and adenopathy neurosarcoidosis Bone lesions	Reticulonodular lung opacities with upper lobe and peri-lymphatic distribution Leptomeningeal enhancement Lacy lytic bone lesions
Scleroderma (diffuse systemic sclerosis)	Raynaud's phenomenon Skin tightening Sclerodactyly Calcinosis cutis Dilated bowel/esophagus Pulmonary hypertension ILD	Soft-tissue calcifications and acro-osteolysis Lack of peristalsis and esophageal dilation NSIP and UIP
Celiac disease	Dermatitis herpetiformis Psoriasis Intestinal manifestations	Small-bowel dilation Reversal of jejunal and ileal folds
Granulomatosis with polyangiitis (Wegner's)	Palpable purpura Subcutaneous nodules Pyoderma-gangrenosum-like ulcerations Lung lesions and hemoptysis Glomerulonephritis Peripheral neuropathy, mononeuritis multiplex Chronic sinusitis and saddle nose deformity	Bilateral cavitary lung lesions with a ground-glass halo sign Mucosal thickening Nasal septal perforation Hyperostosis
Polyarteritis nodosa	Palpable purpura Painful nodules on lower legs Livedo reticularis Medium-sized artery vasculitis	Microaneurysms and constrictions of medium-sized arteritis (beaded appearance)
Behcet's disease	Oral and genital ulcers Ocular findings Vasculitis CNS lesions	Thickening of the aorta and SVC Bilateral pulmonary artery aneurysms Basal ganglia and brainstem lesions
Genetic/Congenital Disorders		
Tuberous sclerosis complex	Facial angiofibroma Hypopigmented macules Shagreen patches Periungual fibromas Osseous abnormalities CNS hamartomas Renal AML Pulmonary LAM	Tubers, RMLs, SENs, SEGAs of brain Focal sclerotic bone lesions Hypertrophic osteoarthropathy Fat-containing renal mass Thin-walled lung cysts
Neurofibromatosis type 1 (NF-1)	Café-au-lait spots Freckling (axillary or inguinal) Lisch nodules Neurofibromas Optic nerve and other gliomas Skeletal abnormalities	Peripheral nerve sheath tumors including cutaneous, spinal, plexiform neuroma Diffuse thickening of the nerve
Sturge–Weber syndrome	Port-wine stains Leptomeningeal capillary malformation Glaucoma	Parieto-occipital cortical hemiatrophy Tram-track calcification Calvarial thickening

Table 1. Cont.

Disorder	Clinical and Dermatologic Findings	Imaging Findings
PHACES syndrome	Craniofacial hemangiomas Posterior fossa malformations Cerebrovascular anomalies Eye anomalies	Ipsilateral cerebellar hemisphere dysplasia Major cerebral vessels dysplasia
Basal cell nevus syndrome	Basal cell carcinomas Palmoplantar pits Skeletal abnormalities Brain abnormalities	Keratocystic odontogenic tumors Ribs and metacarpals abnormalities Medulloblastoma, falx cerebri calcification
Hereditary hemorrhagic telangiectasia	Recurrent epistaxis Multiple telangiectasias Arteriovenous malformations	Bilateral well-defined lung opacities with lobulated shapes Ground-glass nodule
Birt–Hogg–Dube syndrome	Fibrofolliculomas, trichodiscomas, acrochordons Lung cysts (pneumothorax) Renal cysts	Bilateral basilar predominant, thin-walled cysts abutting pleura and pulmonary vessels
McCune–Albright syndrome	Cafe'-au-lait macules Fibrous dysplasia Endocrine dysfunction	Medullary ground-glass lytic lesions with thin cortices Various sclerotic to cystic pattern
Fong (Nail–patella) syndrome	Hypoplastic nails, triangular lunulae Hypoplastic patellae Focal segmental glomerulosclerosisLester iris	Bilateral absence of patellae Posterior iliac horns (Fong's prongs) Subluxation of radial heads
Maffucci syndrome	Multiple enchondromatosis (Ollier disease) Venous malformations	Multiple osteochondromas
Buschke–Ollendorff syndrome	Dermatofibrosis lenticularis disseminata Osteopoikilosis Melorheostosis	Bony islands and multiple sclerotic lesions cause mottled appearance Cortical thickening with undulating bone
Peutz–Jeghers syndrome	Mucocutaneous pigmented macules Hamartomatous polyps	Multiple intraluminal filling defects on barium study
Neoplasm		
Melanotic melanoma	ABCDE features	Enhancing lesions if they contain a sufficient amount of melanin Multiple well-defined lung nodules
Kaposi sarcoma	Erythematous or violaceous macules, plaques, nodules Pulmonary involvement Gastrointestinal involvement	Nodular enhancing masses Peribroncovascular nodules and halo sign

ILD = interstitial lung disease; SI = signal intensities; NSIP = nonspecific interstitial pneumonia; OP = organizing pneumonia; UIP = usual interstitial pneumonia; CNS = central nervous system; SVC = superior vena cava; RML = radial migration lines; SENs = subependymal nodules; SEGAs = subependymal giant cell astrocytomas; ABCDE = asymmetry, irregular border, color variegation, diameter greater than 6 mm, and evolving morphology.

2. Autoimmune/Inflammatory Disorders and Vasculitides

2.1. Dermatomyositis

Dermatomyositis (DM) is a rare autoimmune disease occurring with a bimodal peak incidence of 5–15 at 40–60 years of age with a 2:1 female: male predominance. DM is characterized by skin lesions and myositis [4–6]. Skin lesions in DM are often pruritic or burning, photosensitive, and precede myopathic symptoms in 50% of patients [5,7]. Atrophic dermal papules of dermatomyositis (ADPDM, formerly Gottron papules) are pathognomonic violaceous papules and plaques, sometimes with subtle scale, found on the interphalangeal joints of the hands (Figure 1A) [7]. Additional pathognomonic findings include Gottron sign (erythematous macules or patches over the extensor joints) and the heliotrope rash (periorbital erythema with edema, most often affecting the upper eyelids) [7]. Other characteristic skin findings in DM include V sign (erythematous, confluent papules, and plaques over the lower anterior neck and upper chest), shawl sign (violaceous or erythematous papules and plaques over the posterior shoulders and upper back), calcinosis cutis, and nailfold changes (periungual erythema, capillary loop dilation and dropout, and ragged cuticles) [5–7].

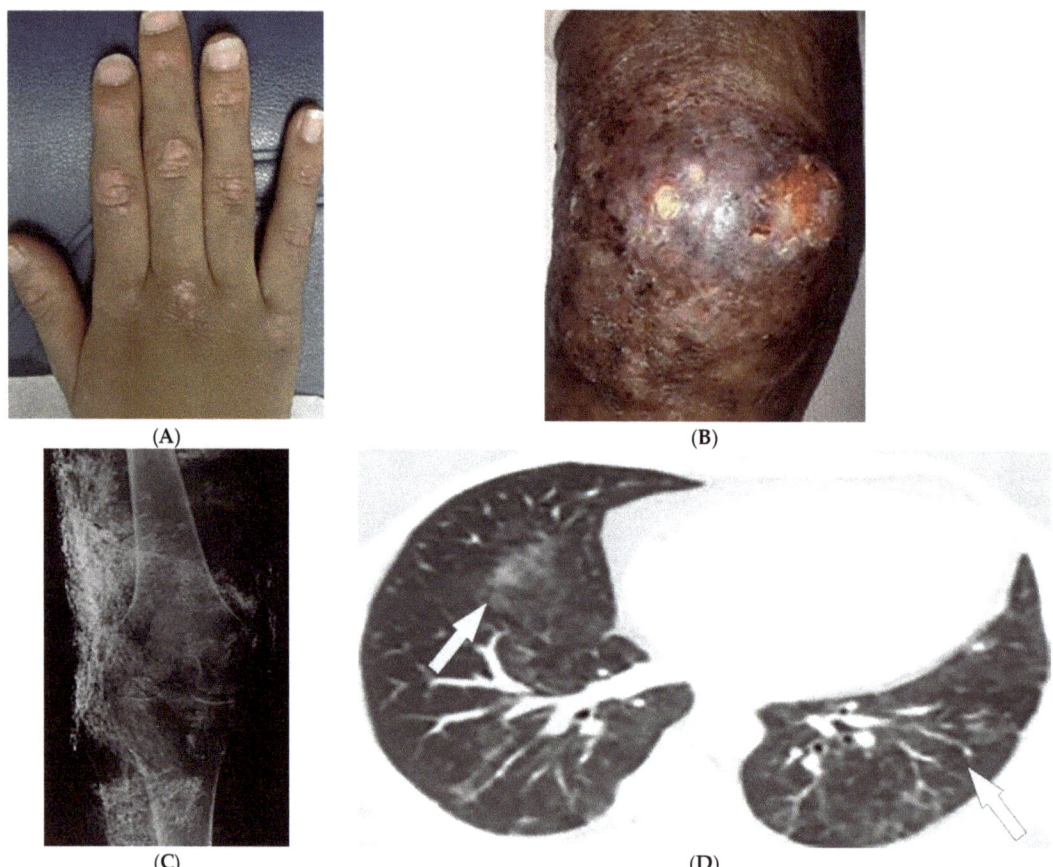

Figure 1. Dermatologic and radiologic images representative of dermatomyositis: (**A**) Flat-topped papules "Gottron's papules" over the dorsum of the hand of a 19-year-old female. (**B**) Skin erythema and ulceration of the knee due to soft-tissue calcifications in a 45-year-old female. (**C**) AP radiograph of the same knee displays sheet-like soft-tissue calcifications. (**D**) Axial chest CT image (lung window) demonstrates patchy bilateral ground-glass opacities (GGOs) indicative of dermatomyositis-associated interstitial lung disease (ILD) (arrows).

A large body of evidence exists substantiating an association between dermatomyositis and malignancy, and newly diagnosed patients should be screened for underlying malignancy. Screening typically involves a comprehensive review of the patient's history, physical examination, and basic labs followed by CT imaging of chest/abdomen/pelvis in cases of high suspicion. Features associated with an increased risk of malignancy include older age at onset (>45), male sex, dysphagia, cutaneous necrosis, cutaneous vasculitis, rapid onset myositis, and elevated inflammatory markers [8,9].

Magnetic resonance imaging (MRI) has become a fundamental noninvasive tool for assessment of myositis. MRI provides information to diagnose subclinical disease, estimate disease chronicity, detect optimal site for biopsy, and evaluates treatment response. However, its application is still limited due to cost and availability [4,9–11]. Multifocal areas of hyperintensities on fluid-sensitive sequences and areas of enhancement on contrast-enhanced fat-saturated T1-weighted images (T1WI) are seen in active disease. Fatty atrophy (chronic disease) is best visualized on T1-weighted sequences [9–11]. Soft-tissue calcifications with varying patterns, including nodular, reticular, amorphous, and sheet-like, occur in up to 70% of patients with DM, predominantly children (Figure 1B). If there is diagnostic uncertainty, plain radiographs are recommended for the initial detection of soft-tissue calcinosis due to their high sensitivity, availability, and low cost (Figure 1C) [4].

Thoracic complications occur in >50% of patients and include interstitial lung disease (ILD), aspiration pneumonia, and hypoventilation [6]. While ILD can present as reticulonodular opacities on radiograph, high-resolution computed tomography (HRCT) of the chest is able to differentiate between predominant patterns with higher diagnostic accuracy. These patterns of ILD, which may coexist (Figure 1D) [4] include (A) nonspecific interstitial pneumonia (NSIP, with imaging characteristics of ground-glass opacification (GGO) with reticulation and traction bronchiectasis), (B) organizing pneumonia (OP, seen as peripheral bilateral consolidation and patchy GGOs) and to a lesser extent (C) usual interstitial pneumonia (UIP, manifesting as peripheral reticulation, traction bronchiectasis, and honeycombing), all with basilar predilection. Another complication of DM is the involvement of pharyngeal muscles, which may result in dysphagia, and aspiration pneumonia. This could be measured by an esophagogram, which is a dynamic fluoroscopic swallow study [4,6].

2.2. Sarcoidosis

Sarcoidosis is a granulomatous disease with unknown etiology and variable prevalence, with a predilection for African American women in their third to fifth decades of life [12–15]. Patients may be asymptomatic or experience a wide spectrum of multiorgan involvement [13,14] demanding radiologic investigation for diagnosis and follow-up [12,13,15]. Twenty to thirty-five percent of patients with sarcoidosis develop skin lesions, which often manifest at the onset of systemic illness and, thus, can provide diagnostic clues. Specific skin lesions are those with epithelioid granulomas without associated inflammation on histopathology (e.g., lupus pernio, Darier–Roussy). Erythema nodosum (EN, reported in up to 25% of cases) consists of tender self-limiting erythematous subcutaneous nodules most commonly present on the shin. Lupus pernio (LP) describes characteristic chronic violaceous indurated papulonodules with central face distribution. It is strongly associated with extracutaneous involvement, specifically pulmonary disease [12,14–16]. Sarcoid may also present as firm, well-demarcated, skin-colored to violaceous papules with a predilection for the face (Figure 2A). Of note, sarcoidosis has been reported to mimic other diseases, including herpes zoster, chronic cutaneous lupus erythematosus, ichthyosis, and psoriasis [17].

Thoracic involvement is seen in nearly 90% of patients with chronic sarcoidosis, and usually presents with symmetric, bilateral, hilar, and right paratracheal adenopathy with amorphous or cloud-like calcified lymph nodes (Figure 2B). Parenchymal involvement and pulmonary embolism are other chest manifestations of sarcoidosis. Parenchymal involvement usually reveals bilateral, symmetric, small, rounded opacities with apical predominance on chest radiography. Irregular (2–5 mm) nodules with perilymphatic predilection causing irregular micronodular thickening of fissures and interlobular septa can be seen on HRCT. Parenchymal involvement can progress to irreversible disease manifesting as mid- to upper lung reticular opacities radiating from the hila (Figure 2C) [13,14,18–20].

Bone involvement mostly affects phalanges and toes with a pathognomonic lacy lytic appearance (Figure 2D), or less commonly, purely lytic lesions. MRI is more sensitive when evaluating appendicular skeleton, axial skeleton, and marrow involvement. MRI can show variable-sized with T1 hypointensities and T2 hyperintensities (Figure 2E). Chronic or healed lesions may present with signal intensities consistent with fat or fibrosis [13–15,18]. Cardiac sarcoidosis accounts for up to 85% of sarcoidosis-related deaths in Japan. Cardiac involvement patterns on late-gadolinium-enhanced cardiac MRI is nonspecific. However, it is mostly seen as patchy and multifocal late gadolinium enhancement in the basal segments of the septum and the lateral wall. On Fluorodeoxyglucose–positron emission tomography (FDG-PET), active inflammation is seen as 18F-FDG uptake with or without a perfusion defect [14].

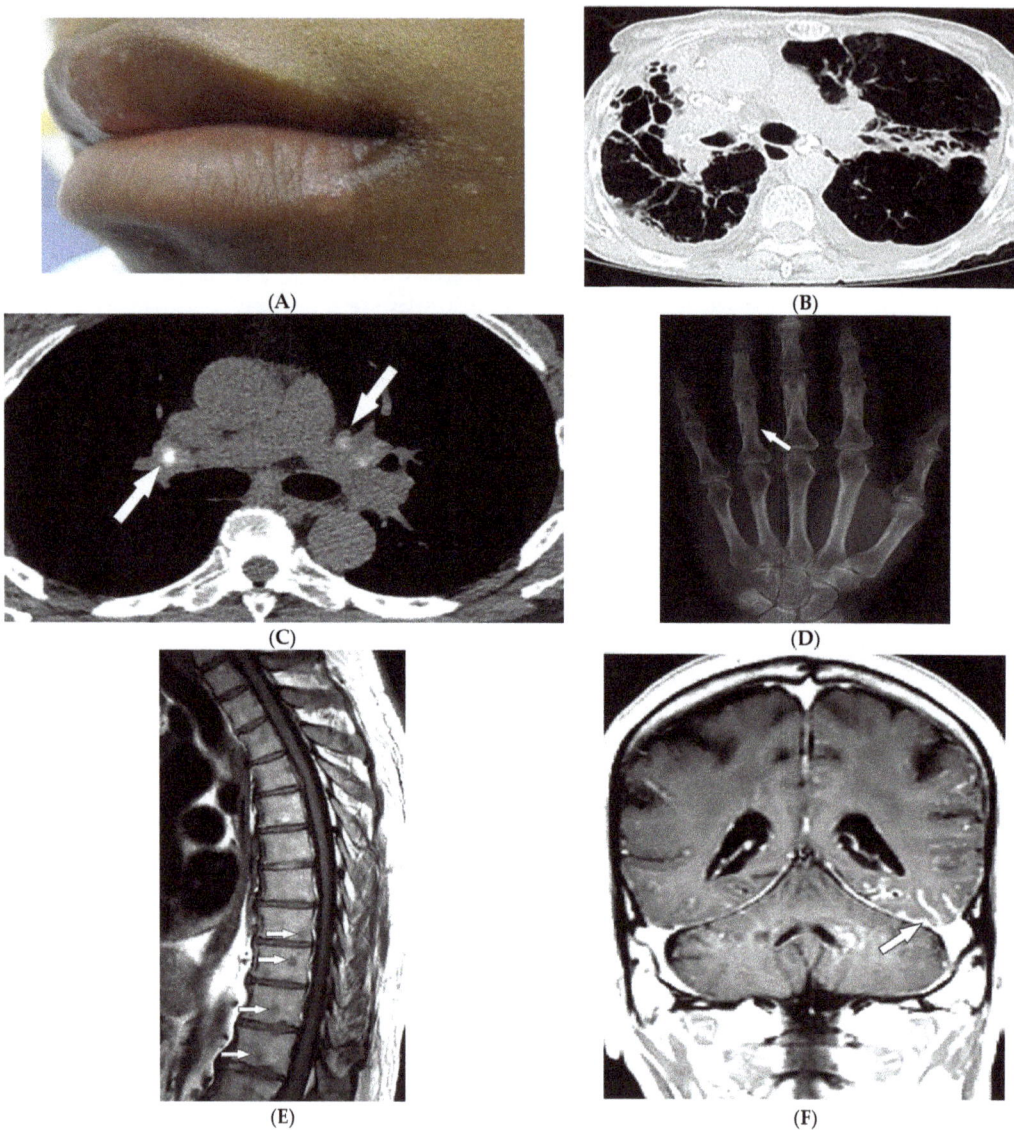

Figure 2. Dermatologic and radiologic images characteristic of sarcoidosis: (**A**) Skin-colored papules on mucosal and cutaneous lips seen in a 19-year-old male with skin sarcoidosis. (**B**) Axial chest HRCT image (lung window) of a 56-year-old male demonstrates multiple areas of bronchiectasis, cysts, and architectural distortion consistent with end-stage pulmonary sarcoidosis. (**C**) Axial chest CT image (soft-tissue window) in a 35-year-old male showing calcified hilar lymph nodes (arrows). (**D**) AP radiograph of the hand of a 45-year-old male demonstrates lacy lytic osseous sarcoid of multiple phalanges (arrow). (**E**) Sagittal T1-weighted image (T1WI) of the thoracic spine in a 40-year-old woman shows multiple well-circumscribed sarcoid marrow lesions (arrows). (**F**) Coronal contrast-enhanced T1WI of the brain of a 42-year-old male shows leptomeningeal enhancement (arrow).

Neurosarcoidosis (NS) can occur in any part of the brain. Cranial neuropathy is the most common CNS presentation, and the optic nerve is the most commonly involved nerve, which may be seen on MRI as thickening of the nerve with abnormal enhancement [13,14,18]. Intraparenchymal findings most commonly present as multiple small T2-hyperintense and T1-hypointense foci within the periventricular white matter. Plaque-like or nodular thickening of the hypothalamus and pituitary gland with T1 isointensity, T2 hypointensity, and marked enhancement may also present on MRI. Leptomeningeal and dural involvement are seen, respectively, as enhancing nodular (Figure 2F) and plaque-like thickening on postcontrast T1-weighted fat-saturated sequences. Dural nodularities also manifest as foci of hypointensity on T2-weighted images (T2WI). In early disease, spinal cord involvement presents as nodular leptomeningeal enhancement along the spinal cord. Late manifestations of cord involvement include elongated eccentric intramedullary T1 hypointensity and T2 hyperintensity with patchy post-contrast enhancement, typically in the cervicothoracic spine, with subsequent cord atrophy [13,14,21].

2.3. Scleroderma

Scleroderma, or systemic sclerosis, is an autoimmune fibrosing disorder, consisting of two subsets: diffuse cutaneous systemic sclerosis (dSSc; a systemic disease characterized by widespread involvement of any organ system with a prevalence of 20/100,000 and peak incidence in females between 30 and 50 years old), and limited cutaneous systemic sclerosis (lcSSc; a disease characterized by manifestations of the CREST syndrome (calcinosis cutis, Raynaud phenomenon, esophageal dysmotility, sclerodactyly (Figure 3A), and telangiectasia). Cases without skin changes but other systemic manifestations have been reported as well and are described as systemic sclerosis sine scleroderma [22–24]. The skin is the main organ involved in scleroderma, and disease subsets are differentiated by the degree of skin involvement [23]. Raynaud's phenomenon, cutaneous sclerosis, nailfold and fingernail alterations, cutaneous ulcerations, telangiectasias, "salt and pepper" hyper/hypopigmentation (Figure 3B), and calcinosis cutis are common skin manifestations seen in scleroderma patients [4,23]. Cutaneous sclerosis begins in the fingers, extends proximally to the metacarpophalangeal joints, and affects the face at an early stage. The skin becomes pale and hairless as the skin folds disappear. The current literature supports using high-frequency ultrasound for quantitative and reliable evaluation of dermal thickness in patients with SSc. Dermal thickness has been shown to be inversely corelated with blood perfusion. Additionally, US elastography has been shown to be of value in the evaluation of the skin in SSc [23,25–29]. Claw hands (Figure 3A), thin lips, sharp nose, and a characteristic "mouse face" appearance can result from this [23].

Morphea, previously called localized cutaneous sclerosis (LSc), is a distinct disorder from systemic sclerosis and causes limited sclerosis of the skin (Figure 3C) with rare subcutaneous tissue and bony involvement. Patients with morphea do not typically have diffuse skin involvement or systemic manifestations. Due to confusion with SSc and to decrease patient anxiety, use of "localized scleroderma" is discouraged [22].

Soft-tissue and musculoskeletal manifestations include hand edema, acro-osteolysis (involving palmar surface with progression to pencil-tip appearance), calcinosis (Figure 3D,E), flexion contractures, and arthralgias [4,23]. Bone resorption may also be seen at the ribs, distal radius and ulna, distal clavicle, and mandible [23]. The GI tract can be involved from the esophagus to anus in patients with SSc. Up to 90% of SSc patients have significant esophageal motility abnormalities. Esophagogram shows a patulous and dilated esophagus, with no peristalsis, and the presence of gastroesophageal reflux [4,23]. Esophageal dilation and shortening below the level of the aortic arch can be seen on the classic chest radiograph. Dilated tubular esophagus without peristalsis with gastro-esophageal junction widening and contrast medium regurgitation back to the esophagus may be seen on barium swallow [29].

Pulmonary involvement is the leading cause of death in SSc and most commonly includes SSc-related ILD (SSc-ILD) and pulmonary hypertension. SSc-ILD is characterized by conventional radiography showing faint bibasilar reticulation to thick peripheral interstitial opacification accompanied by traction bronchiectasis and volume loss [23]. HRCT has a higher sensitivity for detecting SSc-ILD, including mostly NSIP and UIP [6,23]. Reticulation with a predilection for posterior basilar aspects of the lower lobes is seen in both UIP and NSIP (Figure 3F). GGOs and microcytic honeycombing are characteristic of NSIP and UIP, respectively; however, they can be found in both [4,6,23].

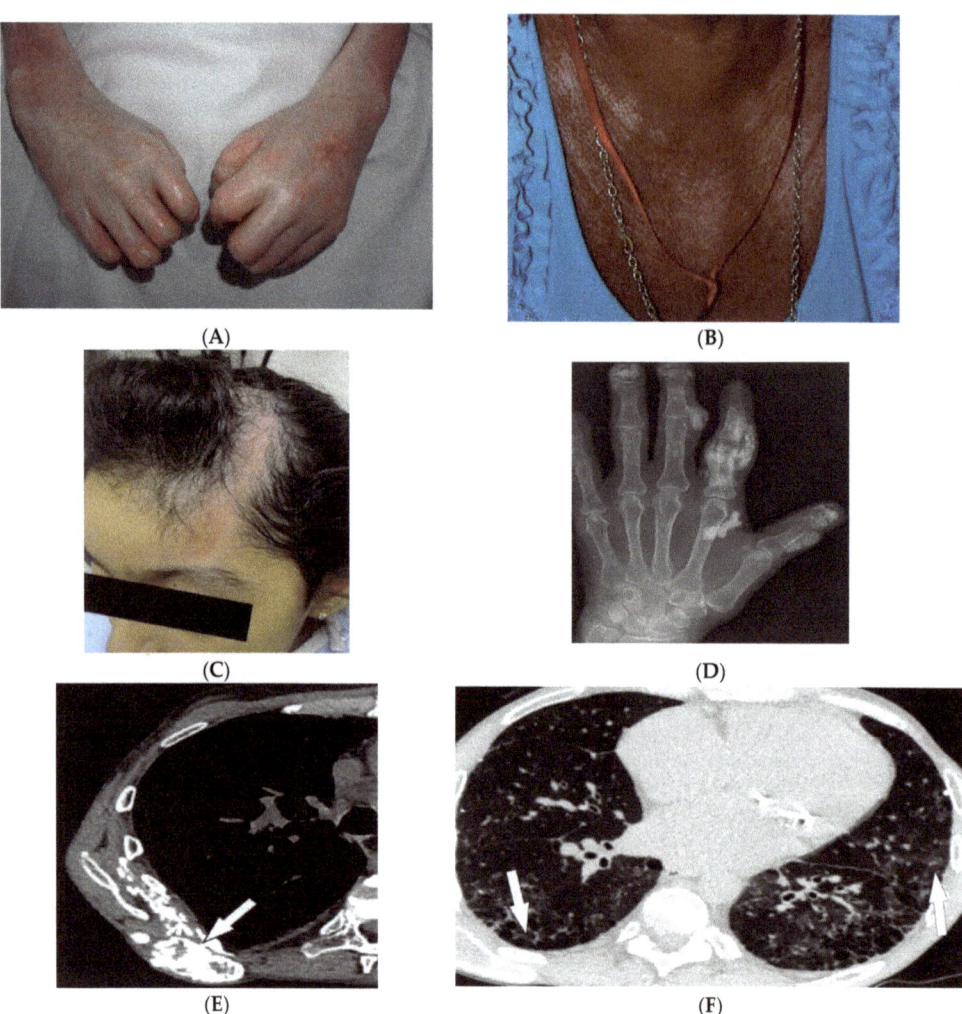

Figure 3. Dermatologic and radiologic images representative of scleroderma: (**A**) Taut shiny skin affecting the arms and hands with associated contractures of the fingers of a 56-year-old female patient with SSc. (**B**) "Salt and pepper" hyper/hypopigmentation of SSc in a 50-year-old female on the chest. (**C**) Indurated bound-down atrophic linear plaque with alopecia on the forehead and scalp of a 19-year-old female consistent with linear morphea. (**D**) AP radiograph of the hand of a 42-year-old female demonstrates soft-tissue calcifications and acro-osteolysis of the scleroderma. (**E**) Axial chest HRCT image (soft-tissue window) in a 42-year-old male shows the right back musculature calcinosis (arrow). (**F**) Axial chest HRCT image (lung window) in 38-year-old male demonstrates fine reticulonodular opacities (arrow) consistent with scleroderma-associated nonspecific interstitial pneumonia (NSIP).

2.4. Celiac Disease

Celiac disease (CD) is an autoimmune disorder reaching a 1% incidence in most populations caused by gluten sensitivity. It is associated with intestinal and extraintestinal manifestations, including osteoporosis, iron deficiency, and skin lesions [30,31]. The most commonly associated skin manifestations are dermatitis herpetiformis (DH) and psoriasis. DH, seen in more than 85% of patients, is a chronic relapsing vesiculobullous skin disease. It is characterized by symmetric, pruritic, erythematous papules, and vesicles with a predilection for the extensor surfaces of the extremities, scalp, and buttocks (Figure 4A). Psoriasis is also associated with CD and is characterized by well-demarcated erythematous, silver-scaled plaques on extensor surfaces [30].

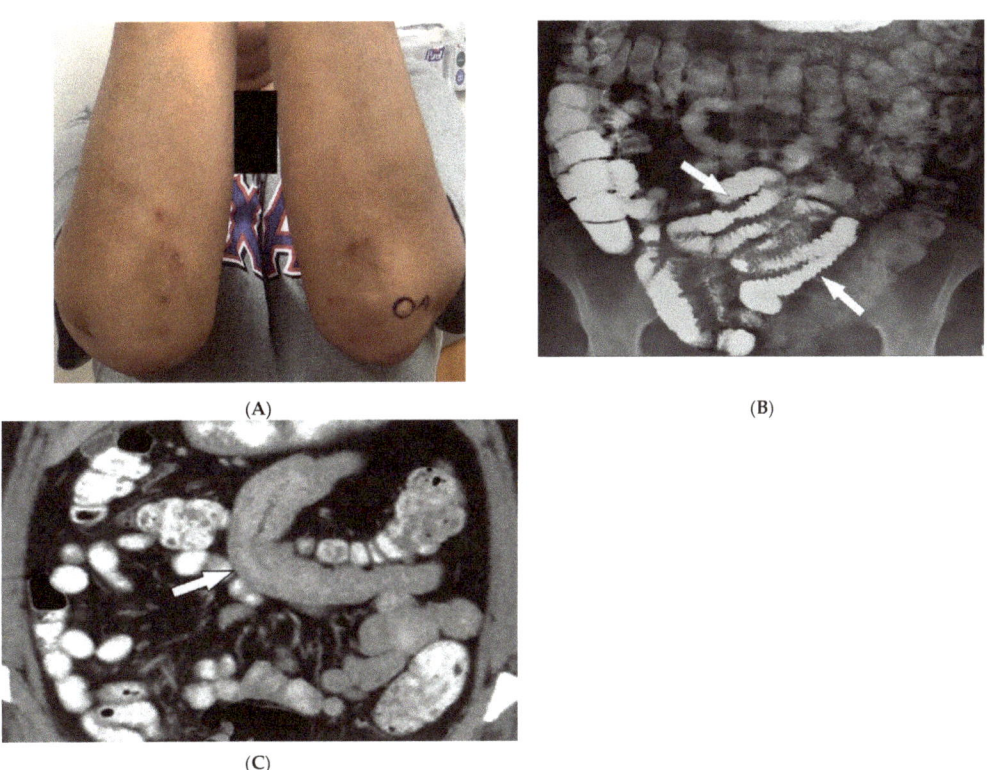

Figure 4. Dermatologic and radiologic images illustrative of Celiac disease: (**A**) Clustered vesicles over the bilateral extensor elbows of a 25-year-old female compatible with dermatitis herpetiformis. (**B**) Fluoroscopic small-bowel follow-through in a 22-year-old female demonstrates reversal of jejunal and ileal folds with more prominent folds in the ileum (arrow). (**C**) CT enterography coronal image (soft-tissue window) in a 42-year-old female shows thickening of the small-bowel folds (arrow).

Intestinal involvement is the leading cause of morbidity, mainly secondary to malabsorption as well as an increased risk for mucosa-associated lymphoid tissue (MALT) lymphoma [25]. Small bowel follow-through under fluoroscopy shows jejunal dilation, fold thickening, decreased jejunal fold with increased ileal fold (so-called "reversal of fold pattern"), hypomotility, and transient intussusceptions (Figure 4B) [32,33]. CT and MRI are more sensitive and can better delineate bowel wall thickening, mesenteric lymphadenopathy, duodenojejunal fatty proliferation, hypervascular mesentery, and hyposplenism. CT enterography (CTE) with intravenous and oral contrast can show ulcers, strictures, mucosal enhancement, increased splanchnic circulation, dilated vasa recta, reversed jejunoileal fold pattern, and ileal fold thickening (Figure 4C) [32–34]. MR enterography (MRE) has shown comparable sensitivity to CTE for the diagnosis of intestinal inflammation and has been used for the diagnosis of CD and its complications, particularly malignancy [31,33].

2.5. Granulomatosis with Polyangiitis

Granulomatosis with polyangiitis (GPA, formerly Wegener's granulomatosis) is a rare necrotizing granulomatous vasculitis, which is associated with positive cytoplasmic antineutrophil cytoplasmic antibodies (c-ANCAs). GPA primarily affects small vessels in the upper and lower respiratory tracts and kidneys, and medium-sized arteries. The peak incidence is from 46 to 60 years of age, with equal prevalence in males and females [34–36]. Skin involvement is seen in about 50% of patients and is polymorphous, including palpable purpura (cutaneous small vessel vasculitis is most common) (Figure 5A), nodules, vesicles, and necrotic lower extremity ulcers on a background of livedo reticularis. Pyoderma-gangrenosum-like ulcerations are a less common finding (Figure 5B) [34].

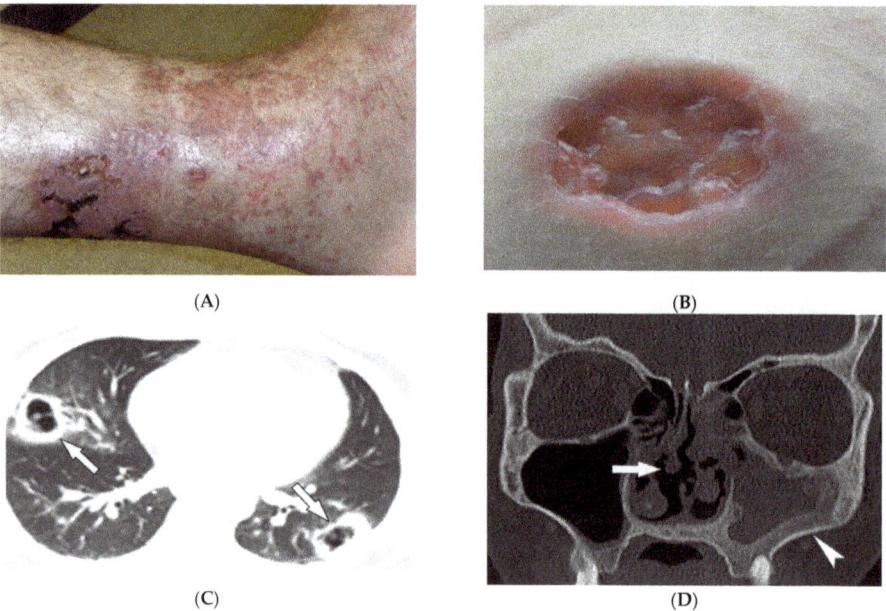

Figure 5. Dermatologic and radiologic images representative of polyangiitis: (**A**) Palpable cutaneous purpura with retiform eschars and ulceration in a 42-year-old male. (**B**) Ulcer with jagged undermined borders in a 26-year-old female with granulomatosis with polyangiitis resembling pyoderma gangrenosum. (**C**) Axial chest HRCT image (lung window) of a 36-year-old male demonstrates bilateral cavitary lung lesions with a ground-glass halo, suggesting surrounding hemorrhage (arrows). (**D**) Coronal maxillofacial CT (bone window) of a 41-year-old female shows sequelae of chronic sinusitis secondary to granulomatous inflammation, including septal perforation (arrow) and left maxillary sinus hyperostosis (arrowheads).

GPA affects the lungs in about 50–90% of patients [35]. Chest radiograph is able to detect large pulmonary nodules. HRCT shows more detailed pathologies, including variable-sized nodules (±cavitation) and GGOs (Figure 5C). Smooth or nodular thickening of the tracheobronchial tree, occasionally multifocal, causes luminal narrowing. The tracheal posterior membrane and subglottic region are most commonly involved [35,36]. Nearly all patients with GPA have ear, nose, and throat involvement at early stages of the disease [35]. Sinonasal involvement manifests as mucosal thickening, bony erosions, and neo-osteogenesis, which together are specific for GPA. Mucosal nodular thickening most commonly involves the maxillary sinuses and is mostly detected on MRI. Erosion and punctuate areas of bone destruction primarily involve the anterior ethmoidal region and is best visualized by CT [35,36]. Saddle nose deformity and perforation of the nasal septum can be present (Figure 5D) [29]. In 6% of patients, contiguous spread of inflammation can lead to the involvement of the skull base, resulting in cranial neuropathy, and is seen as cranial nerve enhancement and thickening on MRI [35,36].

2.6. Polyarteritis Nodosa

Polyarteritis nodosa (PAN) is a rare systemic ANCA-negative vasculitis involving small-to-medium-sized muscular-walled arteries with peak incidence in the fifth to sixth decades of life. The kidneys, skin, peripheral nerves, and gastrointestinal tract are most involved. Tissue biopsy along with clinical and laboratory data is diagnostic for PAN [36–39]. In one-third of patients, cutaneous manifestations are the primary feature of the disease. Common skin manifestations include palpable purpura, livedo reticularis, and nodules (Figure 6A). In addition, some patients might only manifest cutaneous lesions without systemic involvement, termed cutaneous PAN. The most frequent of these manifestations is the presence of nodules on the lower legs, which are often found in different stages of development. Less common skin features include urticaria, superficial phlebitis, distal necrosis, and splinter hemorrhages [39].

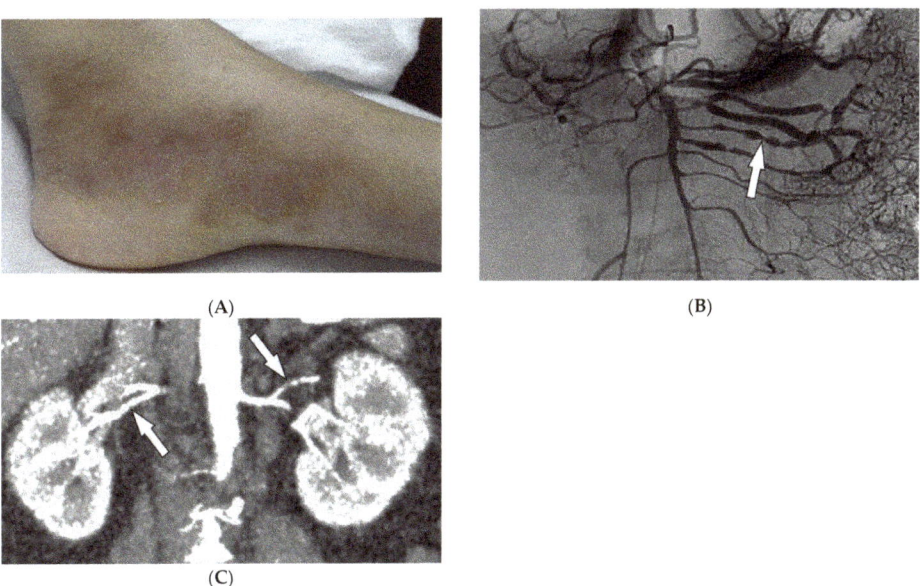

Figure 6. Dermatologic and radiologic images representative of polyarteritis nodosa: (**A**) Painful clustered subcutaneous nodules and plaques on the foot of a 36-year-old female. (**B**) Mesenteric angiogram shows the beaded appearance of multiple mesenteric arteries (arrow). (**C**) Coronal CT angiogram of the abdomen showed a beaded appearance of bilateral renal arteries (arrows).

Imaging can assist with the early diagnosis of PAN. Catheter angiography, CT angiography (CTA), and MR angiography (MRA) can be used to evaluate disease burden, evaluate cases where tissue biopsy is inconclusive or limited, and assess mesenteric (Figure 6B) or renal circulation (Figure 6C). Possible findings include multiple aneurysms (1–5 mm) and irregular constrictions occurring at small- and medium-sized arterial bifurcations. Unlike conventional angiography, CTA and MRA are less invasive and capable of evaluating arterial wall thickening and end-organ damage [36–38].

2.7. Behcet's Disease

Behcet's Disease (BD) is a systemic vasculitis of unknown etiology involving different-sized vessels presenting between the second and fourth decades of life with a higher prevalence around the historical Silk Road. Since various organs may be involved, use of appropriate imaging modalities is mandatory for the assessment of disease extent [40,41]. BD is marked by recurring oropharyngeal ulcers, genital ulcers, and ocular involvement. Earlier onset of mucocutaneous manifestations in BD indicates a worse prognosis [42]. Oral and genital involvement manifests as recurrent painful vesiculopustules evolving into apthous ulcers (Figure 7A,B). Oral ulcerations are often large and appear in groups, with frequent recurrence. Genital ulcers are smaller and occur less frequently. Other common cutaneous lesions include erythema-nodosum-like nodules, pseudofolliculitis, papulopustular lesions, acneiform nodules, and superficial thrombophlebitis (Figure 7C,D) [41,42].

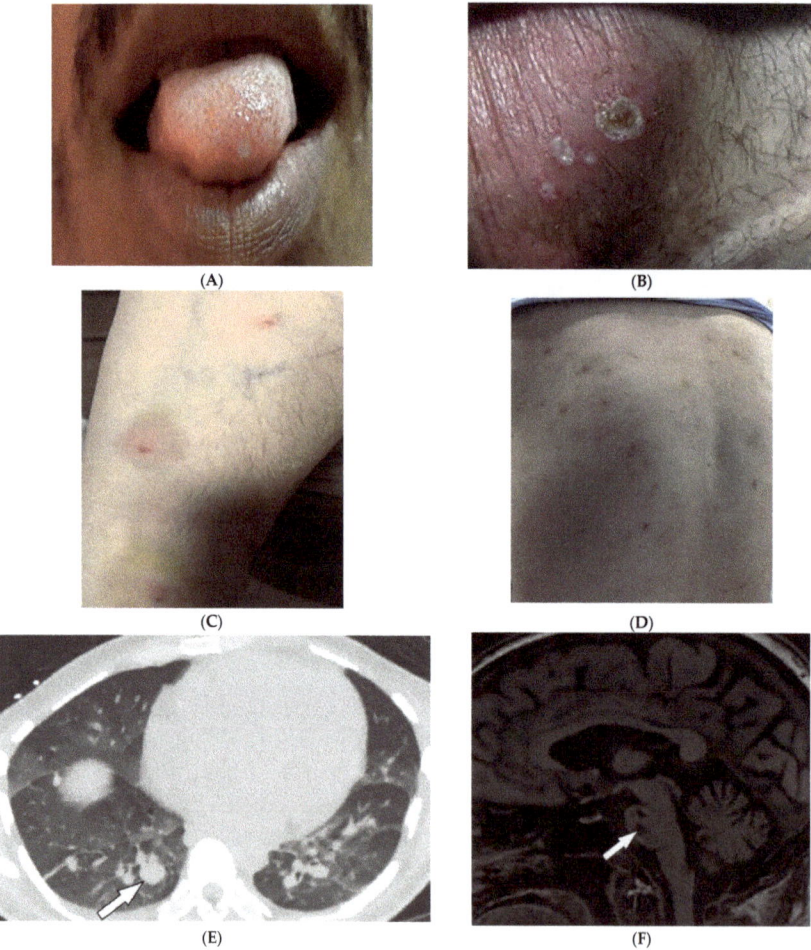

Figure 7. Dermatologic and radiologic images illustrative of Behcet's disease. (**A**) Ulceration on the tongue of a 52-year-old male. (**B**) Scrotal ulcerations and erosions (**C**) Image of the forearm of a 35-year-old male showing a positive pathergy test. (**D**) Acneiform eruption with residual post-inflammatory hyperpigmentation. (**E**) Axial HRCT of the chest with contrast in the lung window shows multiple bilateral pulmonary artery aneurysms (arrow). (**F**) Sagittal FLAIR MRI of the brain displays pontine involvement in neuro-Behçet's disease (arrow).

Vascular involvement in BD includes venous and arterial occlusion and aneurysmal dilation involving the abdominal aorta and pulmonary arteries. Early-stage findings include irregular wall thickening, perivascular fat stranding, and delayed mural enhancement, whereas late-stage features of arterial vasculitis include stenosis and aneurysmal formation on CT and MRI. Multiple, bilateral pulmonary artery aneurysms are a rare but characteristic feature of BD (Figure 7E), which may present as parahilar nodular opacities on chest radiograph. CTA/MRA delineate vessels and collaterals, the presence of thrombus, and evidence of mediastinal involvement [40,43]. CNS disease manifests in 10–50% of patients. Acute attacks initially involve the basal ganglia or brainstem, with extension to the diencephalic structures, and show contrast enhancement and scattered areas of T2 hyperintensity (Figure 7F). Months later, small scattered hyperintense lesions present in the periventricular white matter [40,43].

3. Genetic/Congenital Disorders

3.1. Tuberous Sclerosis Complex

Tuberous sclerosis complex (TSC) is a hamartomatous disease due to a mutation of TSC1/TSC2 genes with a prevalence between 6.8 and 12.4/100,000. It commonly involves the CNS, heart (rhabdomyomas in 50–65% of patients), kidneys, and lungs [2,15,44–47]. A number of skin lesions are diagnostic for TS, including facial angiofibromas (malar hamartomatous red nodules) (Figure 8A), hypopigmented macules ("ash leaf spots" and "confetti" lesions), shagreen patches (grayish-green/light brown lesions in the lumbosacral region), and periungual fibromas ("Koenen tumors", soft periungual nodules) [2,15,45,46].

CNS involvement mostly includes tubers, white matter radial migration lines (RMLs), subependymal nodules (SENs), and subependymal giant cell astrocytomas (SEGAs). Cerebral tubers are commonly multiple and bilateral with frontal lobe predilection. They appear from infancy to adulthood, ranging from T1 hyperintensity to T1 hypointensity and from T2 hypointensity to T2 hyperintensity. Calcified lesions are considered to have T2 hypointensity. On CT, tubers are hypodense [2,46,47]. RMLs, extending outward from the ventricular surface toward the cortex, appear as curvilinear or straight T2/FLAIR hyperintensities on MRI (Figure 8B). SENs are hamartomas usually scattered along the ependymal surface of the lateral ventricles with a predilection for the foramen of Monro; SENs are considered to have T1 hyperintensity and T2 isointensity (hypointensity if calcified). Head CT in children detects more than 80% of calcified SENs. SEGAs are low-grade vascular tumors that are frequently bilateral and located near the foramen of Monro, with the potential to cause severe hydrocephalus. SEGAs are iso- or hyperdense on CT with frequent calcifications and T1 hypo/isointensity and T2 hyperintensity on MR imaging with intense enhancement [2,46,47].

Renal involvement includes angiomyolipomas (AMLs), which are composed of varying amounts of blood vessels, smooth muscle, and fat, and occur in 55–75% of TSC patients, and are commonly multiple and bilateral. On ultrasonography, AMLs are homogeneous or heterogeneous hyperechoic lesions. Propagation velocity artifact is diagnostic for AMLs. CT and MRI are more specific for diagnosis by detection of macroscopic fat. CT scan can detect areas with fat attenuation. On MRI, bulk fat is seen as T1 and T2 hyperintensity, corresponding to T1 and T2 fat-suppressed hypointensity. Peripheral linear signal loss, termed India ink artifact, is seen on T1-weighted opposed-phase images (Figure 8C) [46,47].

Thoracic manifestations include lymphangioleiomyomatosis (LAM; 1–3%). LAM almost exclusively occurs in women, and is characterized by diffuse, thin-walled, well-circumscribed lung cysts of varying sizes and uniform distribution in bilateral lungs (Figure 8D). They are associated with recurrent pneumothoraxes, chylothoraces, and enlarged lymph nodes [2,46,47]. Skeletal manifestations of TS include focal or diffuse, irregular cyst-like lesions, with peripheral sclerosis (found on conventional radiographs or HRCT) and periosteal new bone formation occurring in the short tubular bones, spine, pelvis, and calvaria (hyperostosis of the inner table) [15,47].

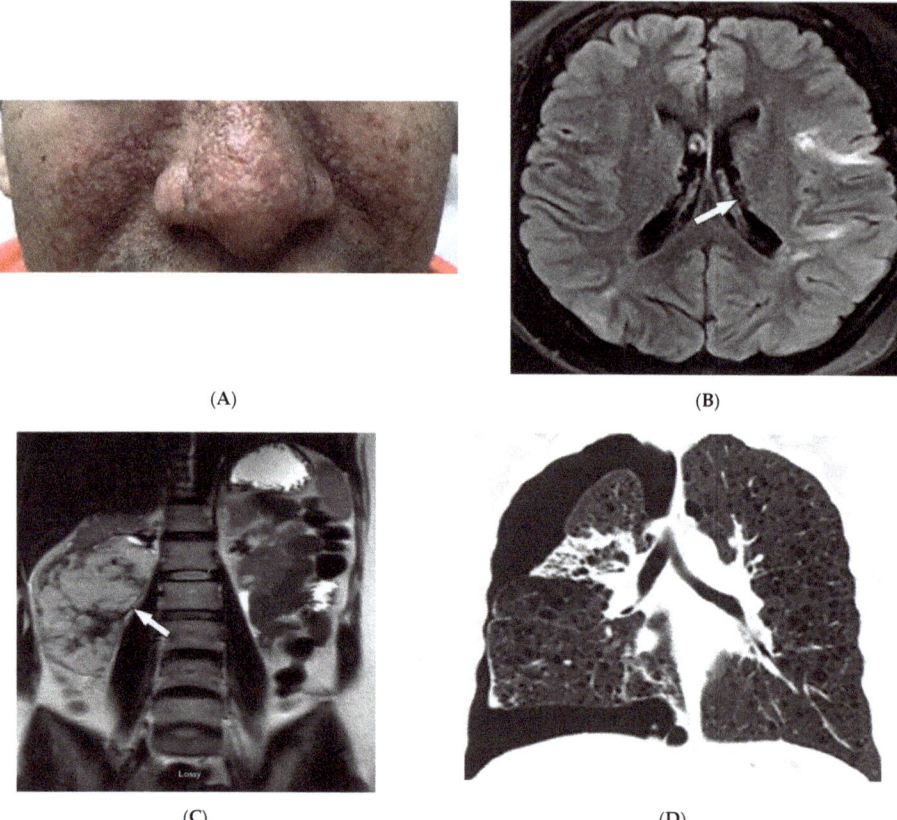

Figure 8. Dermatologic and radiologic images characteristic of tuberous sclerosis (TS): (**A**) Confluent small angiomatous (erythematous, glistening) papules on the cheek and nose of a 44-year-old man consistent with neurofibromas of TS. These lesions were not present during the first few years of life. (**B**) Axial FLAIR MRI of the brain shows linear hyperintensity extending radially from the left subcortical white matter to the gray–white junction, representing subependymal tubers (arrow). (**C**) Coronal T1WI of the abdomen demonstrating a large fat-containing right renal mass, representing angiomyolipoma (arrow). (**D**) Coronal HRCT of the chest demonstrates innumerable thin-walled cysts in a diffuse distribution and a right pneumothorax. Findings are consistent with lymphangioleiomyomatosis (LAM) with spontaneous pneumothorax.

3.2. Neurofibromatosis Type 1

Neurofibromatosis type 1 (NF1, von Recklinghausen's disease) results from a mutation of the neurofibromin gene (incidence 1:2500–1:3000). Manifestations generally occur during the first decade of life [15,48–50]. Hallmark cutaneous manifestations of NF1 include café-au-lait spots (well-defined and homogenous brown macules or patches), freckling (axillary or inguinal) (Figure 9A), Lisch nodules (benign iris hamartomas), and neurofibromas [15,49,50]. Cutaneous neurofibromas are benign tumors that develop during childhood, can occur with pruritis, and range in number from several to thousands of lesions (Figure 9B) [15,50].

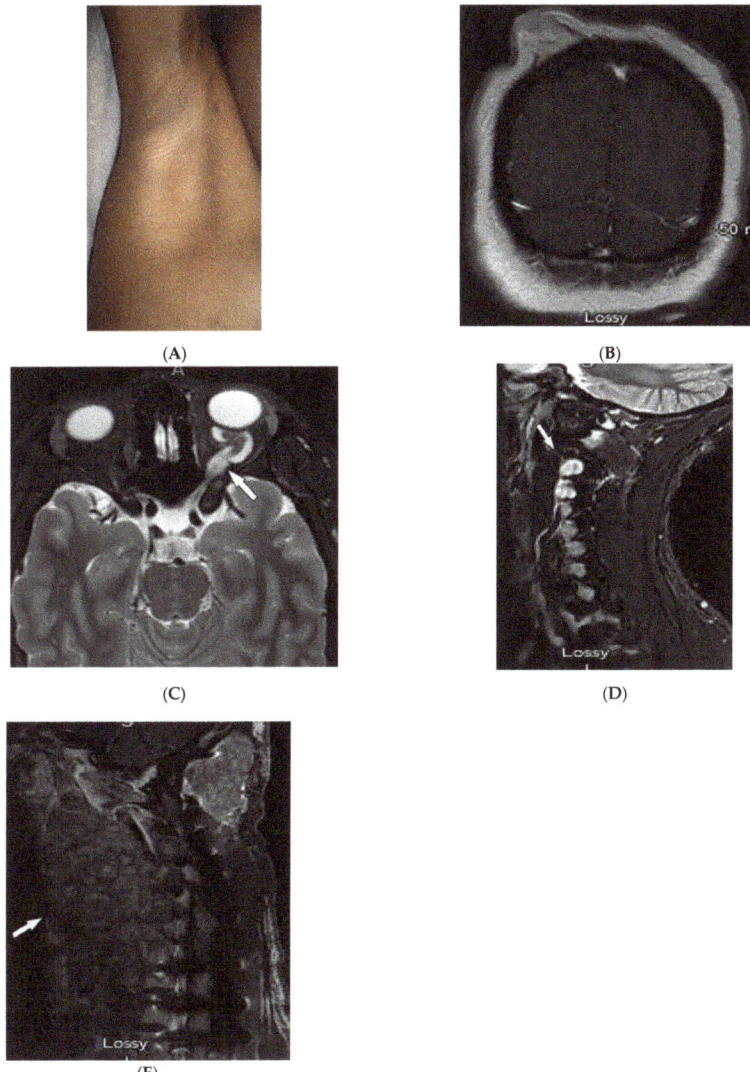

Figure 9. Dermatologic and radiologic images representative of neurofibromatosis type 1 (NF1): (**A**) Café-au-lait macules on the upper arm and multiple small macules on the axillae (axillary "freckling"). (**B**) Coronal post-contrast T1WI of the brain demonstrates diffuse cutaneous neurofibromatosis. (**C**) Axial T2WI of the brain shows diffuse thickening of the left optic nerve (arrow), consistent with optic glioma. (**D**) Sagittal T2WI of cervical spine demonstrates intraneural foraminal neurofibromas (arrow). (**E**) Sagittal T1WI of cervical spine in a 56-year-old male demonstrates plexiform neurofibroma (arrow).

Malignancies, including gliomas and peripheral nerve sheath tumors (PNFs), occur 4–6 times more commonly in NF-1 patients than in the general population. MRI is commonly used for the evaluation of neoplastic lesions [50]. Optic gliomas (pilocytic astrocytoma) are the most common tumor in NF-1 (18%) and can occur bilaterally [15,43,44]. On MRI, gliomas are seen as T1-hypointense and T2-hyperintense with variable contrast enhancement (Figure 9C). Gliomas in NF-1 have also been reported in the cortex, cerebellum, and basal ganglia [50].

Neurofibroma, the most common benign tumor in NF-1, is a peripheral nerve sheath tumor and includes cutaneous, subcutaneous, spinal, and plexiform neurofibromas [15,51]. Spinal neurofibromas, usually originating from cervical peripheral nerves, show T1 hypointensity and T2 hyperintensity with intense contrast enhancement and may contain central necrosis (Figure 9D) [44]. Plexiform neurofibromas grow along nerves longitudinally, may undergo malignant transformation, and can cause hyperostosis of nearby osseous structures [15,50]. On MRI, masses show T1 hypointensity and T2 hyperintensity with variable enhancement and central hypointensity (target sign) (Figure 9E) [49,50]. Some patients with NF-1 develop malignant peripheral nerve sheath tumors that mostly arise from plexiform neurofibromas. Characteristic findings include a large size, lack of a target sign, irregular shape, and unclear margins seen as T1 hyperintensity with inhomogeneous or poor enhancement on MRI [15,49,50]. Structural brain changes include macrocephaly, increased white matter, enlargement of the corpus callosum, cerebral asymmetries, and unidentified bright objects (presenting as T2 hyperintensity without mass effect) [50].

3.3. Sturge–Weber Syndrome

Sturge–Weber syndrome (SWS; encephalotrigeminal angiomatosis) is a sporadic disease characterized by unilateral facial capillary malformation (port-wine stain), eye involvement, and brain abnormalities [47,51,52]. Port-wine stains are blanching dermal venular malformations (pink-to-bright-red patches and plaques) that classically present unilaterally in the first branch of the trigeminal nerve (forehead, eyelids, temple), but occasionally may involve the neck, chest, trunk, and limbs (Figure 10A) [2,51,52].

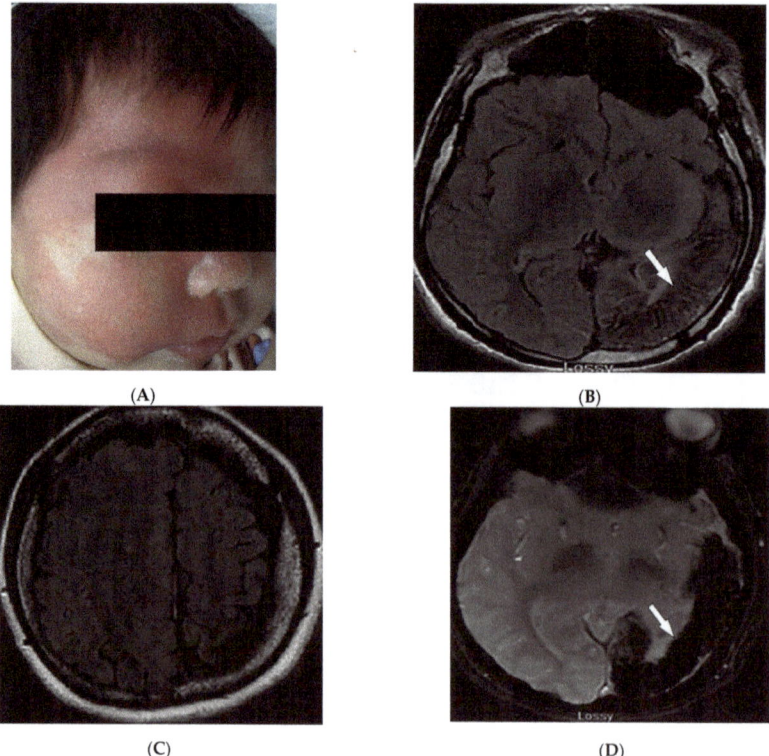

Figure 10. *Cont.*

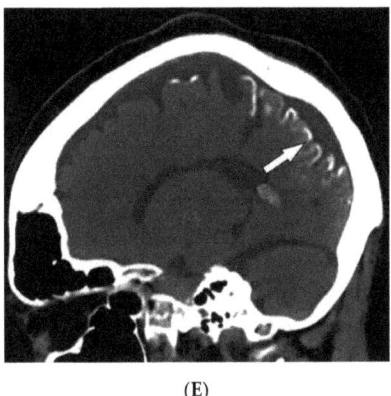

(E)

Figure 10. Dermatologic and radiologic images representative of Sturge–Weber syndrome: (**A**) Sharply marginated port-wine stain involving V1-V2 distribution. (**B**) Axial FLAIR MRI of the brain shows atrophy of the left parietal and occipital lobes (arrow). (**C**) Axial FLAIR MRI of the brain depicts diffuse atrophy of the left cerebral hemisphere. (**D**) Axial susceptibility-weighted MR image of the brain demonstrates corresponding loss of signal in the left parietal and occipital lobes (arrow), likely secondary to microcalcifications. (**E**) Sagittal CT of the brain demonstrates tram-track calcifications of the parasagittal parieto-occipital lobe (arrow) in a 21-year-old male.

In patients with SWS and leptomeningeal venular malformations, characteristic radiologic findings include decreased perfusion of the cortex and white matter with progressive severe ipsilateral parieto-occipital cortical hemiatrophy, calcification, lateral ventricle choroid plexus enlargement, calvarial thickening, and sinus hyperpneumatization [2,46,51,52]. MRI shows extent of the pial angioma [46,51]. Contrast-enhanced T2-weighted FLAIR images improve detection of leptomeningeal disease compared to post-contrast T1-weighted images (Figure 10B,C). Bone marrow signal changes are also observed in the skull or facial bones in the majority of young patients [46]. Calcification is better visualized on CT (Figure 10D) and susceptibility-weighted MR imaging (Figure 10E). Tram-track or railroad-track calcification of the adjacent sulci is also visible on skull radiographs [51,52].

3.4. PHACES Syndrome

PHACES syndrome is a neurocutaneous vascular disorder [53] observed in 2–3% of infantile hemangioma cases with a 9:1 female predilection [52,54]. It is described as posterior fossa malformation, infantile hemangioma (IH), arterial anomalies, cardiac defects, eye, and sternal abnormalities, which rarely all coexist simultaneously [52–54]. Facial hemangiomas are the hallmark of PHACES syndrome. IHs can be absent or present at birth but often are visible by the end of infancy. IHs associated with PHACE syndrome are large (>5 cm) or segmental. Hemangiomas in PHACE syndrome usually occur on the face, affecting regions of facial developmental prominences, especially the cephalic segment [53,54].

Extracutaneous manifestations of PHACES syndrome mostly include structural brain and cerebrovascular anomalies, leading to severe morbidity [46]. Structural brain anomalies include hypoplasia or agenesis of the posterior fossa (Figure 11A,B), cerebrum, corpus callosum, or septum pellucidum [52–54]. Cerebrovascular anomalies include hypoplasia, absence, or an abnormal course of major cerebral vessels, persistent embryonic arteries, and aneurysms. Arterial anomalies are much more common than venular anomalies [53,54]. MRI and MRA of the brain and neck are diagnostic modalities if PHACE syndrome is suspected [53,54].

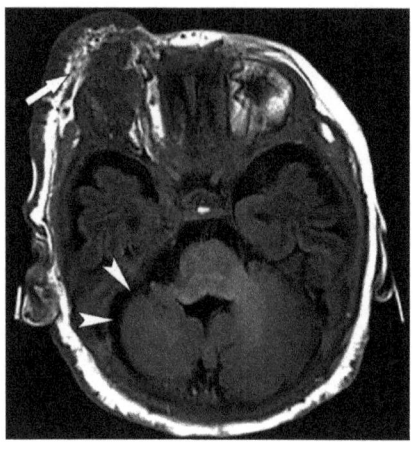 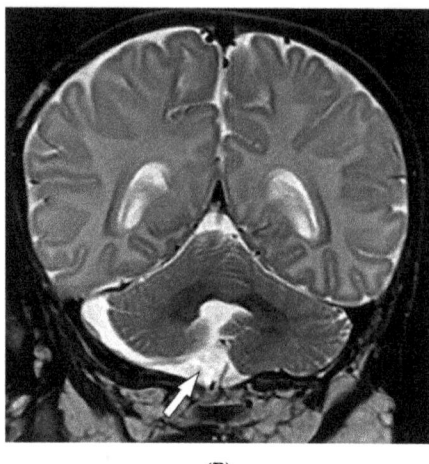

(A) (B)

Figure 11. Radiologic images illustrative of PHACES syndrome: (**A**) Axial T1WI of the brain in a 19-year-old male shows right periorbital cutaneous and deep subcutaneous hemangioma (arrow) and ipsilateral right cerebellar hemisphere hypoplasia (arrowheads). (**B**) Coronal T2WI of the brain on the same patient demonstrates right cerebellar hypoplasia (arrow).

3.5. Nevoid BCC Syndrome (NBCCS)

Nevoid BCC syndrome is an autosomal dominant (AD) disorder also known as basal cell nevus syndrome or Gorlin–Goltz. NBCCS arises from the mutation of PTCH1, PTCH2, or SUFU genes, causing overstimulation of the sonic hedgehog signaling pathway and development of benign and malignant neoplasms [2,15,55]. Patients with NBCCS present primarily in the third decade of life with skin-colored or pigmented dome-shaped basal cell carcinomas resembling benign nevi, with a predilection for sun-exposed areas. Asymmetric palmar and plantar pits (shallow depressions in stratum corneum) are early diagnostic clues present in approximately 85% of patients [2,15].

Keratocystic odontogenic tumors (75% of patients), are aggressive cystic lesions located more frequently in the mandible (Figure 12A) [15]. Other skeletal features include rib abnormalities (bifid, fused, hypoplastic, or splayed) mostly involving the third to fifth ribs (Figure 12B), thoracocervical vertebral fusion, occipitovertebral junction malformations, flame-shaped phalangeal lytic bone lesions, and shortened fourth and fifth metacarpals (Figure 12C) [2,15,49]. Desmoplastic medulloblastoma is an important associated tumor typically positioned laterally in the cerebellar hemispheres. Other imaging findings include early calcification of the falx cerebri (Figure 12D) and osseous bridging of the sella turcica, which are best seen on CT scans [2,15].

3.6. Hereditary Hemorrhagic Telangiectasia

Hereditary hemorrhagic telangiectasia (HHT), also known as Osler–Weber–Rendu syndrome, is an AD disorder. HHT is characterized by recurrent epistaxis, mucocutaneous and visceral telangiectasias, and arteriovenous malformations (AVMs) [56,57]. Epistaxis, caused by nasal mucosa telangiectasia, is the most common manifestation of HHT and is often apparent by age 10. Skin involvement appears by the age of 40 as multiple telangiectasias of the lips, tongue, face, trunk, arms, and fingers (Figure 13A–C) [56,58].

The arteriovenous malformations in HHT are direct connections between the pulmonary artery and vein through a thin-walled aneurysm without any capillary vessels. They often present as well-defined homogeneous opacities and lobulated enlarged arteries and veins on chest radiographs [50,51]. CT shows ground-glass nodules, with solid components and the architecture of the feeding artery and vein (Figure 13D,E). An enhanced phase with thin slice thicknesses is also acquired from the upper abdomen to evaluate the presence of hepatic vascular fistulas (Figure 13F) [58].

3.7. Birt–Hogg–Dube' Syndrome

Birt–Hogg–Dube´ syndrome is an AD disorder caused by mutations in the folliculin tumor suppressor gene. BHD presents with cutaneous lesions, renal tumors, and lung cysts that may lead to spontaneous pneumothorax [59–62]. Cutaneous findings of BHD include fibrofolliculomas and trichodiscomas (benign hamartomas of hair follicles) and acrochordons (skin tags). These findings classically appear in the third and fourth decade of life, often affecting the face, neck, and trunk. Fibrofolliculomas typically appear as 2–4 mm skin and white, smooth, dome-shaped papules, or as comedonal or cystic variants [59,60].

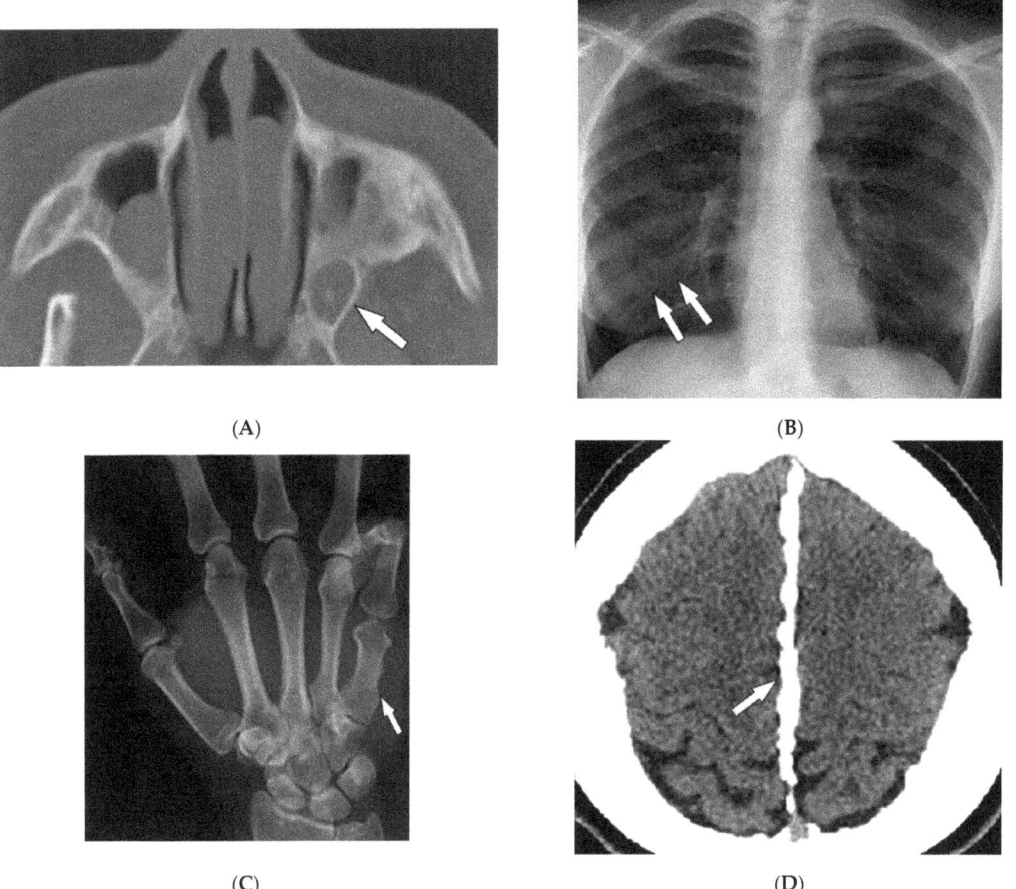

Figure 12. Radiologic images illustrative nevoid basal cell carcinoma syndrome: (**A**) Axial CT of the maxillofacial in bone window in a 24-year-old male demonstrates a left odontogenic keratocyst (arrow). (**B**) Frontal chest radiograph shows multiple bifid ribs (arrows). (**C**) AP radiograph of the hand presents a shortened fifth metacarpal bone (arrow). (**D**) Axial CT of the head in soft-tissue window demonstrates falx calcifications (arrow).

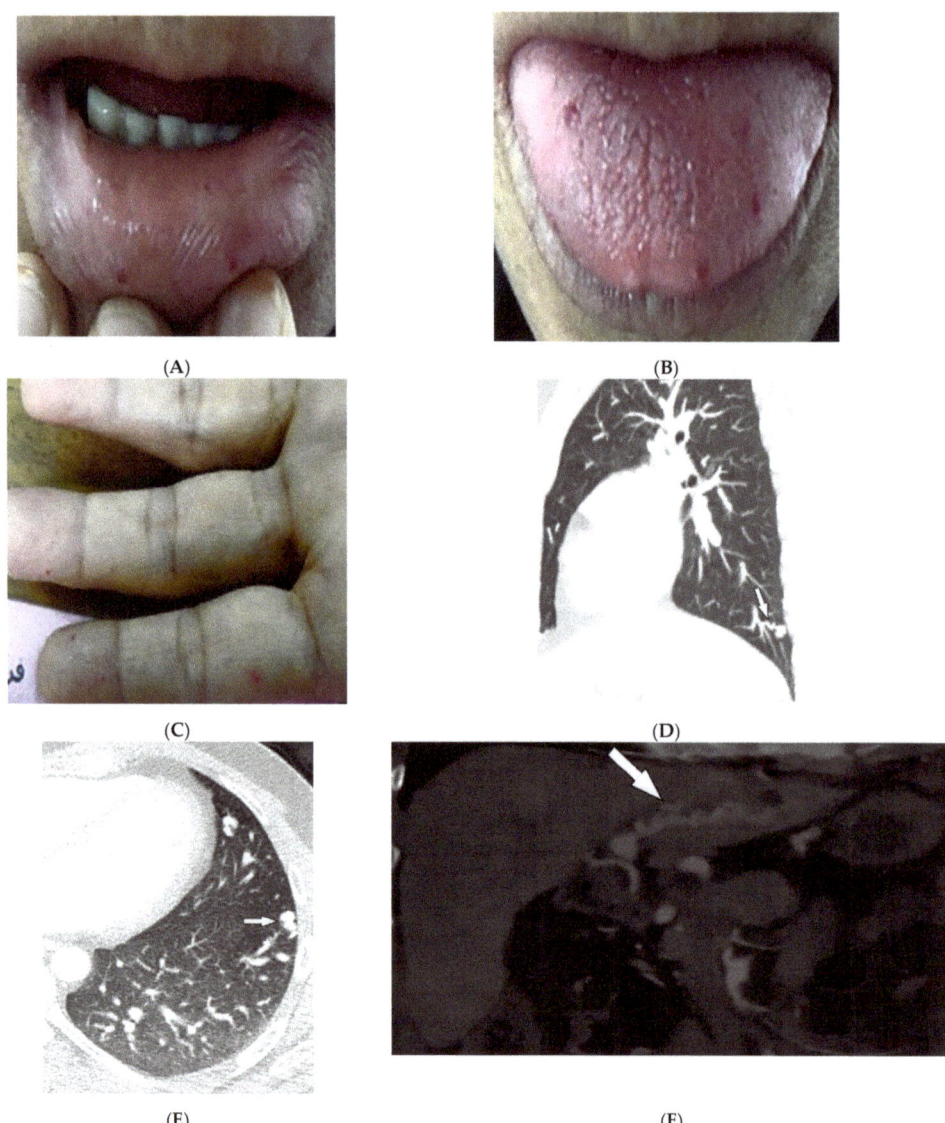

Figure 13. Dermatologic and radiologic images illustrative of hereditary hemorrhagic telangiectasia: (**A**,**B**) Mucosal telangiectasia in a 38-year-old male. (**C**) Telangiectasias over the fingers. (**D**) Sagittal and (**E**) axial contrast-enhanced chest CT of a 17-year-old male demonstrates pulmonary AVM (arrows). (**F**) Coronal contrast-enhanced CT of the abdomen shows hepatoportal AVM (arrow).

Lung cysts on chest CT are characterized by multiple well-defined, thin-walled cysts of various shapes and sizes (<1 cm). These cysts most commonly occur bilaterally with lower and medial lobe predominance. Subpleural (Figure 14A) and fissural cysts, those involving the costophrenic sulci, as well as cysts abutting pulmonary veins or arteries, are helpful in diagnosis. The surrounding lung parenchyma is usually normal [61,62]. The most ominous complication of BHD syndrome is renal cancer occurring in renal cysts (Figure 14B), which should be evaluated by CT or MRI [62].

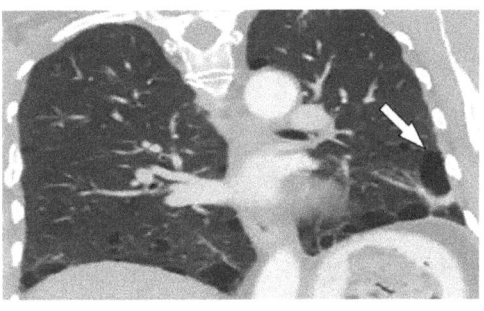 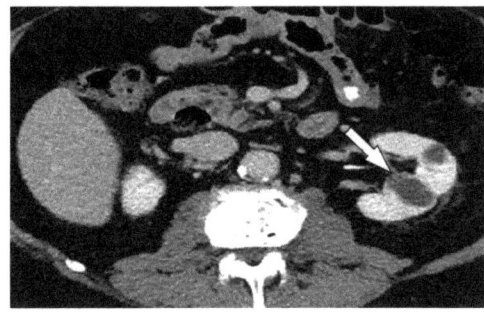

(A) (B)

Figure 14. Radiologic images representative of Birt–Hogg–Dube syndrome: (**A**) Coronal CT of the chest in lung windows in a 44-year-old male demonstrates multiple bilateral basilar predominant lentiform cysts abutting the pleura (arrow). (**B**) Axial contrast-enhanced CT of the abdomen shows two left renal cysts (arrow).

3.8. McCune–Albright Syndrome

McCune–Albright syndrome (MAS) is a rare congenital disorder caused by a mutation in the GNAS1 gene with a mosaic pattern that primarily affects females. MAS is characterized by the clinical triad of fibrous dysplasia (FD; monostotic or polyostotic), skin abnormalities (classical cafe´-au-lait skin pigmentation), and hyperfunctioning endocrinopathies (most commonly precocious puberty) [15,63,64]. MAS presents primarily with skin changes. Shortly after birth, classic cafe´-au-lait macules or patches manifest with jagged irregular borders that have been compared to the coastline of Maine. These lesions often occur in the lumbosacral area and buttocks and tend to be unilateral (ipsilateral to skeletal lesions) [15,64].

Fibrous dysplasia typically presents during childhood and in 50% of cases manifests in the craniofacial bones, pelvis, femur, and tibia. FD extends from the marrow to the cortex as irregular enlargement with polycyclic or multiloculated appearance. Classic imaging findings include medullary ground-glass lytic areas (Figure 15A,B) with thin cortices and endosteal scalloping. The pattern may vary from predominantly sclerotic to cystic. A characteristic sign of FD is the "shepherd's crook" deformity of the femur, which is caused by multiple cortical microfractures [15,63,64]. MRI findings of FD include intermediate-to-low signal intensity on T1WI and intermediate-to-high signal intensity on T2WI and STIR images [63,64].

3.9. Fong Disease

Fong disease, also known as nail–patella syndrome (NPS), is an AD condition affecting mesodermal and ectodermal tissue. NPS is caused by mutations in the LIM homeodomain transcription factor, which results in developmental defects of the glomerular basement membrane (nephropathy), dorsoventral limb structures, nails, and the anterior segment of the eyes [65–69]. Nail dysplasia (triangular nail lunulae) and patellar aplasia or hypoplasia are diagnostic features of NPS. Nail dysplasia usually presents at birth as anonychia, hemianonychia, longitudinal ridging and splitting, and spoon-shaped flaky nails. The thumbs typically show the most severe symptoms [66,69].

Characteristic quartet radiographs findings of "NPS knee" include: patellar aplasia or hypoplasia, anterior surface flattening of the medial femoral condyle, and a short lateral femoral condyle with anterior surface prominence on lateral radiograph (Figure 16A,B). Genu valgus leading to early symptomatic knee arthritis may also occur [66,69]. Luxation of the radial head (Figure 16C) and ("Frog's prongs") posterior iliac horns (Figure 16D) are other common imaging findings of NPS [66–69].

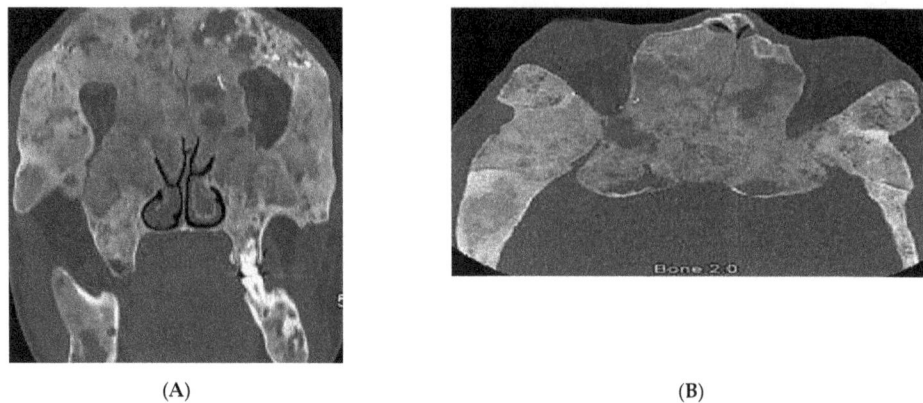

Figure 15. 24-year-old female with McCune–Albright syndrome: (**A**) coronal and (**B**) axial maxillofacial CT demonstrate ground-glass expansile appearance of bony structures, a representation of craniofacial fibrous dysplasia.

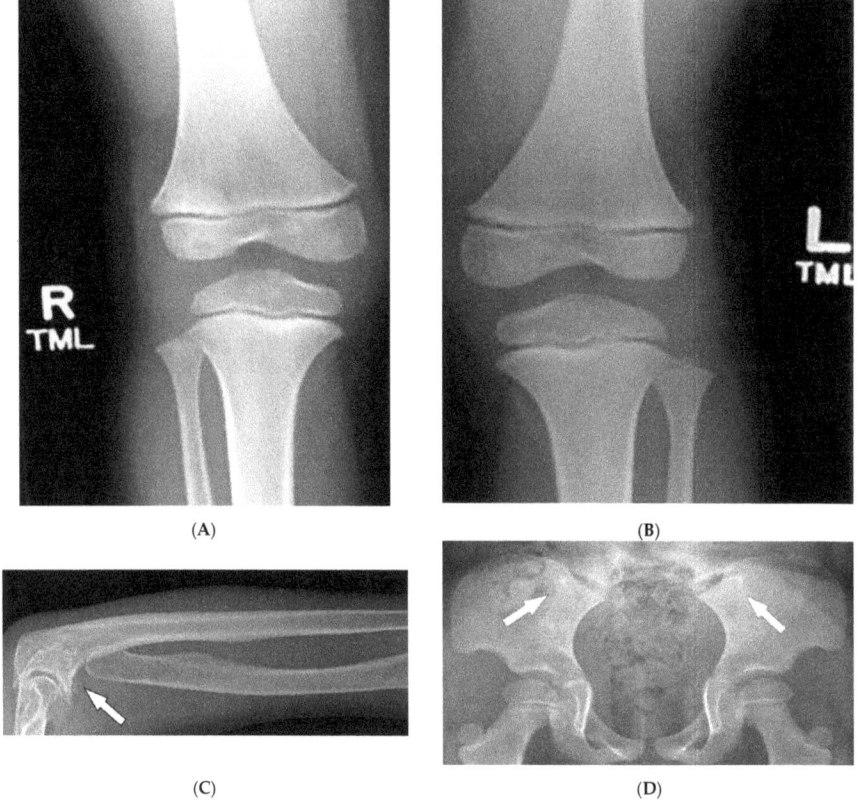

Figure 16. Radiologic images characteristic of Fong (nail–patella) syndrome: (**A**,**B**) AP radiographs of the knees in a 14-year-old male demonstrate a bilateral absence of patellae. (**C**) Radiograph of the forearm in a 56-year-female displays the absence of the radial head (arrow). (**D**) AP radiograph of the pelvis presents bilateral posterior iliac horns (arrows).

3.10. Maffucci Syndrome

Maffucci syndrome (MS) is a congenital nonhereditary disorder of early mesodermal dysplasia, typically appearing before puberty. MS is characterized by multiple enchondromatosis (Ollier disease), venous malformations (hemangiomas and lymphangioma), and malignant transformation [15,70]. Cutaneous lesions of MS are dark blue or skin-colored patches, or nontender nodules, which arise from capillary or cavernous hemangiomas of the subcutaneous tissues. These lesions primarily affect distal extremities (especially hands and feet) and can be associated with pheboliths, which are typical calcifications of the vessels [15,70]. The association between pheboliths and multiple enchondromas on hand radiographs is characteristic of Maffucci syndrome [71].

Enchondromas are benign-appearing radiolucent lesions, occurring asymmetrically on the metacarpals and phalanges of the hands (Figure 17). Radiographs demonstrate expansile remodeling of the adjacent bone with cortical thinning and endosteal scalloping. Tumors outside of the phalanges (commonly involving long bones of the arms and legs) show chondroid matrix mineralization with ring-and-arc calcifications. These lesions may present as a diffusely punctuated or stippled pattern or have a light trabeculation appearance [15,71,72]. The major complication of enchondromatosis is chondrosarcoma. Imaging findings of chondrosarcoma include deep or extensive endosteal scalloping with cortical erosion and periosteal reaction with an enhancing soft-tissue component that is best seen on MRI [71,72].

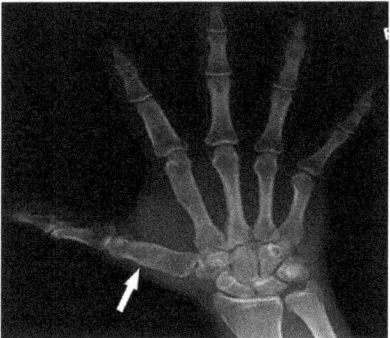

Figure 17. A 30-year-old male with Maffucci syndrome: AP radiograph of the hand demonstrates multiple enchondromas.

3.11. Buschke–Ollendorff Syndrome

Buschke–Ollendorff syndrome (BOS) is a rare, often benign, autosomal dominant skin disorder. BOS is characterized by connective tissue nevi and osteopoikilosis (OPK) sclerotic bony lesions. BOS is caused by a mutation of the LEMD3 gene, affecting bone morphogenesis, and the TGF-b gene, affecting skin elastin formation [15,73–75]. Skin lesions typically appear on the extremities, trunk, lower back, and buttocks within the first year of life. OPK often occurs after puberty at the end of long bones or phalanges, and also in tarsal and carpal spongiosa bones [15,76]. Cutaneous findings of BOS include dermatofibrosis lenticularis disseminate, characterized by symmetrical yellow or skin-colored small papules, or more frequently, larger yellowish nodules with an asymmetrically grouped distribution (Figure 18A) [15,73,75].

OPK are asymptomatic dense "bony islands" (Figure 18B) presenting as numerous well-defined symmetric densities. These lesions are found incidentally on radiographs as sclerotic densities and give the bone a mottled appearance. In some cases, OPK lesions resemble osteoblastic metastases. However, normal bone scintigraphy in OPK excludes other differential diagnoses [15,73–75]. Melorheostosis (Figure 18C), another BOS association, is a dense, irregular, eccentric hyperostosis of the cortex with a distinct demarcation border that causes irregular thickening of cortical bone with a melting wax appearance on imaging [73,76,77].

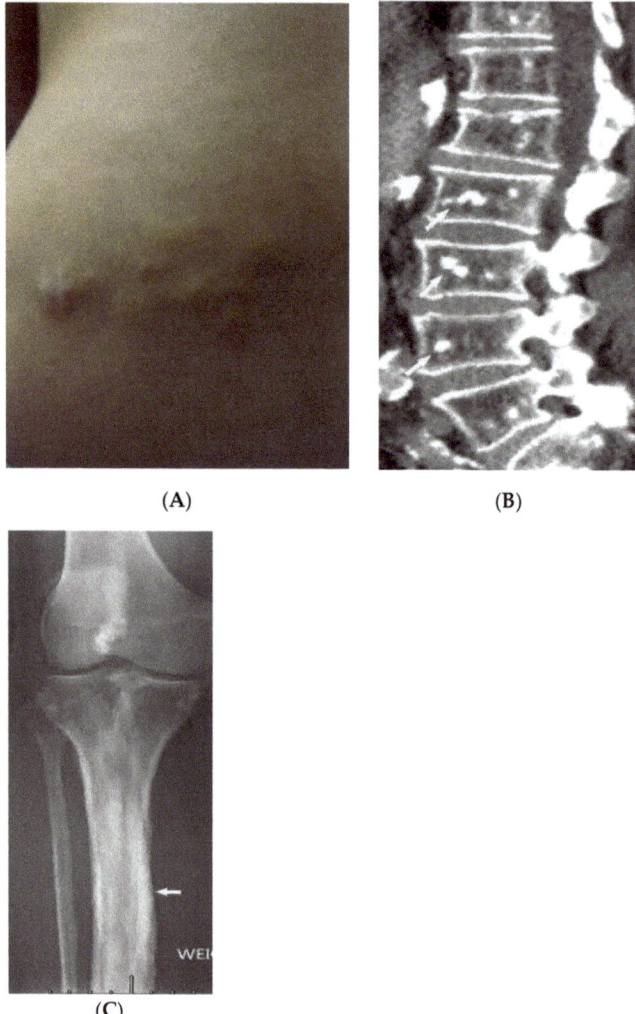

Figure 18. A 60-year-old female with Buschke–Ollendorff syndrome: (**A**) Connective tissue nevi on lower back. (**B**) Sagittal CT of the lumbar spine shows multiple bone islands (arrows). (**C**) AP radiograph of the right knee represents melorheostosis of the tibia (arrow).

3.12. Peutz–Jeghers Syndrome (PJS)

Peutz–Jeghers syndrome (PJS) is a rare AD disease caused by a mutation in the STK11 tumor suppressor gene. PJS is characterized by benign gastrointestinal hamartomatous polyps, mucocutaneous pigmentation, and a high tendency for malignant transformation [78,79]. It is associated with an increased risk of GI malignancies (colon, pancreas, small bowel, gastroesophageal, and stomach) and extraintestinal malignancies (breast, gynecologic, pancreatic, lung, and testis (Figure 19A)) [80–83].

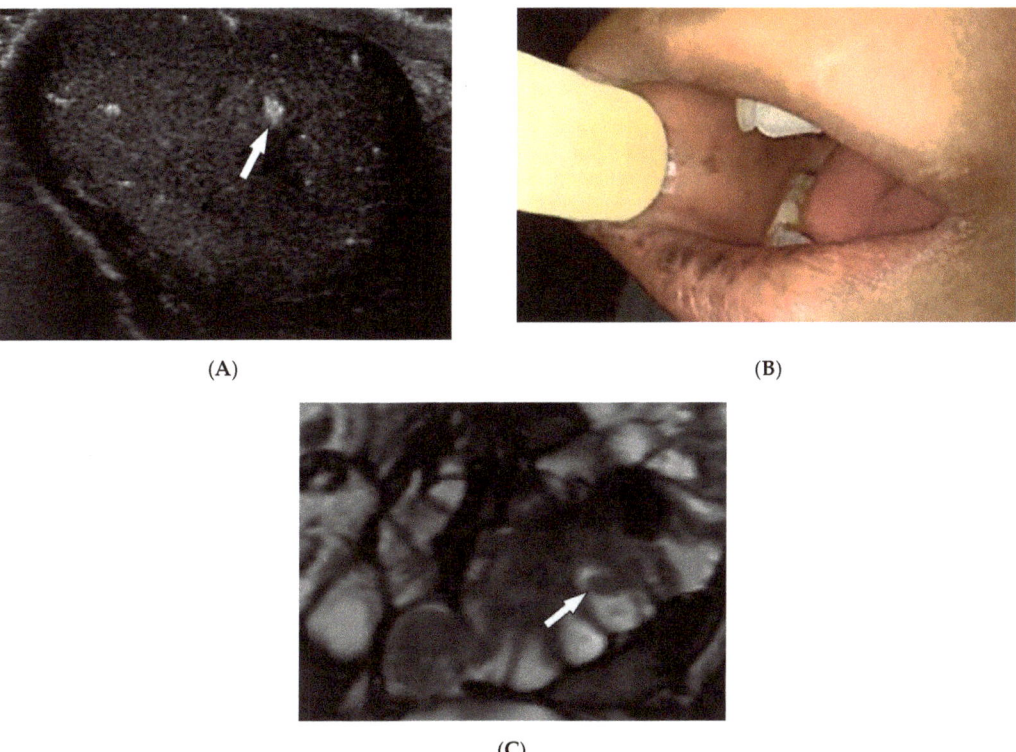

Figure 19. Dermatologic and radiologic images representative of Peutz–Jeghers syndrome: (**A**) Ultrasound of the testis in a 22-year-old male demonstrates testicular lipomatosis (arrow). (**B**) Multiple dark brown lentigines on the mucosal lips and buccal mucosa. (**C**) Coronal MR enterography depicts multiple small-bowel polyps (arrow).

Mucocutaneous pigmented macules often precede GI symptoms, occur in infancy, and are found predominantly around the mouth, nostrils, fingers, toes, and both dorsal and volar aspects of hands and feet. Macules are dark brown or blue-brown (Figure 19B), 1–5 mm in size, and found in 95% of patients with PJS. While cutaneous lesions tend to fade after puberty, oral buccal mucosal pigmentations are usually persistent [81–83]. Clinically, PJS polyps cause colicky abdominal pain and lower GI bleeding. Radiographically, polyps are pedunculated with a typical lobulated pattern at enteroscopy or colonoscopy, presenting as iso- to hyperechoic intraluminal masses on CT and causing multiple nodular filling defects on fluoroscopic study. MR enterography demonstrates T2-isointense intraluminal masses, which are homogeneously enhanced after contrast administration (Figure 19C) [82,83].

4. Neoplasms
4.1. Melanotic Melanoma

Melanoma is a highly invasive cutaneous cancer that is well-known for early metastasis arising from small primary tumors with a 5-year survival rate of 27%. Primary melanomas often arise in sunlight-exposed areas within a pre-existing melanocytic nevus or occur de novo and are divided into pigmented (melanotic) and nonpigmented (amelanotic) subtypes. They may represent one or more of the following ABCDE features: asymmetry, an irregular border, color variegation, a diameter greater than 6mm, and evolving morphology [84–86].

Metastatic melanomas most commonly present near the surgical site of previous lesions as macules, papules, or nodules, or may manifest as firm palpable nodules that may be subcutaneous (Figure 20A). Additionally, melanomas may present as angiomatoid metastasis (soft-tissue mass with hemorrhagic and necrotic components) (Figure 20B) or hematoma-like metastases with ecchymosis [87]. Melanoma often spreads to regional lymph nodes (Figure 20C) via lymphatics but can spread hematogenously to the liver, lung, and brain [85,87]. Brain metastases are best depicted on post-contrast MRI; as melanin reduces T1WI relaxation time, lesions with an adequate amount of melanin represent high SI on T1WI (Figure 20D), which is an uncommon finding in other cancers.

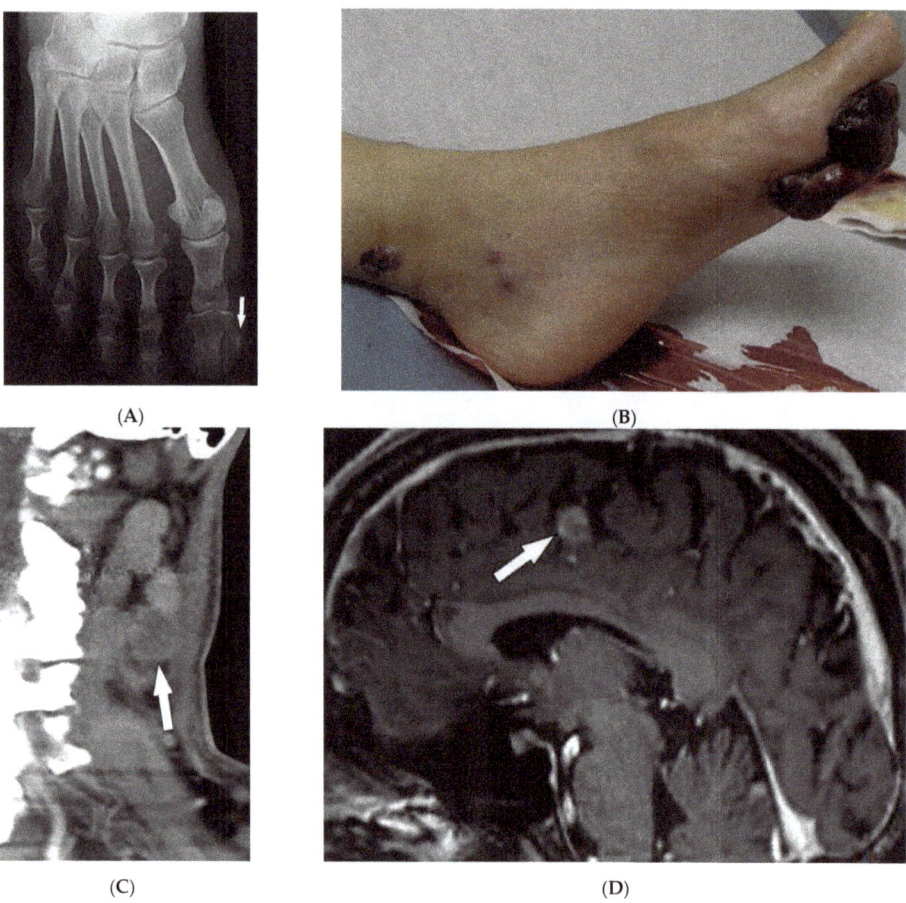

Figure 20. Dermatologic and radiologic images illustrative of melanoma: (**A**) PA radiograph of the foot of a 26-year-old female demonstrated soft-tissue swelling of the great toe with mild calcification medial to the great toe distal phalanx (arrow). (**B**) Large and irregular exophytic plaque on the sole of the left foot. Biopsy confirmed melanoma. (**C**) Sagittal CT of the neck (soft-tissue window) shows a necrotic metastatic lymph node (arrow). (**D**) Sagittal post-contrast T1WI of the brain depicts an enhancing intracranial metastasis (arrow).

Fluorodeoxyglucose–positron emission tomography (FDG-PET) is another modality commonly used in detecting metastatic foci, revealing high FDG uptake due to increased metabolic activity [1,84–87]. A novel machine-learning-based model known as radiomics allows for the translation of the medical images to quantitative data. Radiomic features of

18F-FDG-PET have been investigated in recent studies to predict prognosis in patient with metastatic melanoma before immunotherapy treatment [1,84–88].

4.2. Kaposi Sarcoma

Kaposi sarcoma (KS) is a low-grade endothelial neoplasm associated with human herpesvirus 8 (HHV-8) infection. This vascular tumor affects blood vessels and lymphatic channels, manifesting as one of four clinical subtypes: classic KS (sporadic or Mediterranean), endemic KS (African), iatrogenic KS (immunosuppression-related), and epidemic KS (AIDS–related). KS is currently the most prevalent AIDS-related malignancy. KS skin involvement is polymorphous, ranging from violaceous macules and papules (Figure 21A) to exophytic tumors with associated lymphedema. AIDS-related KS also frequently affects the upper body, head, and neck [88–93]. Twenty-two percent of patients manifest oral cavity lesions as the presenting sign. Oral KS presents simultaneously with cutaneous and visceral involvement in up to 71% of patients with HIV. Lesions are polymorphic and most frequently affect the hard palate, gingiva, and dorsal tongue [92].

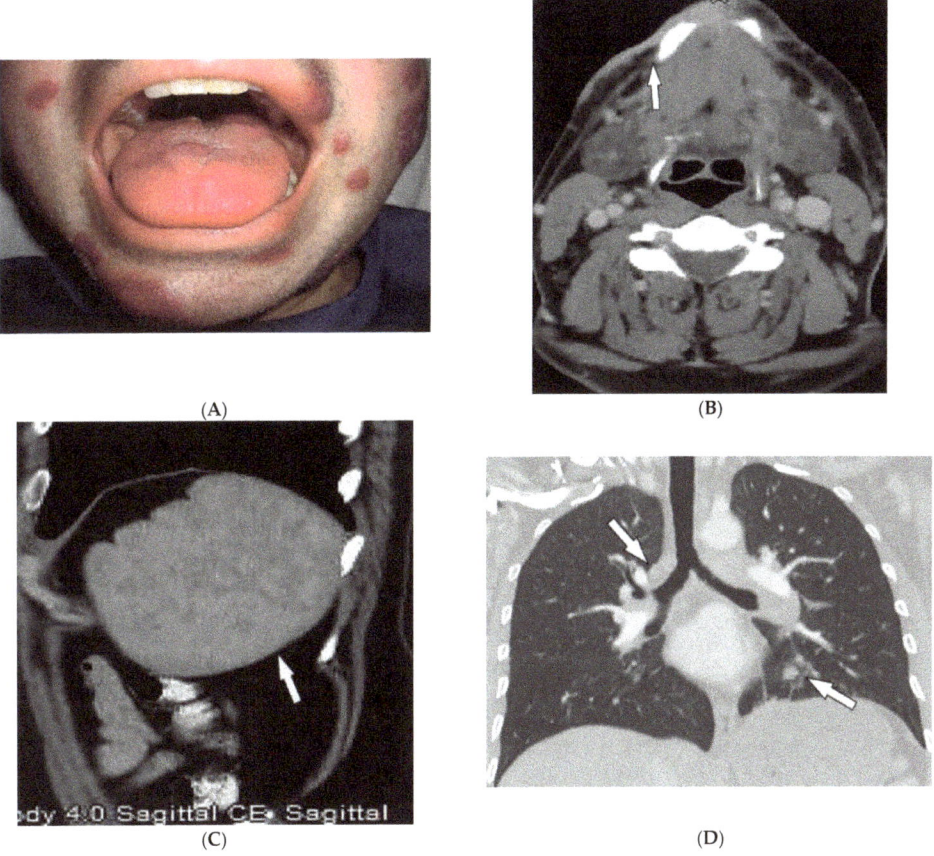

Figure 21. Dermatologic and radiologic images representative of Kaposi sarcoma: (**A**) Red-purple plaques and nodules on the face of a 28-year-old male. (**B**) Axial contrast-enhanced CT of the neck demonstrates diffuse soft-tissue thickening overlying the right mandible (arrow). (**C**) Sagittal contrast-enhanced CT of the abdomen shows splenomegaly (arrow) with heterogeneous enhancement proved to be splenic involvement by Kaposi sarcoma. (**D**) Coronal CT of the chest shows marked peribronchovascular distribution of the tumor with scattered parenchymal nodularity (arrow).

While classic and endemic KS is often restricted to skin manifestations, iatrogenic KS and AIDS-related KS frequently involve visceral organs. The most notable sites of involvement include the GI tract, lymph nodes, lung, and liver (Figure 21B). A characteristic imaging finding of AIDS-related KS is prominent enhancement after contrast injection. Enlarged enhancing lymph nodes are found in 80% of patients with disseminated KS. Hepatosplenomegaly and periportal hyperechoic nodules with associated enhancement on delayed scans are seen on CT and MRI (Figure 21C). Chest CT shows symmetrical ill-defined nodules (Figure 21D) with peribronchovascular distribution (flame-shaped lesions) and surrounding ground-glass opacities (halo sign) [90,91,93].

5. Conclusions

Various systemic conditions have specific or nonspecific dermatologic and imaging features. Simultaneous consideration of imaging findings and dermatologic manifestations helps in more precise imaging interpretation and narrows down the differential diagnosis toward the final diagnosis. Sometimes the cutaneous manifestation of a systemic disease is predictive of systemic involvement, e.g., pulmonary hypertension and ILD in lcSSc vs. dSSc, respectively. Familiarity with the most disease-specific skin lesions help the radiologist pinpoint a specific diagnosis and, consequently, in preventing unnecessary invasive workups and contributing to improved patient care.

Author Contributions: Conceptualization, M.C. and B.M.; methodology, M.C.; validation, F.S.Z., M.S. and H.P.; investigation, F.S.Z., M.S. and H.P.; resources, M.C., N.A., J.H., C.T. and A.D.; data curation, M.S., F.S.Z., M.C. and B.M.; writing—original draft preparation, F.S.Z., M.S. and H.P.; writing—review and editing, N.A., J.H. and A.D.; visualization, N.A., J.H., C.T. and A.D.; supervision, M.C.; project administration, B.M.; All authors have read and agreed to the published version of the manuscript.

Funding: This research received no external funding.

Institutional Review Board Statement: Not applicable.

Informed Consent Statement: Not applicable.

Data Availability Statement: This article is a review and not an original study. All the references are listed.

Acknowledgments: The authors thank Zohre Mehri, and Mona Firoozabadi, for providing dermatologic images.

Conflicts of Interest: The authors declare no relevant conflict of interest.

References

1. Wei, W.; Ehlerding, E.B.; Lan, X.; Luo, Q.; Cai, W. PET and SPECT imaging of melanoma: The state of the art. *Eur. J. Nucl. Med. Mol. Imaging* **2018**, *45*, 132–150. [CrossRef] [PubMed]
2. Fink, A.Z.; Gittler, J.K.; Nakrani, R.N.; Alis, J.; Blumfield, E.; Levin, T.L. Imaging findings in systemic childhood diseases presenting with dermatologic manifestations. *Clin. Imaging* **2018**, *49*, 17–36. [CrossRef] [PubMed]
3. Kanne, J.P.; Donald, R.; Yandow, I.; Haemel, A.K.; Meyer, C.A. Beyond Skin Deep: Thoracic Manifestations of Systemic Disorders Affecting the Skin. *RadioGraphics* **2011**, *31*, 1651–1668. [CrossRef] [PubMed]
4. Kolasinski, S.L.; Chi, A.S.; Lopez-Garib, A.J. Current Perspectives on Imaging for Systemic Lupus Erythematosus, Systemic Sclerosis, and Dermatomyositis/Polymyositis. *Rheum. Dis. Clin. N. Am.* **2016**, *42*, 711–732. [CrossRef] [PubMed]
5. Mainetti, C.; Terziroli Beretta-Piccoli, B.; Selmi, C. Cutaneous Manifestations of Dermatomyositis: A Comprehensive Review. *Clin. Rev. Allergy Immunol.* **2017**, *53*, 337–356. [CrossRef]
6. Ahuja, J.; Arora, D.; Kanne, J.P.; Henry, T.S.; Godwin, J.D. Imaging of Pulmonary Manifestations of Connective Tissue Diseases. *Radiol. Clin. N. Am.* **2016**, *54*, 1015–1031. [CrossRef]
7. Kamperman, R.G.; van der Kooi, A.J.; de Visser, M.; Aronica, E.; Raaphorst, J. Pathophysiological Mechanisms and Treatment of Dermatomyositis and Immune Mediated Necrotizing Myopathies: A Focused Review. *Int. J. Mol. Sci.* **2022**, *23*, 4301. [CrossRef]
8. Ran, J.; Dai, B.; Liu, C.; Zhang, H.; Li, Y.; Hou, B.; Li, X. The diagnostic value of T2 map, diffusion tensor imaging, and diffusion kurtosis imaging in differentiating dermatomyositis from muscular dystrophy. *Acta Radiol.* **2022**, *63*, 467–473. [CrossRef]
9. Kubinova, K.; Dejthevaporn, R.; Mann, H.; Machado, P.M.; Vencovsky, J. The role of imaging in evaluating patients with idiopathic inflammatory myopathies. *Clin. Exp. Rheumatol.* **2018**, *36* (Suppl. S114), 74–81.

10. Schulze, M.; Kötter, I.; Ernemann, U.; Fenchel, M.; Tzaribatchev, N.; Claussen, C.D.; Horger, M. MRI Findings in Inflammatory Muscle Diseases and Their Noninflammatory Mimics. *Am. J. Roentgenol.* **2009**, *192*, 1708–1716. [CrossRef]
11. Smitaman, E.; Flores, D.V.; Gómez, C.M.; Pathria, M.N. MR Imaging of Atraumatic Muscle Disorders. *Radiogr. A Rev. Publ. Radiol. Soc. N. Am. Inc.* **2018**, *38*, 500–522. [CrossRef] [PubMed]
12. Belperio, J.A.; Shaikh, F.; Abtin, F.G.; Fishbein, M.C.; Weigt, S.S.; Saggar, R.; Lynch, J.P. Diagnosis and treatment of pulmonary sarcoidosis: A review. *JAMA* **2022**, *327*, 856–867. [CrossRef] [PubMed]
13. Guidry, C.; Fricke, R.G.; Ram, R.; Pandey, T.; Jambhekar, K. Imaging of Sarcoidosis: A Contemporary Review. *Radiol. Clin. N. Am.* **2016**, *54*, 519–534. [CrossRef] [PubMed]
14. Ganeshan, D.; Menias, C.O.; Lubner, M.G.; Pickhardt, P.J.; Sandrasegaran, K.; Bhalla, S. Sarcoidosis from Head to Toe: What the Radiologist Needs to Know. *Radiogr. Rev. Publ. Radiol. Soc. N. Am. Inc.* **2018**, *38*, 1180–1200. [CrossRef]
15. Lew, P.P.; Ngai, S.S.; Hamidi, R.; Cho, J.K.; Birnbaum, R.A.; Peng, D.H.; Varma, R.K. Imaging of Disorders Affecting the Bone and Skin. *Radiogr. Rev. Publ. Radiol. Soc. N. Am. Inc.* **2014**, *34*, 197–216. [CrossRef]
16. Redissi, A.; Penmetsa, G.K.; Litaiem, N. Lupus pernio. In *StatPearls*; StatPearls Publishing: Treasure Island, FL, USA, 2021.
17. Noe, M.H.; Rosenbach, M. Cutaneous sarcoidosis. *Curr. Opin. Pulm. Med.* **2017**, *23*, 482–486. [CrossRef]
18. Koyama, T.; Ueda, H.; Togashi, K.; Umeoka, S.; Kataoka, M.; Nagai, S. Radiologic Manifestations of Sarcoidosis in Various Organs. *Radiogr. Rev. Publ. Radiol. Soc. N. Am. Inc.* **2004**, *24*, 87–104. [CrossRef]
19. Sève, P.; Pacheco, Y.; Durupt, F.; Jamilloux, Y.; Gerfaud-Valentin, M.; Isaac, S.; Boussel, L.; Calender, A.; Androdias, G.; Valeyre, D.; et al. Sarcoidosis: A clinical overview from symptoms to diagnosis. *Cells* **2021**, *10*, 766. [CrossRef]
20. Ruaro, B.; Confalonieri, P.; Santagiuliana, M.; Wade, B.; Baratella, E.; Kodric, M.; Berria, M.; Jaber, M.; Torregiani, C.; Bruni, C.; et al. Correlation between Potential Risk Factors and Pulmonary Embolism in Sarcoidosis Patients Timely Treated. *J. Clin. Med.* **2021**, *10*, 2462. [CrossRef]
21. Barreras, P.; Stern, B.J. Clinical features and diagnosis of neurosarcoidosis–review article. *J. Neuroimmunol.* **2022**, *368*, 577871. [CrossRef]
22. Chapin, R.; Hant, F.N. Imaging of scleroderma. *Rheum. Dis. Clin. N. Am.* **2013**, *39*, 515–546. [CrossRef] [PubMed]
23. Kowalska-Kępczyńska, A. Systemic Scleroderma—Definition, Clinical Picture and Laboratory Diagnostics. *J. Clin. Med.* **2022**, *11*, 2299. [CrossRef] [PubMed]
24. Abbas, L.F.; O'Brien, J.C.; Goldman, S.; Pezeshk, P.; Chalian, M.; Chhabra, A.; Jacobe, H.T. A Cross-sectional Comparison of Magnetic Resonance Imaging Findings and Clinical Assessment in Patients With Morphea. *JAMA Dermatol.* **2020**, *156*, 590–592. [CrossRef] [PubMed]
25. Ruaro, B.; Sulli, A.; Pizzorni, C.; Paolino, S.; Smith, V.; Alessandri, E.; Trombetta, A.C.; Alsheyyab, J.; Cutolo, M. Correlations between blood perfusion and dermal thickness in different skin areas of systemic sclerosis patients. *Microvasc. Res.* **2018**, *115*, 28–33. [CrossRef] [PubMed]
26. Sulli, A.; Ruaro, B.; Cutolo, M. Evaluation of blood perfusion by laser speckle contrast analysis in different areas of hands and face in patients with systemic sclerosis. *Ann. Rheum. Dis.* **2014**, *73*, 2059–2061. [CrossRef]
27. Dzwigala, M.; Sobolewski, P.; Maslinska, M.; Yurtsever, I.; Szymanska, E.; Walecka, I. High-resolution ultrasound imaging of skin involvement in systemic sclerosis: A systematic review. *Rheumatol. Int.* **2021**, *41*, 285–295. [CrossRef]
28. Hughes, M.; Bruni, C.; Cuomo, G.; Delle Sedie, A.; Gargani, L.; Gutierrez, M.; Lepri, G.; Ruaro, B.; Santiago, T.; Suliman, Y.; et al. The role of ultrasound in systemic sclerosis: On the cutting edge to foster clinical and research advancement. *J. Scleroderma Relat. Disord.* **2021**, *6*, 123–132. [CrossRef]
29. Chatzinikolaou, S.L.; Quirk, B.; Murray, C.; Planche, K. Radiological findings in gastrointestinal scleroderma. *J. Scleroderma Relat. Disord.* **2020**, *5*, 21–32. [CrossRef]
30. Abenavoli, L.; Dastoli, S.; Bennardo, L.; Boccuto, L.; Passante, M.; Silvestri, M.; Proietti, I.; Potenza, C.; Luzza, F.; Nisticò, S.P. The Skin in Celiac Disease Patients: The Other Side of the Coin. *Medicina* **2019**, *55*, 578. [CrossRef]
31. Tennyson, C.A.; Semrad, C.E. Small bowel imaging in celiac disease. *Gastrointest. Endosc. Clin. N. Am.* **2012**, *22*, 735–746. [CrossRef]
32. Sheedy, S.P.; Barlow, J.M.; Fletcher, J.G.; Smyrk, T.C.; Scholz, F.J.; Codipilly, D.C.; Al Bawardy, B.F.; Fidler, J.L. Beyond moulage sign and TTG levels: The role of cross-sectional imaging in celiac sprue. *Abdom. Radiol.* **2017**, *42*, 361–388. [CrossRef] [PubMed]
33. Paolantonio, P.; Tomei, E.; Rengo, M.; Ferrari, R.; Lucchesi, P.; Laghi, A. Adult celiac disease: MRI findings. *Abdom. Imaging* **2007**, *32*, 433–440. [CrossRef] [PubMed]
34. Marzano, A.V.; Raimondo, M.G.; Berti, E.; Meroni, P.L.; Ingegnoli, F. Cutaneous Manifestations of ANCA-Associated Small Vessels Vasculitis. *Clin. Rev. Allergy Immunol.* **2017**, *53*, 428–438. [CrossRef] [PubMed]
35. Singhal, M.; Gupta, P.; Sharma, A. Imaging in small and medium vessel vasculitis. *Int. J. Rheum. Dis.* **2019**, *22* (Suppl. S1), 78–85. [CrossRef]
36. Schmidt, W.A. Imaging in vasculitis. *Best Pract. Res. Clin. Rheumatol.* **2013**, *27*, 107–118. [CrossRef]
37. Howard, T.; Ahmad, K.; Swanson, J.A.; Misra, S. Polyarteritis nodosa. *Tech. Vasc. Interv. Radiol.* **2014**, *17*, 247–251. [CrossRef]
38. Chasset, F.; Frances, C. Cutaneous Manifestations of Medium- and Large-Vessel Vasculitis. *Clin. Rev. Allergy Immunol.* **2017**, *53*, 452–468. [CrossRef]
39. Diaz-Perez, J.L.; De Lagran, Z.M.; Diaz-Ramon, J.L.; Winkelmann, R.K. Cutaneous polyarteritis nodosa. *Semin. Cutan. Med. Surg.* **2007**, *26*, 77–86. [CrossRef]

40. Mehdipoor, G.; Davatchi, F.; Ghoreishian, H.; Arjmand Shabestari, A. Imaging manifestations of Behcet's disease: Key considerations and major features. *Eur. J. Radiol.* **2018**, *98*, 214–225. [CrossRef]
41. Elbendary, A.; Abdel-Halim, M.R.; Ragab, G. Updates in cutaneous manifestations of systemic vasculitis. *Curr. Opin. Rheumatol.* **2022**, *34*, 25–32. [CrossRef]
42. Chae, E.J.; Do, K.-H.; Seo, J.B.; Park, S.H.; Kang, J.-W.; Jang, Y.M.; Lee, J.S.; Song, J.-W.; Song, K.-S.; Lee, J.H.; et al. Radiologic and Clinical Findings of Behçet Disease: Comprehensive Review of Multisystemic Involvement. *Radiogr. Rev. Publ. Radiol. Soc. N. Am. Inc.* **2008**, *28*, e31. [CrossRef] [PubMed]
43. Vural, S.; Boyvat, A. The skin in Behçet's disease: Mucocutaneous findings and differential diagnosis. *JEADV Clin. Pract.* **2022**, *1*, 11–20. [CrossRef]
44. Krishnan, A.; Kaza, R.K.; Vummidi, D.R. Cross-sectional Imaging Review of Tuberous Sclerosis. *Radiol. Clin. N. Am.* **2016**, *54*, 423–440. [CrossRef] [PubMed]
45. Nguyen, Q.D.; DarConte, M.D.; Hebert, A.A. The cutaneous manifestations of tuberous sclerosis complex. *Am. J. Med. Genet. Part C Semin. Med. Genet.* **2018**, *178*, 321–325. [CrossRef] [PubMed]
46. Umeoka, S.; Koyama, T.; Miki, Y.; Akai, M.; Tsutsui, K.; Togashi, K. Pictorial review of tuberous sclerosis in various organs. *Radiogr. A Rev. Publ. Radiol. Soc. N. Am. Inc.* **2008**, *28*, e32. [CrossRef]
47. Vézina, G. Neuroimaging of phakomatoses: Overview and advances. *Pediatric Radiol.* **2015**, *45* (Suppl. S3), S433–S442. [CrossRef]
48. Razek, A. MR imaging of neoplastic and non-neoplastic lesions of the brain and spine in neurofibromatosis type I. *Neurol. Sci. Off. J. Ital. Neurol. Soc. Ital. Soc. Clin. Neurophysiol.* **2018**, *39*, 821–827. [CrossRef]
49. Salamon, J.; Mautner, V.F.; Adam, G.; Derlin, T. Multimodal Imaging in Neurofibromatosis Type 1-associated Nerve Sheath Tumors. *RoFo Fortschr. Auf Geb. Rontgenstrahlen Nukl.* **2015**, *187*, 1084–1092. [CrossRef]
50. Hernández-Martín, A.; Duat-Rodríguez, A. An Update on Neurofibromatosis Type 1: Not Just Café-au-Lait Spots, Freckling, and Neurofibromas. An Update. Part I. Dermatological Clinical Criteria Diagnostic of the Disease. *Actas Dermo-Sifiliogr.* **2016**, *107*, 454–464. [CrossRef]
51. Abdel Razek, A.A. Vascular neurocutaneous disorders: Neurospinal and craniofacial imaging findings. *Jpn. J. Radiol.* **2014**, *32*, 519–528. [CrossRef]
52. Puttgen, K.B.; Lin, D.D. Neurocutaneous vascular syndromes. Child's nervous system. *ChNS Off. J. Int. Soc. Pediatric Neurosurg.* **2010**, *26*, 1407–1415. [CrossRef]
53. Rotter, A.; Samorano, L.P.; Rivitti-Machado, M.C.; Oliveira, Z.N.P.; Gontijo, B. PHACE syndrome: Clinical manifestations, diagnostic criteria, and management. *An. Bras. Dermatol.* **2018**, *93*, 405–411. [CrossRef] [PubMed]
54. Barros, F.S.; Marussi, V.H.R.; Amaral, L.L.F.; Da Rocha, A.J.; Campos, C.M.; Freitas, L.F.; Huisman, T.A.G.M.; Soares, B.P. The Rare Neurocutaneous Disorders: Update on Clinical, Molecular, and Neuroimaging Features. *Top. Magn. Reson. Imaging TMRI* **2018**, *27*, 433–462. [CrossRef] [PubMed]
55. Subramanyam, S.B.; Sujata, D.N.; Sridhar, K.; Pushpanjali, M. Nevoid Basal cell carcinoma syndrome: A case report and review. *J. Maxillofac. Oral Surg.* **2015**, *14*, 11–15. [CrossRef] [PubMed]
56. Dupuis-Girod, S.; Cottin, V.; Shovlin, C. The lung in hereditary hemorrhagic telangiectasia. *Respiration* **2017**, *94*, 315–330. [CrossRef] [PubMed]
57. Azma, R.; Dmytriw, A.A.; Biswas, A.; Pollak, M.; Ratjen, F.; Amirabadi, A.; Branson, H.M.; Kulkarni, A.V.; Dirks, P.; Muthusami, P. Neurovascular Manifestations in Pediatric Patients With Hereditary Haemorrhagic Telangiectasia. *Pediatric Neurol.* **2022**, *129*, 24–30. [CrossRef] [PubMed]
58. Guttmacher, A.E.; Marchuk, D.A.; White, R.I., Jr. Hereditary hemorrhagic telangiectasia. *N. Engl. J. Med.* **1995**, *333*, 918–924. [CrossRef]
59. Contegiacomo, A.; Del Ciello, A.; Rella, R.; Attempati, N.; Coppolino, D.; Larici, A.R.; Di Stasi, C.; Marano, G.; Manfredi, R. Pulmonary arteriovenous malformations: What the interventional radiologist needs to know. *Radiol. Med.* **2019**, *124*, 973–988. [CrossRef]
60. Tong, Y.; Schneider, J.A.; Coda, A.B.; Hata, T.R.; Cohen, P.R. Birt–Hogg–Dubé syndrome: A review of dermatological manifestations and other symptoms. *Am. J. Clin. Dermatol.* **2018**, *19*, 87–101. [CrossRef]
61. Agarwal, P.P.; Gross, B.H.; Holloway, B.J.; Seely, J.; Stark, P.; Kazerooni, E.A. Thoracic CT findings in birt-hogg-dube syndrome. *Am. J. Roentgenol.* **2011**, *196*, 349–352. [CrossRef]
62. Lee, J.E.; Cha, Y.K.; Kim, J.S.; Choi, J.-H. Birt-Hogg-Dubé syndrome: Characteristic CT findings differentiating it from other diffuse cystic lung diseases. *Diagn. Interv. Radiol.* **2017**, *23*, 354. [CrossRef]
63. Ferreira, E.C.; Brito, C.C.; Domingues, R.C.; Bernardes, M.; Marchiori, E.; Gasparetto, E.L. Whole-body MR imaging for the evaluation of mcCune-albright syndrome. *J. Magn. Reson. Imaging Off. J. Int. Soc. Magn. Reson. Med.* **2010**, *31*, 706–710. [CrossRef]
64. Defilippi, C.; Chiappetta, D.; Marzari, D.; Mussa, A.; Lala, R. Image diagnosis in McCune-Albright syndrome. *J. Pediatric Endocrinol. Metab.* **2006**, *19*, 561–570. [CrossRef]
65. Bongers, E.M.; Gubler, M.-C.; Knoers, N.V. Nail-patella syndrome. Overview on clinical and molecular findings. *Pediatric Nephrol.* **2002**, *17*, 703–712. [CrossRef] [PubMed]
66. KZuberi, H.Z.; Angirekula, A.; Akram, M.R.; Kooner, K.S. Nail-Patella Syndrome: Optical Coherence Tomography Angiography Findings. *Case Rep. Ophthalmol.* **2022**, *13*, 227–233. [CrossRef] [PubMed]

67. Al-Dawsari, N.; Al-Mokhadam, A.; Al-Abdulwahed, H.; Al-Sannaa, N. Nail-Patella Syndrome: A Report of a Saudi Arab Family with an Autosomal Recessive Inheritance. *J. Cutan. Med. Surg.* **2015**, *19*, 595–599. [CrossRef] [PubMed]
68. Witzgall, R. Nail-patella syndrome. *Pflügers Arch. Eur. J. Physiol.* **2017**, *469*, 927–936. [CrossRef]
69. Tigchelaar, S.; Rooy Jd Hannink, G.; Koëter, S.; van Kampen, A.; Bongers, E. Radiological characteristics of the knee joint in nail patella syndrome. *Bone Jt. J.* **2016**, *98*, 483–489. [CrossRef] [PubMed]
70. Ann-Louise McDermott, F.; Sunil, N.D.; Chavda, S.V.; Morgan, D. Maffucci's syndrome: Clinical and radiological features of a rare condition. *J. Laryngol. Otol.* **2001**, *115*, 845–847.
71. Dasgeb, B.; Morris, M.A.; Ring, C.M.; Mehregan, D.; Mulligan, M.E. Musculoskeletal and overgrowth syndromes associated with cutaneous abnormalities. *Br. J. Radiol.* **2016**, *89*, 20160521. [CrossRef]
72. Silve, C.; Jüppner, H. Ollier disease. *Orphanet J. Rare Dis.* **2006**, *1*, 37. [CrossRef] [PubMed]
73. Pope, V.; Dupuis, L.; Kannu, P.; Mendoza-Londono, R.; Sajic, D.; So, J.; Yoon, G.; Lara-Corrales, I. Buschke–Ollendorff syndrome: A novel case series and systematic review. *Br. J. Dermatol.* **2016**, *174*, 723–729. [CrossRef] [PubMed]
74. Korkmaz, M.F.; Elli, M.; Özkan, M.B.; Bilgici, M.C.; Dağdemir, A.; Korkmaz, M.; Tosun, F.C.; Dağdemir, A. Osteopoikilosis: Report of a familial case and review of the literature. *Rheumatol. Int.* **2015**, *35*, 921–924. [CrossRef] [PubMed]
75. Kawamura, A.; Ochiai, T.; Tan-Kinoshita, M.; Suzuki, H. Buschke–Ollendorff syndrome: Three generations in a Japanese family. *Pediatric Dermatol.* **2005**, *22*, 133–137. [CrossRef]
76. Nevin, N.C.; Thomas, P.S.; Davis, R.I.; Cowie, G.H. Melorheostosis in a family with autosomal dominant osteopoikilosis. *Am. J. Med. Genet.* **1999**, *82*, 409–414. [CrossRef]
77. Ruaro, B.; Sulli, A.; Alessandri, E.; Ravera, F.; Cutolo, M. Coexistence of osteopoikilosis with seronegative spondyloarthritis and Raynaud's phenomenon: First case report with evaluation of the nailfold capillary bed and literature review. *Reumatismo* **2012**, *64*, 335–339. [CrossRef]
78. Tomas, C.; Soyer, P.; Dohan, A.; Dray, X.; Boudiaf, M.; Hoeffel, C. Update on imaging of Peutz-Jeghers syndrome. *World J. Gastroenterol. WJG* **2014**, *20*, 10864. [CrossRef]
79. Katabathina, V.S.; Menias, C.O.; Khanna, L.; Murphy, L.; Dasyam, A.K.; Lubner, M.G.; Prasad, S.R. Hereditary gastrointestinal cancer syndromes: Role of imaging in screening, diagnosis, and management. *RadioGraphics* **2019**, *39*, 1280–1301. [CrossRef]
80. Tabriz, H.M.; Obohat, M.; Vahedifard, F.; Eftekharjavadi, A. Survey of Mast Cell Density in Transitional Cell Carcinoma. *Iran. J. Pathol.* **2021**, *16*, 119. [CrossRef]
81. Thrash, B.; Patel, M.; Shah, K.R.; Boland, C.R.; Menter, A. Cutaneous manifestations of gastrointestinal disease: Part II. *J. Am. Acad. Dermatol.* **2013**, *68*, 211.e1–211.e33. [CrossRef]
82. Beggs, A.; Latchford, A.; Vasen, H.F.; Moslein, G.; Alonso, A.; Aretz, S.; Bertario, L.; Blanco, I.; Bulow, S.; Burn, J.; et al. Peutz–Jeghers syndrome: A systematic review and recommendations for management. *Gut* **2010**, *59*, 975–986. [CrossRef]
83. Giardiello, F.M.; Trimbath, J.D. Peutz-Jeghers syndrome and management recommendations. *Clin. Gastroenterol. Hepatol.* **2006**, *4*, 408–415. [CrossRef]
84. Patnana, M.; Bronstein, Y.; Szklaruk, J.; Bedi, D.G.; Hwu, W.J.; Gershenwald, J.E.; Prieto, V.G.; Ng, C.S. Multimethod imaging, staging, and spectrum of manifestations of metastatic melanoma. *Clin. Radiol.* **2011**, *66*, 224–236. [CrossRef]
85. Schmid, R.; Schmidt, S.K.; Detsch, R.; Horder, H.; Blunk, T.; Schrüfer, S.; Schubert, D.W.; Fischer, L.; Thievessen, I.; Heltmann-Meyer, S.; et al. A New Printable Alginate/Hyaluronic Acid/Gelatin Hydrogel Suitable for Biofabrication of In Vitro and In Vivo Metastatic Melanoma Models. *Adv. Funct. Mater.* **2022**, *32*, 2107993. [CrossRef]
86. Vyas, R.; Selph, J.; Gerstenblith, M.R. (Eds.) Cutaneous manifestations associated with melanoma. In *Seminars in Oncology*; Elsevier: Amsterdam, The Netherlands, 2016.
87. Flaus, A.; Habouzit, V.; de Leiris, N.; Vuillez, J.P.; Leccia, M.T.; Simonson, M.; Perrot, J.L.; Cachin, F.; Prevot, N. Outcome Prediction at Patient Level Derived from Pre-Treatment 18F-FDG PET Due to Machine Learning in Metastatic Melanoma Treated with Anti-PD1 Treatment. *Diagnostics* **2022**, *12*, 388. [CrossRef]
88. Vahedifard, F.; Hassani, S.; Afrasiabi, A.; Esfe, A.M. Artificial intelligence for radiomics; diagnostic biomarkers for neuro-oncology. *World J. Adv. Res. Rev.* **2022**, *14*, 304–310. [CrossRef]
89. Karabajakian, A.; Ray-Coquard, I.; Blay, J.Y. Molecular Mechanisms of Kaposi Sarcoma Development. *Cancers* **2022**, *14*, 1869. [CrossRef]
90. Restrepo, C.S.; Martínez, S.; Lemos, J.A.; Carrillo, J.A.; Lemos, D.F.; Ojeda, P.; Koshy, P. Imaging manifestations of Kaposi sarcoma. *Radiographics* **2006**, *26*, 1169–1185. [CrossRef]
91. Schwartz, R.A.; Micali, G.; Nasca, M.R.; Scuderi, L. Kaposi sarcoma: A continuing conundrum. *J. Am. Acad. Dermatol.* **2008**, *59*, 179–206. [CrossRef]
92. Fatahzadeh, M. Kaposi sarcoma: Review and medical management update. *Oral Surg. Oral Med. Oral Pathol. Oral Radiol.* **2012**, *113*, 2–16. [CrossRef]
93. Pesqué, L.; Delyon, J.; Lheure, C.; Baroudjian, B.; Battistella, M.; Merlet, P.; Lebbé, C.; Vercellino, L. Yield of FDG PET/CT for Defining the Extent of Disease in Patients with Kaposi Sarcoma. *Cancers* **2022**, *14*, 2189. [CrossRef] [PubMed]

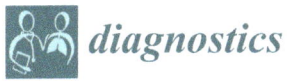

Review

Emerging Targets for the Treatment of Osteoarthritis: New Investigational Methods to Identify Neo-Vessels as Possible Targets for Embolization

Reza Talaie [1], Pooya Torkian [1,*], Alexander Clayton [1], Stephanie Wallace [1], Hoiwan Cheung [2], Majid Chalian [2] and Jafar Golzarian [1]

[1] Vascular and Interventional Radiology, Department of Radiology, University of Minnesota, Minneapolis, MN 55455, USA; rtalaie@umn.edu (R.T.); aclayton@umn.edu (A.C.); walla649@umn.edu (S.W.); jafar@umn.edu (J.G.)
[2] Department of Radiology, Division Musculoskeletal Imaging and Intervention, University of Washington, Seattle, WA 98195, USA; hcheung@uw.edu (H.C.); mchalian@uw.edu (M.C.)
* Correspondence: ptorkian@umn.edu; Tel.: +1-612-626-5566

Abstract: Osteoarthritis (OA) is the major cause of disability, affecting over 30 million US adults. Continued research into the role of neovascularization and inflammation related to osteoarthritis in large-animal models and human clinical trials is paramount. Recent literature on the pathogenetic model of OA has refocused on low-level inflammation, resulting in joint remodeling. As a result, this has redirected osteoarthritis research toward limiting or treating joint changes associated with persistent synovitis. The overall goal of this review is to better understand the cellular and tissue-specific mechanisms of inflammation in relation to a novel OA treatment modality, Genicular Artery Embolization (GAE). This article also assesses the utility and mechanism of periarticular neovascular embolization for the treatment of OA with a particular emphasis on the balance between pro-angiogenic and anti-angiogenic cytokines, inflammatory biomarkers, and imaging changes.

Keywords: osteoarthritis; genicular artery embolization; embolization

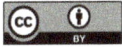

1. Introduction

Traditionally considered a "wear and tear" phenomena of the bone and cartilage, osteoarthritis (OA) is increasingly understood to represent sequela of chronic inflammatory processes [1]. As our basic understanding of osteoarthritis pathology broadens, so too do potential treatment targets. Prior literature has identified that the neovascularization of joint tissues plays a significant role in the pathology of OA and is a suggested target for future treatment [2]. Continued research into the role of neovascularization and inflammation related to osteoarthritis in large-animal models and human clinical trials is paramount. Recent literature has shifted the pathogenetic model of OA to refocus on low-level inflammation, resulting in joint remodeling [3]. Chronic inflammation alters chondrocyte function, shifting normal cell signaling to pro-inflammatory cytokines, which in turn promotes angiogenesis [3]. Multiple small animal models have demonstrated that the degree of angiogenesis correlates with more severe OA [4–11]. These new vessels may in turn function as a conduit for continued joint inflammation and new neuronal migration [2]. These nerves are sensitized to pain due to their subjection to hypoxia, inflammation, and mechanical stress within the joint [12]. This new understanding of the pathophysiology of OA has served as a target opportunity for new treatment modalities to address gaps in clinical needs. Development in the pathogenetic model of OA has redirected research in its treatment and shifted the focus to limiting or treating joint changes associated with persistent synovitis.

Okuno et al. have employed targeted neo-vessel embolization to successfully treat symptomatic osteoarthritis with durable therapeutic response [13]. Early results of geniculate artery embolization (GAE) demonstrate improved patient pain and function [14–20]. GAE is hypothesized to limit inflammation and pain in OA via embolization of neo-vessels. Treatments of neovascularization in osteoarthritis show promise with GAE but will require robust randomized clinical trials before the utility of this procedure can be fully established. The overall goal of this review is to better understand the cellular and tissue-specific mechanisms of inflammation in relation to a novel OA treatment modality, GAE. We assess the utility and mechanism of periarticular neovascular embolization for the treatment of OA with a particular emphasis on understanding the balance between the pro and anti-angiogenic cytokines, inflammatory biomarkers, and imaging changes.

2. Global Prevalence, Natural History, Risk Factors, Pathophysiology, and Treatment of OA

2.1. Epidemiology and Economic Burden of OA

Of all types of arthritis, osteoarthritis (OA) is the most common, affecting over 30 million US adults [21]. The radiographic incidence of symptomatic knee OA has an incidence of 4.3% in men and 8.1% in women of all ages. It has been shown that the overall prevalence of radiographic OA reaches 37.1% [22] with nearly half of people with symptomatic OA experiencing physical disability. As the population ages, the incidence, prevalence, and economic burden of its treatment and disability will increase [23]. In the United States, the number of individuals over the age of 65 is projected to rise to 78 million by 2035 from 49.2 million in 2016 [24]. The prevalence of total knee arthroplasty (TKA) was demonstrated to be 4.7 million individuals in 2010 with the overall trend being of increasing prevalence over time [25]. This comes at no small cost, with the annual total hospitalization charges for TKA nearly quadrupling from $8.1 billion in 1998 to $38.5 billion in 2011 [26]. The average lifetime direct medical cost for treatment of those diagnosed with OA is estimated to be $12,400 or 10% of all estimated direct medical expenses for those individuals. Most of those costs affect the 54% of OA patients who undergo TKA, which on average costs $20,293, and for patients who require revision surgery, resulting in additional costs averaging $29,388. Non-surgical regimens are estimated between $494 and $684 annually [27]. The skyrocketing costs of an aging population coupled with expanded TKA eligibility have led Losina et al. to conclude that there is legitimate need for more effective non-operative therapies [27].

2.2. Natural History, Prognosis, and Imaging of OA

Patients with knee OA can present with joint pain, stiffness, bony crepitus, joint edema, and physical deformities. Radiographic findings include narrowing of the joint compartment, osteophytes, and subchondral sclerosis [28]. Current non-operative treatment is limited to physical therapy, oral anti-inflammatories, and intra-articular corticosteroid/hyaluronic acid injections. Non-steroidal anti-inflammatories (NSAIDs) are well tolerated but are not without risk, as they may cause acute renal failure, gastritis, or interfere with platelet aggregation [29]. Arthroplasty comes with its own risks of perioperative morbidity and mortality [30,31]; hence, this is reserved for severe OA, resulting in significant lifestyle limitations.

2.3. Pathophysiology: Understanding of the Balance between Pro and Anti-Angiogenic Cytokines, Inflammatory Biomarkers

While the pathophysiology of knee osteoarthritis has traditionally been described in the context of inflammation and joint space narrowing, new evidence in the literature suggests that abnormal blood vessel formation may also play a role. Osteoarthritic pain is thought to be caused by joint space inflammation, abnormal innervation of synovial structures and increased sensitization of the central and peripheral nervous systems (Figure 1).

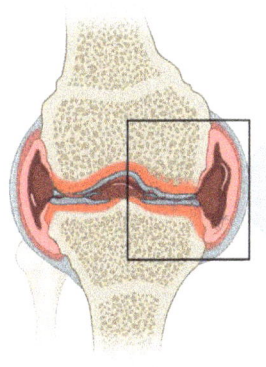
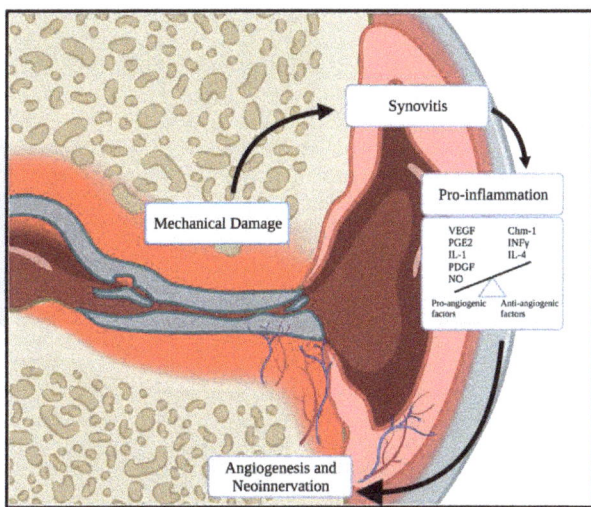

VEGF= vascular endothelial growth factor; PGE2= prostaglandin E2; IL-1= Interleukin-1; PDGF= platelet derived growth factor; NO= nitric oxide; Chm-1= chondromodulin-1; INFγ= interferon gamma; IL-4= Interleukin-4

Figure 1. Understanding of the balance between pro and anti-angiogenic cytokines, inflammatory biomarkers.

Synovitis may damage underlying tissues by altering chondrocyte function, while increased angiogenesis and bony remodeling contribute to chronic inflammation in OA [1]. Angiogenesis is the process by which new capillaries are formed from pre-existing blood vessels and plays an important role in physiologic wound healing. Pathologic angiogenesis can result in chronic inflammatory conditions and the metastatic spread of tumors [1]. Vasculogenesis, a consequence of angiogenesis, occurs when circulating angioblasts differentiate into endothelial cells. Matrix metalloproteinases (MMP) and other cytokines establish an environment for the new arterioles and venules to form in the perivascular space [32]. Vascular endothelial growth factor (VEGF) and platelet-derived growth factor (PDGF) help maintain blood vessel stability after MMPs create new ostia by destroying part of the existing endothelium [1]. The process by which endothelial cells proliferate and localize to avascular spaces are known as "angiogenic sprouting" [3]. In osteoarthritis, neo-vessels may contribute to persistent inflammation by maintaining oxygen and nutrients to abnormal endothelial cells as well as giving pro-inflammatory cytokines access to the local microenvironment [3].

Recent attention has focused on the local microenvironment as it pertains to osteoarthritis. Like generic inflammation, regulatory molecules and cytokines function in a complex, sophisticated manner to stimulate and/or inhibit angiogenesis [1]. Compounds that upregulate angiogenesis include prostaglandin E2 (PGE2), histamine, VEGF, interleukin-1 (IL-1), PDGF, and nitric oxide (NO) [1]. VEGF is itself stimulated by pro-inflammatory cytokines, such as IL-1, interleukin 17 (IL-17), tumor necrosis factor alpha (TNF-alpha), NO, and reactive oxygen species [33]. Some factors that inhibit angiogenesis in the synovium include chondromodulin-1, interferon gamma (IFN-gamma), interleukin-4 (IL-4), and tissue inhibitors of MMP-1 and 2 [1]. Chondromodulin 1 and U-995 have been shown to not only discourage angiogenesis but to prevent endothelial cell production and migration [32]. Normally, pro-inflammatory and anti-inflammatory cytokines exist in a complex, homeostatic environment. In certain inflammatory conditions, the balance is tilted toward pro-inflammatory cytokines. While conventionally associated with other inflammatory diseases, this net catabolic context may exist in processes that have traditionally been understood as non-inflammatory, such as osteoarthritis [3].

Articular cartilage is an avascular tissue. The blood supply to the cartilage is derived from the adjacent, vascular synovium. Cartilage is a critical component of the joint, as it helps to evenly distribute high mechanical forces and maintain the structure of the joint as a unit [28]. Chondrocytes are specifically resistant to angiogenesis, as they secrete antiangiogenic factors, such as troponin 1, chondromodulin 1, and matrix metalloproteinase inhibitors [33]. Normal cartilage is composed of type II collagen. In early osteoarthritis, there is loss of the proteoglycans and glycosaminoglycans that are normally found in the extracellular matrix of the chondrocytes. Type X collagen may be involved in the pathophysiology of endochondral ossification in knee OA. Type I collagen is also present in vascularized, osteoarthritic knee joint cartilage [34].

Nerve tissue tends to parallel vascular structures. The synovium and subchondral bone contain sensory nerves, which consist of unmyelinated C fibers. This nervous tissue functions along with the neuropeptides Substance P and calcitonin gene-related peptide [28]. Mechanical forces, hypoxia, and inflammation may increase nerve sensitivity to pain [12]. Hypoxic conditions stimulate the release of collagen prolyl 4-hydroxylase (P4Halpha(I)) and hypoxia-inducible factor (HIF-1 alpha) [35]. Normal cartilage is not innervated; however, with pathological vascularization, the perivascular tissue and cartilage may become innervated and more sensitive to pain [28]. Chondrocytes have been found to possess not only receptors for substance P and calcitonin generated peptide but also adrenergic receptors and vasoactive intestinal peptide (VIP) receptors. Peripheral nerve fibers are normally found in periosteal tissue and trabecular bone. These fibers are involved physiologically in normal developmental processes, such as endochondral ossification and limb formation. Additionally, they provide sympathetic and sensory innervation, which assists with healing fractures [36]. Pathologically, the sensory and sympathetic neurotransmitters may have a role in inflammatory arthropathies, such as rheumatoid arthritis [36]. Sensory and sympathetic nerve fibers are concentrated in human cartilage associated with tibiofemoral osteoarthritis and marginal osteophytes. The abnormal nerve fibers have been observed accompanying abnormal vasculature originating from subchondral bone, extending into the cartilaginous tissue [36].

2.4. A Review of Translational Animal Models

Larger animal model studies have shown angiogenic invasion to be statistically increased in OA knee joints across the osteochondral junction [8]. McDougall et al. showed increased angiogenesis in the medial collateral ligament (MCL) in induced OA joints compared to sham joints in rabbits [9]. Jansen et al. showed that following bilateral ACL transections in rabbits, VEGF was present in the joint cartilage but not present in the cartilage of control animals [10]. Bray et al. showed a five-fold increase in blood flow to the meniscus at four weeks post injury, which was statistically significant compared to control and sham-operated animals [11].

2.5. GAE: Anatomy of Genicular Arteries

GAE requires a fundamental knowledge of knee vascular anatomy, along with its variations, for effectively and safely identifying the embolizing target [37,38]. Three main vessels provide the vascular supply to the knee. The descending genicular artery (DGA) branching from the femoral artery supplies the superior knee, the anterior tibial recurrent artery (ATRA) branching from the anterior tibial artery supplies the inferior knee, and the genicular arteries arising from the popliteal artery supply the remainder of the knee joint [39]. Because the medial aspect of the joint is the weight-bearing portion of the knee, the medial knee joint compartment is more commonly affected by OA than the lateral compartment [37,40,41]. Consequently, the medial genicular branches of the popliteal artery and the DGA branches are of particular importance, as these vessels are common targets for GAE [37]. Several studies, however, have shown the high degree of variation in genicular vessels and DGA [39,40,42–47]. A recent cadaver study by Sighary et al. noted that although the most common genicular artery pattern was independent branches of the superior medial (SMGA), superior lateral (SLGA), inferior medial (IMGA), inferior lateral (ILGA), and medial genicular artery (MGA) from the popliteal artery, 72% of cadavers had genicular artery variations [39]. Most variants were related to the origin of the MGA, which is consistent with previous studies [48,49]. Additionally, the same cadaver study noted anatomical variations of the DGA and its muscular (MB), articular (AB), and saphenous branches (SB). Previous plastic surgery literature has created a DGA classification system of seven subtypes [47,50]. Shighary et al., however, utilized a three-subtype classification system of DGA that is more oriented toward GAE. In this, the MB was excluded because it can easily be identified during GAE and is not likely to be a site of nontarget embolization. In addition, the medial epicondyle and the origin of the DGA from the femoral artery were used as landmarks for classification and can be easily visualized during GAE. Type A classification was defined as the division of the AB and SB above the midpoint of the medial epicondyle and origin of the DGA, and Type B was defined as the division below this midpoint. Type C classification was defined as separate AB and SB origins from the femoral artery [39]. Results showed 72% of DGAs were classified as Type B, 24% were classified as Type A, and 4% were classified as Type C [39]. Angiographic studies also correlate with these cadaveric findings. In a recent study by Bagla et al., angiographic findings from 39 GAE procedures showed anatomical variations of the medial and lateral genicular arteries [38]. Three medial branches (DGA, SMGA, and IMGA) and three lateral branches (SLGA, ILGA, and ATRA) were analyzed. As opposed to previous classification systems that focused primarily on the MGA [39,42,43], Bagla et al. created a new classification system of genicular artery anatomy that excluded the MGA due to its limited perfusion of the knee. For the medial aspect of the knee, M1 was classified as the presence of all three medial branches, whereas M2 was classified as the presence of two of the three medial branches. For the lateral knee, the presence of all three lateral branches was classified as L1 while L2 was classified as the presence of two of the three. This provides a classification system clinically oriented toward consistent reporting for GAE and better predicting anastomotic networks [38].

Anastomotic networks between the genicular arteries provide additional complex variation to the vascular network of the knee. Bagla et al. observed anastomoses in 26.4% of genicular arteries, with highest rates between the musculoarticular branch of the DGA and the SMGA/SLGA [38]. Other cadaver studies have observed anastomoses between the DGA and SMGA and between the IMGA and medial sural artery [41]. Although the clinical impact of these anastomoses was not discussed, Little et al. noted the impact vessel anastomoses within the knee vasculature network can have on nontarget embolization [18]. In their prospective pilot study, three cases were reported to have significant retrograde flow through geniculate anastomoses from the target artery to the popliteal artery, increasing the risk of embolization of nontarget sites. As a result, these patients were not embolized [18]. Additionally, GAE poses a particular challenge for coil embolizing anastomotic vessels to prevent nontarget embolization. The knee joint, patella, distal femur, and proximal tibia receive blood from the geniculate arteries [51]. Combined GAE and coil embolization for nontarget embolization prevention could result in osteonecrosis, which would provide poor GAE outcomes and future osseous complications [18]. Additionally, the genicular arteries provide a collateral network of vessels in peripheral vascular disease [18,43].

Knowledge of knee vascular anatomy is essential for minimizing risk of GAE. A common side effect of GAE is skin discoloration secondary to cutaneous ischemia from nontarget embolization of cutaneous arteries. Okuno et al. reported that four patients experienced transient color change of the overlying skin of the treated knee that spontaneously resolved by 1 month follow-up [13]. Bagla et al. observed a similar adverse event after GAE, with 13 of 20 patients noting skin discoloration that self-resolved within 3 months of GAE [14]. O'Grady et al. and other studies have observed cutaneous supply from the DGA and SLGA [41,50,52]. Additionally, unavoidable cutaneous branches are present on the ILGA and IMGA [41]. Little et al. minimized the nontarget embolization of cutaneous arteries by utilizing ice packs to constrict cutaneous vessels temporarily [18]. As a result, the

GENESIS study observed a much lower 12.5% [18] rate of skin discoloration compared to 65% [14] and 57% [13] in previous studies. Common origins are also important to consider for minimizing the risk of nontarget embolization. Common trunks involving the MGA are especially important, as nontarget embolization may result in damage to the cruciate ligaments [37,41,43,53]. O'Grady et al. observed three variants of vessels with a common origin of the MGA: the SMGA (5 out of 20 cadavers), SLGA (4 out of 20 cadavers), and both the SMGA and SLGA (1 out of 20) [41]. Sighary et al. observed similar results with 45 out of 196 cadavers having an SMGA and MGA common trunk, 31 out of 204 having an SLGA and MGA common trunk, and 20 out of 204 having an MGA common trunk with SLGA and MLGA [39]. MSGA and LSGA common trunks must also be considered, as nontarget embolization of the contralateral side could result [38]. Overall, a comprehensive knowledge of the knee vascular network is essential for GAE. Recognition of normal and variant anatomy as well as anastomotic connections can help minimize risks associated with GAE and reduce procedure time.

2.6. A Continued Need for OA Treatment

Advancements in the pathogenetic model of OA has redirected research into its treatment and shifted the focus to limiting or treating joint changes associated with persistent synovitis. Okuno et al. has published four studies in human subjects showing that targeted neovessel embolization successfully treated symptomatic osteoarthritis with durable therapeutic response. Twenty-five patients with radiographic and clinical findings of knee osteoarthritis underwent the angiography and embolization of identifiable neo-vessels. These vessels tended to be associated with the synovium, infrapatellar fat pad, medial meniscus, medial joint capsule, and the periosteum adjacent to the medial condyle. They were identified as "excessive, disorganized" vascular structures, which often demonstrated arteriovenous shunting and early venous drainage [16]. Neo-vessels were embolized using 10–70 micrometer imipenem/cilastatin (IPM/CS) particles or 75 micrometer microspheres loaded with the same drug. Patients reported substantial pain relief and improvement in symptoms after embolization. Interestingly, some patients experienced clinical improvement minutes after the procedure, whereas others reported clinical improvement several weeks to months after treatment [17].

Continued follow-up with magnetic resonance imaging in treated patients demonstrated significantly improved synovitis. These results suggest that embolization may function to treat pain and modify disease progression. While the clinical results are promising, the effect of embolization on laboratory, histological and imaging findings of OA are not well understood. Imaging studies have similarly coalesced on the association between OA and synovitis. Separate from any study related to GAE, but speaking more broadly of synovitis, Macfarlane et al. recently stated, "changes in synovitis, whether persistently extensive or intermittent, are associated with cartilage damage over time." They ultimately conclude, "Since synovitis is a potentially modifiable intraarticular feature, further research is warranted to assess whether treatment of synovitis mitigates cartilage destruction" [54]. Results from the Multicenter Osteoarthritis Study (MOST) have created compelling evidence of synovitis as an independent cause of OA as well as a potential modifiable contributor to the disease [55]. As it relates to pain, there is early evidence that there is a direct correlation between the Western Ontario and McMaster Universities Osteoarthritis Index (WOMAC) pain scale and synovitis [56].

3. New Opportunities in the Treatment of OA

There remains a sizable portion of knee OA patients who do not respond to non-operative therapy and are not considered good surgical candidates due to associated comorbidities or early disease stage. Therapeutic embolization for osteoarthritis has had promising early results [14–20,57,58]. Heller et al. reviewed the technical success, defined as embolization of at least one target genicular artery, and clinical success of GAE [37]. According to Heller et al., the technical success of GAE has been reported to range from

84 to 100%, and GAE has shown clinical success based on WOMAC [13,14], KOOS [15,18], and VAS scores [13,14,18,57]. A recent meta-analysis by Torkian et al. also validated the therapeutic success of GAE on OA [59]. In the 11 included studies, GAE resulted in significant improvement of VAS and WOMAC scores. After two years, VAS scores improved by 80% from pre to postembolization, and WOMAC scores improved by 85%. Additionally, the number of patients who used pain medication for OA reduced following GAE [59]. Of note, Torkian et al. also reported a 25.2% overall complication rate of GAE, the most common being transient cutaneous ischemia. Other adverse events reported include access-site hematomas, redness of the skin, and transient fever [59].

Despite the technical and clinical success of therapeutic embolization, the mechanism of action is not well understood. Okuno et al. have shown that targeted geniculate artery embolization resulted in statistically significant pain relief at 1-month, 4-month, and 12-month follow-up [17]. Midterm results demonstrated decreased WOMAC scores following geniculate artery embolization from an average baseline score of 43 +/− 8.3 to an average post-treatment score of 14 +/− 17 at 24 months [13]. Results also showed improved functionality and decreased pain symptoms of the knee for up to 4 years follow-up [13]. However, in these same patients, there was no significant improvement in the imaging appearance of their osteoarthritis on knee MRI as calculated by their WORMS scores nearly two years after treatment. Whole-Organ Magnetic Resonance Scoring (WORMS) suggests that although GAE results in a significant reduction in clinical symptoms, the imaging findings of osteoarthritis remain unchanged. Although the overall WORMS score did not improve in OA patients following GAE, the MRI appearance of synovitis was one imaging finding that did improve following GAE [13]. Similarly, a significant improvement in synovitis following GAE was observed in an interim analysis of GENESIS by Little et al. from WORMS [18]. Of note, Little et al. also found a significant deterioration in osteophytes and bone attrition from WORMS analysis, which was not previously reported. This was explained by the significantly higher median BMI (35) of the four patients who had a significant deterioration in osteophytes and bone attrition compared to the median BMI (25.2) of patients in the cohort included by Okuno et al. [13,18,60]. These four patients did, however, report improvement in the KOOS pain subscale. The overall results from Little et al. showed a significant decrease in mean visual analog scale (VAS) from 60 to 36 and 45 at 3 months and 1 year, respectively, and a significant improvement in the pain, other symptoms, function in sport and recreation, and knee-related quality of life subscales of the Knee Injury and Osteoarthritis Outcome Score (KOOS) questionnaire [18].

Early evidence shows that GAE is a straightforward procedure with less comorbidity relative to TKA that decreases pain via interruption of the inflammatory pathways and may also have a disease-modifying effect on the cartilage itself. These findings demonstrate the potential for neo-vessels as a target for disease-modifying treatment of OA as it relates to inflammation and synovitis [61–63]. Basic science, animal models, imaging studies, and early human trials demonstrate a link between synovitis, synovial angiogenesis, and OA. Our expanding knowledge of OA warrants further investigation of neo-vessels as a treatment target utilizing embolization therapy. In addition, prior literature has shown knee embolization to be a safe procedure with low complication rates, which has previously been used in other settings such as hemarthrosis [64–68].

Given the clinical need for effective non-surgical treatments of OA, evidence linking synovial neovascularization and the development of osteoarthritis, and clinical improvement in OA symptoms following GAE, future studies should seek to better understand the mechanisms involved in this burgeoning treatment modality. It has been nearly two decades since it was demonstrated during unanesthetized knee arthroscopy that "the anterior synovial tissues, fat pad, and capsule were exquisitely sensitive to the mechanical loading stimulus of the probe" [69], and in the interim, basic science research more accurately characterized the physiologic and pathologic basis of knee pain. Still, "further mechanisms by which transcatheter arterial embolization relieves patients' symptoms remain obscure" [17], demanding further study in animal models and ultimately, in humans.

4. Challenges and Recommendation

Understanding the inflammatory response to embolotherapy of OA will better guide treatment strategies. Although GAE has shown promise in treating intractable OA pain resistant to conservative management, the disease modification mechanism of embolization in OA remains poorly understood. The pathogenesis of OA results from a disturbance in the intra-articular microenvironment homeostasis toward a pro-inflammatory state associated with neovascularity and angiogenesis. These neo-vessels are suspected to be responsible for hyperalgesia in OA patients. However, the causality of these neo-vessels with respect to OA is not proven nor is the mechanism of action for GAE completely understood. The current animal models have only proven an association between microscopic neo-vessels and joints affected by OA. Identifying a similar type of macroscopic radiographically evident neo-vessel in an OA animal model would further elucidate the pathophysiology of this phenomenon in humans. Ultimately, continued study of intra-arterial joint embolization may lead to improved clinical outcomes for OA patients who do not respond to optimized non-operative therapy and are not considered surgical candidates. Geniculate artery embolization has shown promising early results for the management of mild to moderate OA of the knee, but expanded randomized controlled trials are needed to better evaluate its potential role in OA treatment. In a recent multicenter, randomized controlled trail, Bagla et al. showed that GAE significantly reduced pain and improved disability in patients with mild to moderate OA compared to patients of the sham group [58]. In addition, the Neovascularization Embolization for knee Osteoarthritis (NEO) trial is a randomized sham-controlled trial that is currently analyzing the safety of GAE for treating OA [70,71]. Correa et al. recently proposed the Genicular Artery embolization Using imipenem/Cilastatin vs. microspHere for knee Osteoarthritis (GAUCHO) trail, a randomized control trial, to compare impinem/cilstatin vs. microspheres in GAE for OA treatment [72]. While reducing patient pain is the chief concern in OA treatment, additional quantitative studies are needed to elucidate the downstream changes in biophysical factors and inflammatory cytokine cascade following GAE treatment. Additional human clinical trials coupled with expanded animal research on GAE will result in greater scientific understanding of the role of arterial embolization as a potential target treatment of osteoarthritis and may identify future targets for therapy. Appropriate indications and clinical application of embolization will be best informed via a thorough understanding of the effects of embolization on laboratory, histological and imaging correlates of OA.

Funding: This study was not supported by any funding.

Institutional Review Board Statement: This article does not contain any studies with human participants or animals performed by any of the authors.

Informed Consent Statement: Not applicable.

Conflicts of Interest: The authors declare that they have no conflict of interest.

References

1. Bonnet, C.S. Osteoarthritis, angiogenesis and inflammation. *Rheumatology* **2005**, *44*, 7–16. [CrossRef] [PubMed]
2. Mapp, P.I.; Walsh, D.A. Mechanisms and targets of angiogenesis and nerve growth in osteoarthritis. *Nat. Rev. Rheumatol.* **2012**, *8*, 390–398. [CrossRef]
3. Costa, C.; Incio, J.; Soares, R. Angiogenesis and chronic inflammation: Cause or consequence? *Angiogenesis* **2007**, *10*, 149–166. [CrossRef] [PubMed]
4. Cruz, R.; Ramírez, C.; Rojas, O.I.; Casas-Mejía, O.; Kouri, J.B.; Vega-López, M.A. Menisectomized miniature Vietnamese pigs develop articular cartilage pathology resembling osteoarthritis. *Path. Res. Pract.* **2015**, *211*, 829–838. [CrossRef]
5. Mapp, P.I.; Walsh, D.A.; Bowyer, J.; Maciewicz, R.A. Effects of a metalloproteinase inhibitor on osteochondral angiogenesis, chondropathy and pain behavior in a rat model of osteoarthritis. *Osteoarthr. Cartil.* **2010**, *18*, 593–600. [CrossRef] [PubMed]
6. Xie, L.; Lin, A.S.; Kundu, K.; Levenston, M.E.; Murthy, N.; Guldberg, R.E. Quantitative imaging of cartilage and bone morphology, reactive oxygen species, and vascularization in a rodent model of osteoarthritis. *Arthritis Rheum.* **2012**, *64*, 1899–1908. [CrossRef]

7. Talaie, R.; Richards, M.; Krug, H.; Dorman, C.; Noorbaloochi, S.; Golzarian, J. 4:12 PM Abstract No. 209 Neovascularization in knee osteoarthritis: A new mouse model using micro computed tomography to delineate pathological vascular remodeling. *J. Vasc. Interv. Radiol.* **2018**, *29*, S91. [CrossRef]
8. Saito, M.; Sasho, T.; Yamaguchi, S.; Ikegawa, N.; Akagi, R.; Muramatsu, Y.; Mukoyama, S.; Ochiai, N.; Nakamura, J.; Nakagawa, K.; et al. Angiogenic activity of subchondral bone during the progression of osteoarthritis in a rabbit anterior cruciate ligament transection model. *Osteoarthr. Cartil.* **2012**, *20*, 1574–1582. [CrossRef] [PubMed]
9. McDougall, J.J.; Bray, R.C. Vascular volume determination of articular tissues in normal and anterior cruciate ligament-deficient rabbit knees. *Anat. Rec.* **1998**, *251*, 207–213. [CrossRef]
10. Jansen, H.; Meffert, R.H.; Birkenfeld, F.; Petersen, W.; Pufe, T. Detection of vascular endothelial growth factor (VEGF) in moderate osteoarthritis in a rabbit model. *Ann. Anat.* **2012**, *194*, 452–456. [CrossRef] [PubMed]
11. Bray, R.C.; Smith, J.A.; Eng, M.K.; Leonard, C.A.; Sutherland, C.A.; Salo, P.T. Vascular response of the meniscus to injury: Effects of immobilization. *J. Orthop. Res.* **2001**, *19*, 384–390. [CrossRef]
12. Ashraf, S.; Walsh, D.A. Angiogenesis in osteoarthritis. *Curr. Opin. Rheumatol.* **2008**, *20*, 573–580. [CrossRef]
13. Okuno, Y.; Korchi, A.M.; Shinjo, T.; Kato, S.; Kaneko, T. Midterm Clinical Outcomes and MR Imaging Changes after Transcatheter Arterial Embolization as a Treatment for Mild to Moderate Radiographic Knee Osteoarthritis Resistant to Conservative Treatment. *J. Vasc. Interv. Radiol.* **2017**, *28*, 995–1002. [CrossRef]
14. Bagla, S.; Piechowiak, R.; Hartman, T.; Orlando, J.; Del Gaizo, D.; Isaacson, A. Genicular artery embolization for the treatment of knee pain secondary to osteoarthritis. *J. Vasc. Interv. Radiol.* **2020**, *31*, 1096–1102. [CrossRef] [PubMed]
15. Landers, S.; Hely, R.; Page, R.; Maister, N.; Hely, A.; Harrison, B.; Gill, S. Genicular artery embolization to improve pain and function in early-stage knee osteoarthritis-24-month pilot study results. *J. Vasc. Interv. Radiol.* **2020**, *31*, 1453–1458. [CrossRef] [PubMed]
16. Okuno, Y.; Oguro, S.; Iwamoto, W.; Miyamoto, T.; Ikegami, H.; Matsumura, N. Short-term results of transcatheter arterial embolization for abnormal neovessels in patients with adhesive capsulitis: A pilot study. *J. Shoulder Elbow Surg.* **2014**, *23*, e199–e206. [CrossRef]
17. Okuno, Y.; Korchi, A.M.; Shinjo, T.; Kato, S. Transcatheter Arterial Embolization as a Treatment for Medial Knee Pain in Patients with Mild to Moderate Osteoarthritis. *Cardiovasc. Intervent. Radiol.* **2014**, *38*, 336–343. [CrossRef] [PubMed]
18. Little, M.W.; Gibson, M.; Briggs, J.; Speirs, A.; Yoong, P.; Ariyanayagam, T.; Davies, N.; Tayton, E.; Tavares, S.; MacGill, S.; et al. Genicular artery embolization in patients with osteoarthritis of the knee (GENESIS) using permanent microspheres: Interim analysis. *Cardiovasc. Intervent. Radiol.* **2021**, *44*, 931–940. [CrossRef]
19. Sun, C.H.; Gao, Z.L.; Lin, K.; Yang, H.; Zhao, C.Y.; Lu, R.; Wu, L.Y.; Chen, Y. Efficacy analysis of selective genicular artery embolization in the treatment of knee pain secondary to osteoarthritis. *Zhonghua Yi Xue Za Zhi* **2022**, *102*, 795–800. [CrossRef]
20. Casadaban, L.C.; Mandell, J.C.; Epelboym, Y. Genicular Artery Embolization for Osteoarthritis Related Knee Pain: A Systematic Review and Qualitative Analysis of Clinical Outcomes. *Cardiovasc. Intervent. Radiol.* **2021**, *44*, 1–9. [CrossRef] [PubMed]
21. Osteoarthritis (OA). Secondary Osteoarthritis (OA). Available online: https://www.cdc.gov/arthritis/basics/osteoarthritis.htm (accessed on 1 January 2021).
22. Felson, D.T.; Zhang, Y.; Hannan, M.T.; Naimark, A.; Weissman, B.N.; Aliabadi, P.; Levy, D. The incidence and natural history of knee osteoarthritis in the elderly, The Framingham Osteoarthritis Study. *Arthritis Rheum.* **1995**, *38*, 1500–1505. [CrossRef] [PubMed]
23. Martel-Pelletier, J.; Barr, A.J.; Cicuttini, F.M.; Conaghan, P.G.; Cooper, C.; Goldring, S.R.; Jones, G.; Teichtahl, A.J.; Pelletier, J.P. Osteoarthritis. *Nat. Rev. Dis. Primers* **2016**, *2*, 16072. [CrossRef]
24. Older People Projected to Outnumber Children for First Time in U.S. History. Available online: https://www.census.gov/programs-surveys/popproj.html (accessed on 1 January 2021).
25. Maradit Kremers, H.; Larson, D.R.; Crowson, C.S.; Kremers, W.K.; Washington, R.E.; Steiner, C.A.; Jiranek, W.A.; Berry, D.J. Prevalence of Total Hip and Knee Replacement in the United States. *J. Bone Jt. Surg. Am.* **2015**, *97*, 1386–1397. [CrossRef]
26. United States Bone and Joint Initiative. *The Burden of Musculoskeletal Diseases in the United States (BMUS)*, 3rd ed.; United States Bone and Joint Initiative: Rosemont, IL, USA, 2014. Available online: http://www.boneandjointburden.org (accessed on 1 January 2021).
27. Losina, E.; Paltiel, A.D.; Weinstein, A.M.; Yelin, E.; Hunter, D.J.; Chen, S.P.; Klara, K.; Suter, L.G.; Solomon, D.H.; Burbine, S.A.; et al. Lifetime medical costs of knee osteoarthritis management in the United States: Impact of extending indications for total knee arthroplasty. *Arthritis Care Res.* **2015**, *67*, 203–215. [CrossRef]
28. Walsh, D.A. Angiogenesis in osteoarthritis and spondylosis: Successful repair with undesirable outcomes. *Curr. Opin. Rheumatol.* **2004**, *16*, 609–615. [CrossRef]
29. Davies, N.M.; Reynolds, J.K.; Undeberg, M.R.; Gates, B.J.; Ohgami, Y.; Vega-Villa, K.R. Minimizing risks of NSAIDs: Cardiovascular, gastrointestinal and renal. *Expert Rev. Neurother.* **2006**, *6*, 1643–1655. [CrossRef]
30. Gill, G.S.; Mills, D.; Joshi, A.B. Mortality Following Primary Total Knee Arthroplasty. *J. Bone Jt. Surg. Am.* **2003**, *85*, 432–435. [CrossRef] [PubMed]
31. Belmont, P.J.J.; Goodman, G.P.; Waterman, B.R.; Bader, J.O.; Schoenfeld, A.J. Thirty-Day Postoperative Complications and Mortality Following Total Knee Arthroplasty: Incidence and Risk Factors Among a National Sample of 15,321 Patients. *J. Bone Jt. Surg. Am.* **2014**, *96*, 20–26. [CrossRef]

32. Ballara, S.C.; Miotla, J.M.; Paleolog, E.M. New vessels, new approaches: Angiogenesis as a therapeutic target in musculoskeletal disorders. *Int. J. Exp. Pathol.* **2001**, *80*, 235–250. [CrossRef]
33. Murata, M.; Yudoh, K.; Masuko, K. The potential role of vascular endothelial growth factor (VEGF) in cartilage. *Osteoarthr. Cartil.* **2008**, *16*, 279–286. [CrossRef]
34. Fenwick, S.A.; Gregg, P.J.; Rooney, P. Osteoarthritic cartilage loses its ability to remain avascular. *Osteoarthr. Cartil.* **1999**, *7*, 441–452. [CrossRef] [PubMed]
35. Adesida, A.B.; Grady, L.M.; Khan, W.S.; Millward-Sadler, S.J.; Salter, D.M.; Hardingham, T.E. Human meniscus cells express hypoxia inducible factor-1α and increased SOX9 in response to low oxygen tension in cell aggregate culture. *Arthritis Res. Ther.* **2007**, *9*, R69. [CrossRef] [PubMed]
36. Grässel, S.G. The role of peripheral nerve fibers and their neurotransmitters in cartilage and bone physiology and pathophysiology. *Arthritis Res. Ther.* **2014**, *16*, 1–13. [CrossRef] [PubMed]
37. Heller, D.B.; Beggin, A.E.; Lam, A.H.; Kohi, M.P.; Heller, M.B. Geniculate Artery Embolization: Role in Knee Hemarthrosis and Osteoarthritis. *RadioGraphics* **2022**, *42*, 289–301. [CrossRef] [PubMed]
38. Bagla, S.; Piechowiak, R.; Sajan, A.; Orlando, J.; Canario, D.A.H.; Isaacson, A. Angiographic Analysis of the Anatomical Variants in Genicular Artery Embolization. *J. Clin. Interv. Radiol. ISVIR* **2022**, *6*, 18–22. [CrossRef]
39. Sighary, M.; Sajan, A.; Walsh, J.; Márquez, S. Cadaveric Classification of the Genicular Arteries, with Implications for the Interventional Radiologist. *J. Vasc. Interv. Radiol.* **2022**, *33*, 437–444.e1. [CrossRef] [PubMed]
40. Jones, R.K.; Chapman, G.J.; Findlow, A.H.; Forsythe, L.; Parkes, M.J.; Sultan, J.; Felson, D.T. A new approach to prevention of knee osteoarthritis: Reducing medial load in the contralateral knee. *J. Rheomatol.* **2013**, *40*, 309–315. [CrossRef]
41. O'Grady, A.; Welsh, L.; Gibson, M.; Briggs, J.; Speirs, A.; Little, M. Cadaveric and Angiographic Anatomical Considerations in the Genicular Arterial System: Implications for Genicular Artery Embolisation in Patients with Knee Osteoarthritis. *Cardiovasc. Intervent. Radiol.* **2022**, *45*, 80–90. [CrossRef]
42. Yang, K.; Park, J.H.; Jung, S.J.; Lee, H.; Choi, I.J.; Lee, J.H. Topography of the middle genicular artery is associated with the superior and inferior genicular arteries. *Int. J. Morphol.* **2017**, *35*, 913–918. [CrossRef]
43. Shahid, S.; Saghir, N.; Cawley, O.; Saujani, S. A cadaveric study of the branching pattern and diameter of the genicular arteries: A focus on the middle genicular artery. *J. Knee Surg.* **2015**, *28*, 417–424. [CrossRef]
44. García-Pumarino, R.; Franco, J.M. Anatomical variability of descending genicular artery. *Ann. Plast. Surg.* **2014**, *73*, 607–611. [CrossRef] [PubMed]
45. Xu, Q.; Zheng, X.; Li, Y.; Zhu, L.; Ding, Z. Anatomical study of the descending genicular artery chimeric flaps. *J. Investig. Surg.* **2020**, *33*, 422–427. [CrossRef]
46. Salaria, H.; Atkinson, R. Anatomic study of the middle genicular artery. *J. Orthop. Surg.* **2008**, *16*, 47–49. [CrossRef]
47. Ziegler, T.; Kamolz, L.P.; Vasilyeva, A.; Schintler, M.; Neuwirth, M.; Parvizi, D. Descending genicular artery. Branching patterns and measuring parameters: A systematic review and meta-analysis of several anatomical studies. *J. Plast. Reconstr. Aesthet. Surg.* **2018**, *71*, 967–975. [CrossRef]
48. Bettaiah, A.; Venkat, S.; Saraswathi, G. A study of variations in the branching pattern of popliteal artery and its clinical perspective. *Int. J. Res. Med. Sci.* **2016**, *4*, 3584–3589. [CrossRef]
49. Singla, R.; Kaushal, S.; Chabbra, U. Popliteal artery branching pattern: A cadaveric study. *Eur. J. Anat.* **2012**, *16*, 157–162.
50. Dubois, G.; Lopez, R.; Puwanarajah, P.; Noyelles, L.; Lauwers, F. The corticoperiosteal medial femoral supracondylar flap: Anatomical study for clinical evaluation in mandibular osteoradionecrosis. *Surg. Radiol. Anat.* **2010**, *32*, 971–977. [CrossRef]
51. Bowers, Z.; Nassereddin, A.; Sinkler, M.A.; Bordoni, B. *Anatomy, Bony Pelvis and Lower Limb, Popliteal Artery*; StatPearls Publishing: Treasure Island, FL, USA, 2021.
52. Parvizi, D.; Vasilyeva, A.; Wurzer, P.; Tuca, A.; Lebo, P.; Winter, R.; Clayton, R.P.; Rappl, T.; Schintler, M.V.; Kamolz, L.P.; et al. Anatomy of the vascularized lateral femoral condyle flap. *Plast. Reconstr. Surg.* **2016**, *137*, 1024e–1032e. [CrossRef]
53. Duthon, V.B.; Barea, C.; Abrassart, S.; Fasel, J.H.; Fritschy, D.; Ménétrey, J. Anatomy of the anterior cruciate ligament. *Knee Surg. Sports Traumatol. Arthrosc.* **2006**, *14*, 204–213. [CrossRef] [PubMed]
54. MacFarlane, L.A.; Yang, H.; Collins, J.E.; Jarraya, M.; Guermazi, A.; Mandl, L.A.; Martin, S.D.; Wright, J.; Losina, E.; Katz, J.N.; et al. Association of Changes in Effusion-Synovitis With Progression of Cartilage Damage Over Eighteen Months in Patients With Osteoarthritis and Meniscal Tear. *Arthritis Rheumatol.* **2019**, *71*, 73–81. [CrossRef] [PubMed]
55. Felson, D.T.; Niu, J.; Neogi, T.; Goggins, J.; Nevitt, M.C.; Roemer, F.; Torner, J.; Lewis, C.E.; Guermazi, A.; Group, M.I. Synovitis and the risk of knee osteoarthritis: The MOST Study. *Osteoarthr. Cartil.* **2016**, *24*, 458–464. [CrossRef] [PubMed]
56. Wallace, G.; Cro, S.; Dore, C.; King, L.; Kluzek, S.; Price, A.; Roemer, F.; Guermazi, A.; Keen, R.; Arden, N. Associations Between Clinical Evidence of Inflammation and Synovitis in Symptomatic Knee Osteoarthritis: A Cross-Sectional Substudy. *Arthritis Care Res.* **2017**, *69*, 1340–1348. [CrossRef] [PubMed]
57. Lee, S.H.; Hwang, J.H.; Kim, D.H.; So, Y.H.; Park, J.; Cho, S.B.; Kim, J.E.; Kim, Y.J.; Hur, S.; Jae, H.J. Clinical outcomes of transcatheter arterial embolisation for chronic knee pain: Mild-to-moderate versus severe knee osteoarthritis. *Cardiovasc. Intervent. Radiol.* **2019**, *42*, 1530–1536. [CrossRef] [PubMed]
58. Bagla, S.; Piechowiak, R.; Hartman, T.; Orlando, J.; Lipscomb, M.; Benefield, T.; Isaacson, A. Multicenter prospective, randomized, sham-controlled study of genicular artery embolization. *J. Vasc. Interv. Radiol.* **2020**, *31*, S6. [CrossRef]

59. Torkian, P.; Golzarian, J.; Chalian, M.; Clayton, A.; Rahimi-Dehgolan, S.; Tabibian, E.; Talaie, R. Osteoarthritis-Related Knee Pain Treated With Genicular Artery Embolization: A Systematic Review and Meta-analysis. *Orthop. J. Sports Med.* **2021**, *9*, 23259671211021356. [CrossRef]
60. Zheng, H.; Chen, C. Body mass index and risk of knee osteoarthritis: Systematic review and meta-analysis of prospective studies. *BMJ Open* **2015**, *5*, e007568. [CrossRef]
61. De Lange-Brokaar, B.J.; Ioan-Facsinay, A.; Yusuf, E.; Kroon, H.M.; Zuurmond, A.M.; Stojanovic-Susulic, V.; Nelissen, R.G.; Bloem, J.L.; Kloppenburg, M. Evolution of synovitis in osteoarthritic knees and its association with clinical features. *Osteoarthr. Cartil.* **2016**, *24*, 1867–1874. [CrossRef]
62. Scanzello, C.R.; Goldring, S.R. The role of synovitis in osteoarthritis pathogenesis. *Bone* **2012**, *51*, 249–257. [CrossRef]
63. Siebuhr, A.S.; Bay-Jensen, A.C.; Jordan, J.M.; Kjelgaard-Petersen, C.F.; Christiansen, C.; Abramson, S.B.; Attur, M.; Berenbaum, F.; Kraus, V.; Karsdal, M.A. Inflammation (or synovitis)-driven osteoarthritis: An opportunity for personalizing prognosis and treatment? *Scand. J. Rheumatol.* **2016**, *45*, 87–98. [CrossRef]
64. Kolber, M.K.; Shukla, P.A.; Kumar, A.; Zybulewski, A.; Markowitz, T.; Silberzweig, J.E. Endovascular Management of Recurrent Spontaneous Hemarthrosis After Arthroplasty. *Cardiovasc. Intervent. Radiol.* **2017**, *40*, 216–222. [CrossRef]
65. Weidner, Z.D.; Hamilton, W.G.; Smirniotopoulos, J.; Bagla, S. Recurrent Hemarthrosis Following Knee Arthroplasty Treated with Arterial Embolization. *J. Arthroplast.* **2015**, *30*, 2004–2007. [CrossRef] [PubMed]
66. Bagla, S.; Rholl, K.S.; van Breda, A.; Sterling, K.M.; van Breda, A. Geniculate artery embolization in the management of spontaneous recurrent hemarthrosis of the knee: Case series. *J. Vasc. Interv. Radiol.* **2013**, *24*, 439–442. [CrossRef]
67. Van Baardewijk, L.J.; Hoogeveen, Y.L.; van der Geest, I.C.M.; Schultze Kool, L.J. Embolization of the geniculate arteries is an effective treatment of recurrent hemarthrosis following total knee arthroplasty that can be safely repeated. *J. Arthroplast.* **2018**, *33*, 1177–1180. [CrossRef] [PubMed]
68. Given, M.F.; Smith, P.; Lyon, S.M.; Robertson, D.; Thomson, K.R. Embolization of spontaneous hemarthrosis post total knee replacement. *Cardiovasc. Intervent. Radiol.* **2008**, *31*, 986–988. [CrossRef] [PubMed]
69. Dye, S.F.; Vaupel, G.L.; Dye, C.C. Conscious neurosensory mapping of the internal structures of the human knee without intraarticular anesthesia. *Am. J. Sports Med.* **1998**, *26*, 773–777. [CrossRef]
70. Van Zadelhoff, T.A.; Moelker, A.; Bierma-Zeinstra, S.M.; Bos, K.P.; Krestin, G.P.; Oei, E.H. Safety of Genicular Artery Embolization for the Treatment of Knee Osteoarthritis: Data from the NEO Trial. *Osteoarthr. Cartil.* **2022**, *30*, S427. [CrossRef]
71. Van Zadelhoff, T.A.; Moelker, A.; Bierma-Zeinstra, S.M.A.; Bos, P.K.; Krestin, G.P.; Oei, E.H. Genicular artery embolization as a novel treatment for mild to moderate knee osteoarthritis: Protocol design of a randomized sham-controlled clinical trial. *Trials* **2022**, *23*, 1–8. [CrossRef]
72. Correa, M.P.; Motta-Leal-Filho, J.M.; Lugokeski, R.; Mezzomo, M.; Leite, L.R. GAUCHO-Trial Genicular Artery Embolization Using Imipenem/Cilastatin vs. Microsphere for Knee Osteoarthritis: A Randomized Controlled Trial. *Cardiovasc. Intervent. Radiol.* **2022**, 1–8. [CrossRef] [PubMed]

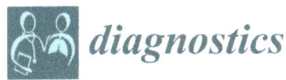

Review

A Review of Posteromedial Lesions of the Chest Wall: What Should a Chest Radiologist Know?

Sara Haseli [1], Bahar Mansoori [2], Mehrzad Shafiei [1], Firoozeh Shomal Zadeh [1], Hamid Chalian [3], Parisa Khoshpouri [1], David Yousem [4] and Majid Chalian [1,*]

1 Department of Radiology, Division of Musculoskeletal Imaging and Intervention, University of Washington, Seattle, WA 98105, USA; sarahaseli@gmail.com (S.H.); mshafie@uw.edu (M.S.); shomal@uw.edu (F.S.Z.); khoshpouriparisa@gmail.com (P.K.)
2 Department of Radiology, Division of Abdominal Imaging, University of Washington, Seattle, WA 98105, USA; mansoori@uw.edu
3 Department of Radiology, Division of Cardiothoracic Imaging, University of Washington, Seattle, WA 98105, USA; Hamid.Chalian@hsc.utah.edu
4 Russell H. Morgan Department of Radiology and Radiological Sciences, Division of Neuroradiology, Johns Hopkins Medical Center, Baltimore, MD 21287, USA; dyousem1@jhu.edu
* Correspondence: mchalian@uw.edu; Tel.: +1-(206)-598-2405

Abstract: A heterogeneous group of tumors can affect the posteromedial chest wall. They form diverse groups of benign and malignant (primary or secondary) pathologies that can arise from different chest wall structures, i.e., fat, muscular, vascular, osseous, or neurogenic tissues. Chest radiography is very nonspecific for the characterization of chest wall lesions. The modality of choice for the initial assessment of the chest wall lesions is computed tomography (CT). More advanced cross-sectional modalities such as magnetic resonance imaging (MRI) and positron emission tomography (PET) with fluorodeoxyglucose are usually used for further characterization, staging, treatment response, and assessment of recurrence. A systematic approach based on age, clinical history, and radiologic findings is required for correct diagnosis. It is essential for radiologists to be familiar with the spectrum of lesions that might affect the posteromedial chest wall and their characteristic imaging features. Although the imaging findings of these tumors can be nonspecific, cross-sectional imaging helps to limit the differential diagnosis and determine the further diagnostic investigation (e.g., image-guided biopsy). Specific imaging findings, e.g., location, mineralization, enhancement pattern, and local invasion, occasionally allow a particular diagnosis. This article reviews the posteromedial chest wall anatomy and different pathologies. We provide a combination of location and imaging features of each pathology. We will also explore the role of imaging and its strengths and limitations for diagnosing posteromedial chest wall lesions.

Keywords: chest wall; posteromedial; lesion; imaging; benign; malignant

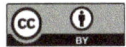

1. Introduction

Chest wall tumors are uncommon causes of thoracic neoplasms, which are less common than soft tissue or bony neoplasms elsewhere. Unfamiliarity with the complex posteromedial chest wall anatomy and radiologic features of related neoplasms is a diagnostic dilemma for radiologists [1]. These tumors are heterogeneous with nonspecific clinical manifestations and different imaging characteristics, which make their diagnosis challenging. Either a benign or malignant nature and primary or secondary origin are probable [2–4]. Primary chest wall neoplasms originate from chest wall structures, e.g., bony thorax, cartilage, muscle, fat, blood vessels, and nerve sheath [3,5]. Secondary chest wall neoplasms include direct invasion from adjacent malignancies (lung or breast carcinomas) or distant metastasis [2].

The posteromedial aspect of the chest wall has complex anatomy due to the presence of intercostal nerves, sympathetic chain, and vascular structures. Many neoplasms originate from these structures [6]. Some of them may be almost exclusive to this location. Neurogenic tumors are more commonly arising from the posteromedial chest wall as they originate from autonomic ganglia, paraganglia, or nerve sheets. So, they account for the majority of lesions found in the posterior mediastinum and chest wall [7]. Many of these lesions have specific imaging characteristics that help make precise diagnoses and avoid invasive sampling. In other conditions with nonspecific imaging appearance, cross-sectional imaging plays an essential role in limiting the differential diagnosis and defining the further investigation, e.g., imaging-guided biopsy. So, it is crucial for radiologists to be familiar with these diverse group of lesions and their imaging characteristics [4,8].

Previous studies mostly focused on the assessment of malignant lesions of the chest wall. None of them specifically evaluated the lesions of the posteromedial chest wall [9–11]. Only one review article investigated the paravertebral masses in the thoracic boundary. This study categorized lesions into neurogenic tumors, non-neurologic tumors, and non-neoplastic masses [6]. To the best of our knowledge, our review is the only one focusing on the posteromedial aspect of the chest wall, addressing nearly all of the lesions that could be found in this anatomic location. This article reviews the posteromedial chest wall anatomy and different pathologies. We illustrated the imaging features of each lesion, e.g., the location, presence of calcification, adjacent bone destruction, the pattern of enhancement, and appearance on magnetic resonance imaging and positron emission tomography. We also explored the role of imaging and its strengths and limitations for diagnosing posteromedial chest wall lesions.

2. Posteromedial Chest Wall Anatomy

In this article, we focus on the posteromedial segment of the thoracic wall. The medial aspect of the posterior chest wall consists of multiple components detailed below (Figure 1):

1. Osseous/cartilaginous parts: 12 thoracic spine vertebrae, 12 ribs, and intervertebral discs.
2. Muscles: Intercostal muscles (external, internal, and innermost), subcostalis, and transverse thoracic.
3. Nerves: intercostal nerves, dorsal root ganglions, and sympathetic trunk.
4. Vascular tissues: Intercostal vessels feed above components.
5. Subcutaneous fat: beneath the superficial fascia and builds the padding for underlying muscles and bones.
6. Superficial fascia and skin: acting as protecting layers [5,12].

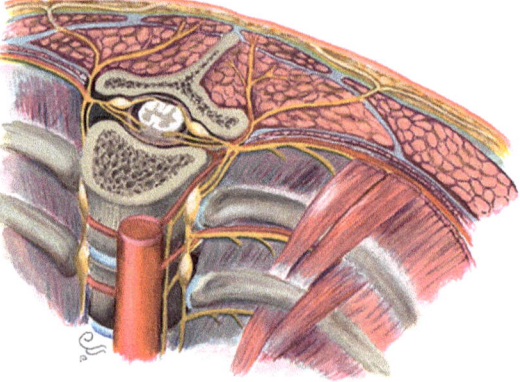

Figure 1. Posteromedial thorax anatomy, consisting of multiple components: skeletal components, muscles, nerves, ligaments, subcutaneous fat, fascia, skin, and vascular feeding tissues.

3. Classification of Posteromedial Chest Wall Lesions

Chest wall neoplasms are heterogonous lesions, and there is a lack of universally accepted classification. So, these neoplasms are usually classified according to the tissue of origin Table 1.

Table 1. Posteromedial chest wall tumors classification based on site of origin.

Origin	Malignant Neoplasm	Benign Neoplasm
Osseous and cartilaginous lesions - Rib - Thoracic spine	Osteosarcoma: - Osseous osteosarcoma - Extraosseous osteosarcoma Chondrosarcoma Ewing sarcoma: - Ewing sarcoma of bone - Extraosseous Ewing sarcoma Bone lymphoma Askin tumor Multiple myeloma Solitary plasmocytoma of bone	Osteochondroma Aneurysmal bone cyst Fibrous dysplasia of bone Ossifying fibromyxoid tumor Giant cell tumor Chondromyxoid fibroma Enchondroma Langerhans cell histiocytosis
Vascular lesions - Aorta - Intercostal vessels	Angiosarcoma Kaposi sarcoma	Lymphangioma Hemangioma
Adipose tumors	Liposarcoma	Lipoma Spindle cell lipoma
Neurogenic tumors - Intercostal nerve - Sympathetic nerve	Malignant peripheral nerve sheath tumor Neuroblastoma	Schwannoma Neurofibroma Ganglioneuroma Paraganglioma Meningocele
Lung and pleural lesions invading the chest wall	Mesothelioma Drop metastasis of thymic malignancy Lung malignancy with chest wall invasion	Localized fibrous tumor of pleura Empyema necessitans
Cutaneous lesions	Dermatofibrosarcoma protuberance	Cavernous hemangioma Epidermal inclusion cyst
Fibrous and muscle tumors	Undifferentiated pleomorphic sarcoma	Fibromatosis
Miscellaneous tumors	Neurofibrosarcoma	Extramedullary hematopoiesis Castleman disease Monoclonal immunoglobulin deposition diseases (MIDDs)
Secondary tumors	Bone metastasis	NA

4. Role of Imaging

Chest radiography is usually the first imaging modality performed when chest wall lesions are clinically suspected, although it can provide some nonspecific information [4]. More specific cross-sectional modalities such as computed tomography (CT) and magnetic resonance imaging (MRI) are warranted for better tissue characterization and assessment of lesion extension [2]. Obtaining high-resolution images as well as a short acquisition time makes CT the modality of choice for the initial evaluation of chest wall lesions. Although CT is more precise in assessing bone lesions, MRI has a superior contrast resolution, revealing more details regarding tissue characterization and tumor extension [2,4,6]. 18F-Fluorodeoxyglucose positron emission tomography/computed tomography (18F-FDG PET/CT) is another complementary modality beneficial in initial staging, evaluation of response to treatment, and tumor recurrence [2,13].

On the other hand, recent advances in deep learning and artificial intelligence (AI) provide the ability of automatic classification, disease detection, and segmentation. Chest radiography and CT scan are excellent candidates for developing deep learning algorithms [14]. AI has the potential to detect visual information and perform quantitative analyses. Besides, radiomics can be used to characterize the benign or malignant nature of a lesion and predict the prognosis and probability of response to treatment of the malignant lesions (Figure 2) [14,15].

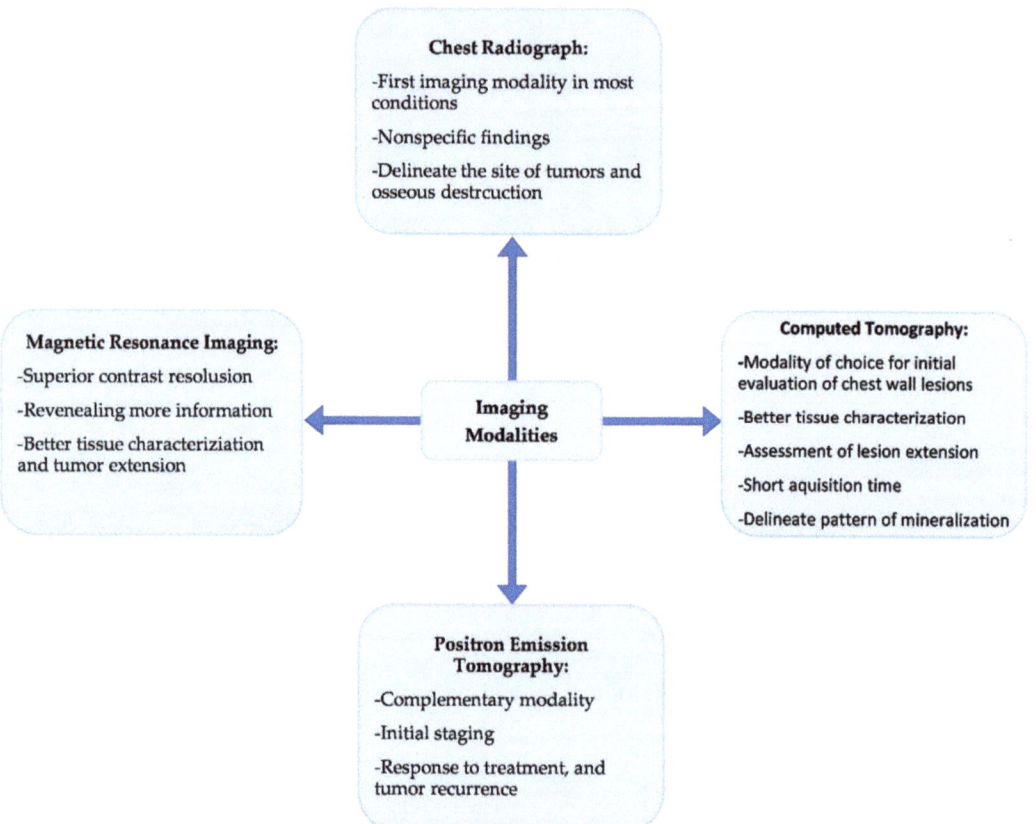

Figure 2. Tree graph of the most commonly used modalities for posteromedial chest wall lesions.

5. Malignant Bone Tumors

Radiologic characteristics of malignant bone tumors are summarized in Table 2.

5.1. Osteosarcoma

Chest wall osteosarcoma is a high-grade tumor accounting for 10–15% of primary chest wall malignancies, which can arise from rib or scapula with an extrapleural component. It has a poor prognosis as the lung and lymph nodes metastases are more frequent than extremities osteosarcoma [1,2].

A sclerotic lesion with higher central calcification is the most common appearance of osteosarcoma on radiography. Cortical destruction, expansile remodeling, and periosteal reaction are other common findings. CT can show soft-tissue destruction with variable types of calcifications such as cloudy, ivory-like, or dense (Figure 3) [1,2]. On MRI, the soft tissue component of osteosarcoma shows low to intermediate intensity on T1-weighted and hyperintensity on T2-weighted images. Foci of matrix mineralization have low signal intensity on both T1-weighted and T2-weighted images. Osteosarcoma demonstrates heterogeneous postcontrast enhancement. Invasion of deeper structures, pathologic fracture, and spinal canal invasion also have been described [1,2].

Table 2. Imaging manifestations of posteromedial chest wall osseous lesions.

Tumor Type	Imaging Findings	
	CT	MRI
Malignant		
Osteosarcoma	Dense central calcification, expansile bone remodeling, periosteal reaction, pathologic fracture. Sparing of the intervertebral disk while decreasing the height of the vertebral body. Lung and nodal metastasis	T1W: low to intermediate signal (high signal in hemorrhage) T2W: hyperintense Mineralization: hypointense on both T1W and T2W T1W FS + C: heterogeneous enhancement
Ewing sarcoma	Lytic bone destruction with ill-defined border, rare calcification, heterogenous paraspinal soft tissue with soft tissue larger than osseous component	T1W: iso to hyperintense to the muscle (high signal in hemorrhage) T2W: heterogeneous to hyperintense T1W FS + C: intense homogenous or heterogeneous enhancement
Chondrosarcoma	Well-defined mass: soft tissue+ mineralization Calcification: rings and arcs, stippled or dense Invasion of adjacent structures	T1W: variable, iso to hypointense to muscle T2W: overall hyperintense Mineralization: hypointense on both T1W and T2W T1WFS + C: heterogeneous enhancement
Multiple Myeloma	Osteolytic lesion with endosteal scalloping, diffuse osteopenia, multiple small lesions with mottled appearance, and osteoporotic fracture	Five patterns of marrow involvement: normal, focal, diffuse, combined diffuse and focal pattern, salt and pepper appearance. T1W: hypointense (significantly in the later phase of the disease) T2W: intermediate to hyperintense DWI: hyperintense T1WFS + C: enhancement expected
Solitary Plasmacytoma of the Bone	Extrapleural mass with well-circumscribed margin and "soap bubble" appearance and rare calcification, multicystic expansion	T1W: hypointense T2W: hyperintense
Benign		
Aneurysmal bone cyst	Well-defined expansile osteolytic lesion with thin marginal sclerosis and typical fluid-fluid level with internal septation	Fluid-fluid level T1W: hyperintense secondary to subacute age of internal hemorrhage T1W FS + C: can be seen in solid component of secondary ABCs
Fibrous dysplasia	Well-defined intramedullary osteolytic lesion with fusiform bony expansion and endosteal scalloping with preservation of cortical contour, sclerotic margin, trabeculation, and cortical thickening, "Ground glass" appearance, sometimes completely radiolucent or sclerotic	T1W: hypointense T2W: variable low to high signal depending on varying amounts of fibrous tissue
Giant cell tumor	Osteolytic lesion with bone expansion, cortical thinning, and heterogeneous soft-tissue attenuation with area of hemorrhage or necrosis	T1W, T2W: low to intermediate intensity representative of the abundant internal amount of hemosiderin and collagen
Enchondroma	Focally expansile well-demarcated osteolytic lesion, with or without cortical bulging, matrix calcification	T1W: significantly hypointense T2W: significantly hyperintense T1WFS + C: contrast uptake is uncommon unless in the small enchondromas or peripheral enhancement. Internal calcification: hypointense in all sequences
Chondromyxoid fibroma	Cortical expansion with lobulated border, abundant peripheral sclerosis, and rarely internal matrix calcification	T1W: isointense with hypointense rim T2W: intermediate to significantly hyperintense with hypointense rim T1WFS + C: diffuse moderate to intense enhancement
Chondroblastoma	Oval or round well-circumscribed lesion with internal mineralization and variable aggressiveness. Radiography is more accurate than MRI for diagnosis.	T1W: homogenously hypointense T2W: heterogeneously signal intensity with common peri-tumoral marrow edema, ABC changes, and periosteal reaction resembling malignant bone lesions.
Paget's disease of the rib	Osseous expansion, cortical thickening, and trabecular coarsening	Blastic phase: hypointense on both T1W and T2W images Lytic phase: speckled hypointense on T1W and hyperintense on T2W, T1WFS + C enhancement

T1W = T1-weighted, T2W = T2-weighted, FS = fat saturated, C = contrast; DWI = Diffusion weighted imaging.

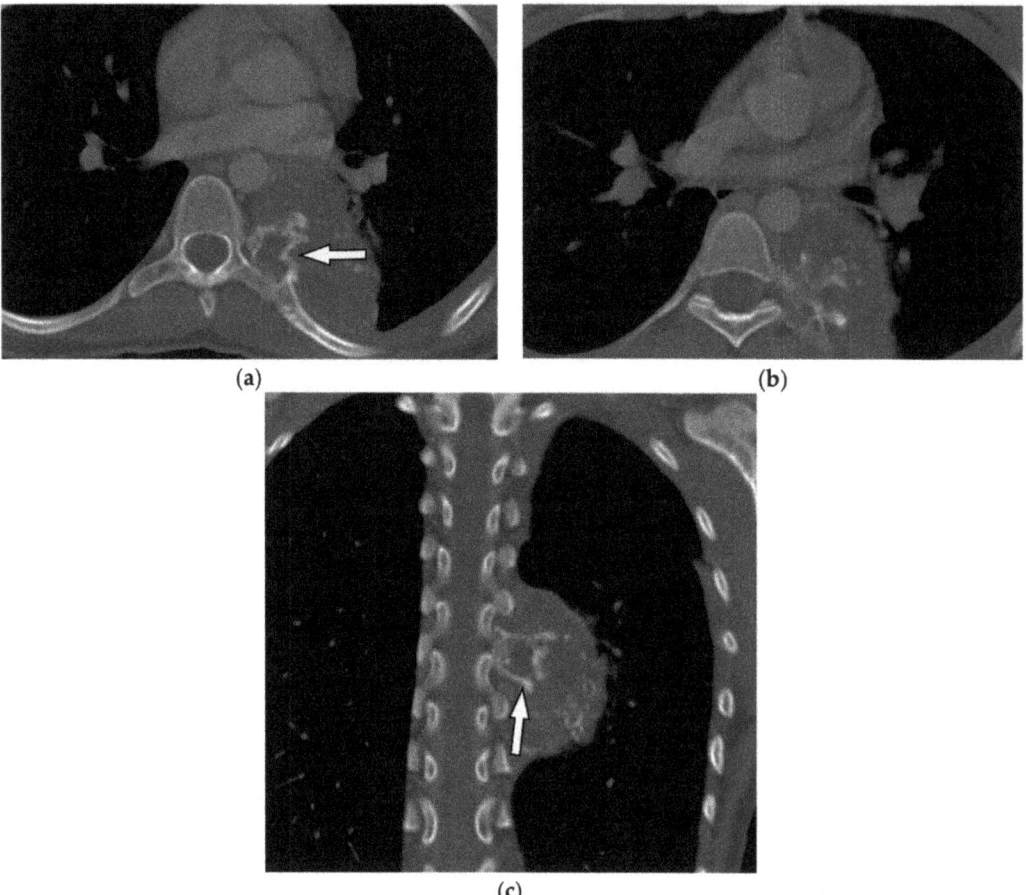

Figure 3. An 18-year-old woman with vague chest pain. The axial plane CT in the bone window obtained at the level of four chambers shows large destructive soft tissue mass within the posteromedial aspect of the chest wall on the left side with internal ossification that has a "sunburst" appearance (arrow) (**a**,**b**). The coronal view also shows the same large destructive soft tissue mass with internal calcification (arrow), which is denser centrally (**c**).

5.2. Ewing Sarcoma

Chest wall Ewing sarcoma is the most common primary chest wall tumor in children, typically arising from ribs or, less frequently, scapula, clavicle, and sternum. Painful chest wall mass with fever and malaise are the most common presentations [16].

On CT, Ewing sarcoma appears as a destructive paraspinal soft tissue mass with internal necrosis and hemorrhage. Calcification is rarely reported, and the soft tissue component is usually larger than the osseous component [11]. It appears iso to hyperintense on T1-weighted and heterogeneous to hyperintense on T2-weighted MRI sequences. Intense homogenous or heterogeneous post-contrast enhancement is expected. Extraosseous Ewing sarcoma, usually seen in older patients, manifests as a large non-calcified mass within the paravertebral location (Figure 4) [17]. 18F-FDG PET/CT is a valuable complementary tool enabling accurate identification of adjacent invasion and distant metastasis [18,19].

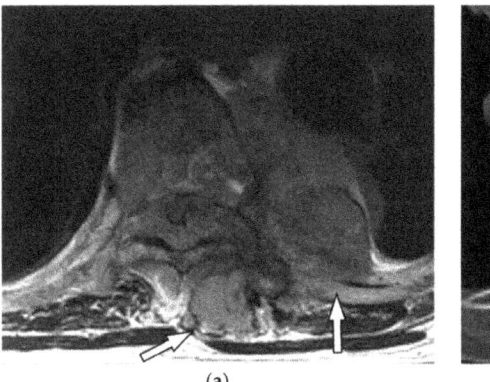 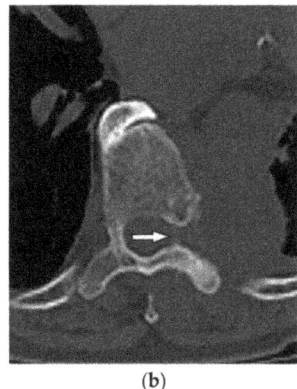

Figure 4. A 28-year-old man with bilateral leg weakness. The axial non-contrast-enhanced CT in the bone window (**a**) demonstrates a destructive mass in the posteromedial aspect of the chest wall on the left side, with a prominent soft tissue component with the left lateral vertebral body, pedicle, and lamina destruction (arrow). Axial T1W (**b**) MRI shows an inhomogeneous mass with iso to hyperintense signal intensity to paraspinal muscle with extension and invasion to left lateral recess, adjacent chest wall muscles, and rib (arrow).

5.3. Chondrosarcoma

Chondrosarcoma is the most common primary neoplasm of the chest wall accounting for 30% of malignant lesions [2]. It develops as either primary or malignant degeneration of preexisting benign lesions. It usually occurs between the 4th to 7th decades with a male predilection [1].

The typical CT appearance is a well-defined destructive mass with a mixture of soft tissue and mineralized components with stippled, dense, flocculent, rings, or arcs patterns. The invasion of adjacent structures has also been described [17]. On MR imaging, background cartilage shows iso- to hypointensity on T1-weighted and hyperintensity on T2-weighted images. The area of mineralization is low signal on both T1-weighted and T2-weighted images. Heterogeneous post-contrast enhancement is seen especially at the periphery of lesions with linear or septa-like patterns [17]. It is supposed that 18F-FDG PET/CT can play a complementary role in characterizing the chondrosarcoma from chondroma (Figure 5) [20].

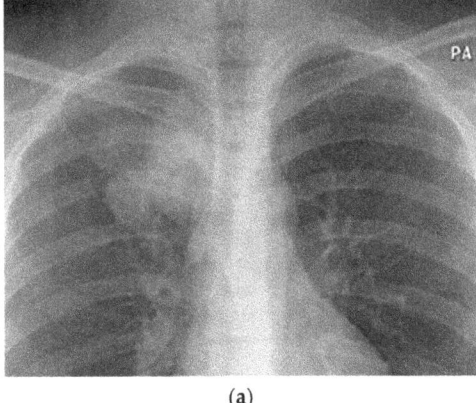 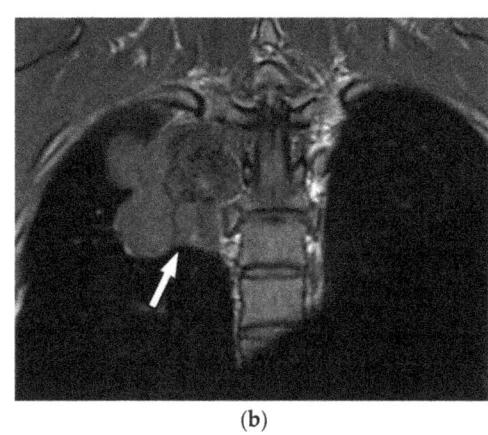

Figure 5. *Cont.*

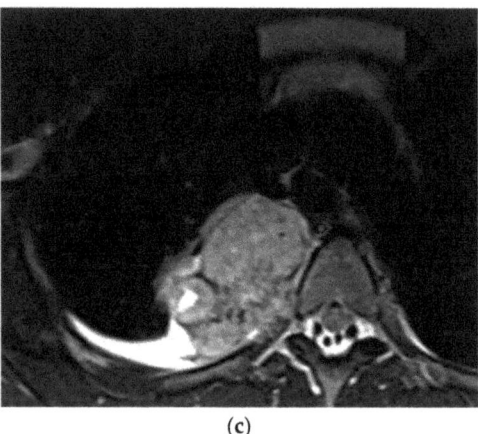

(c)

Figure 5. A 35-year-old man with chronic vague chest pain. (**a**) Frontal chest radiograph shows a right-sided lobulated mass with a cervicothoracic sign indicating the retro mediastinal location of the lesions. (**b**) Coronal T1W image shows lobulated paraspinal mass isointense to muscle (arrow). (**c**) Axial T2W fat-saturated image demonstrates heterogeneous high signal intensity with lobulated margin and internal foci of low signal intensity representing calcifications seen on CT (not shown). There is no neural foraminal extension.

6. Malignant Plasma Cell Tumors

6.1. Multiple Myeloma

Multiple myeloma (MM) is an infiltrative bone marrow disorder and concurrent bone lesion predominantly involving the axial skeleton, including vertebral bodies, skull, pelvis, and ribs [21].

Multiple myeloma radiologic features are osteolytic lesion with endosteal scalloping, diffuse osteopenia, multiple small lesions with mottled appearance, and osteoporotic fracture. In contrast to bone metastasis, the sclerotic halo is absent in MM, explaining the lower accuracy of scintigraphy compared to skeletal survey. Whole-body low dose CT was recommended as the initial survey for diagnosing osteolytic lesions of MM, which improved identification of extraosseous involvement and cortical disruption. STIR and T2-weighted imaging are the most sensitive sequences for depicting marrow signal changes. The T1-weighted sequence is useful for the evaluation of marrow infiltration [21,22].

Solitary Plasmacytoma of the Bone

Solitary plasmacytoma (SBP) of bone is an uncommon plasma cell neoplasm with localized bony growth. There are few case reports on solitary plasmacytoma of the rib [23,24].

Its radiologic appearance varies from purely non-expansile osteolytic to multicystic mass with bony expansion. CT may reveal extrapleural mass with a well-circumscribed margin and "soap bubble" appearance in advanced cases (Figure 6a,b). MRI shows T1-hypointensity and T2-hyperintensity (Figure 6c) [16,25]. SBP tends to show metabolic activity on 18F-FDG PET/CT, which seems to be a risk of multiple myeloma transformation (Figure 6d,e) [26].

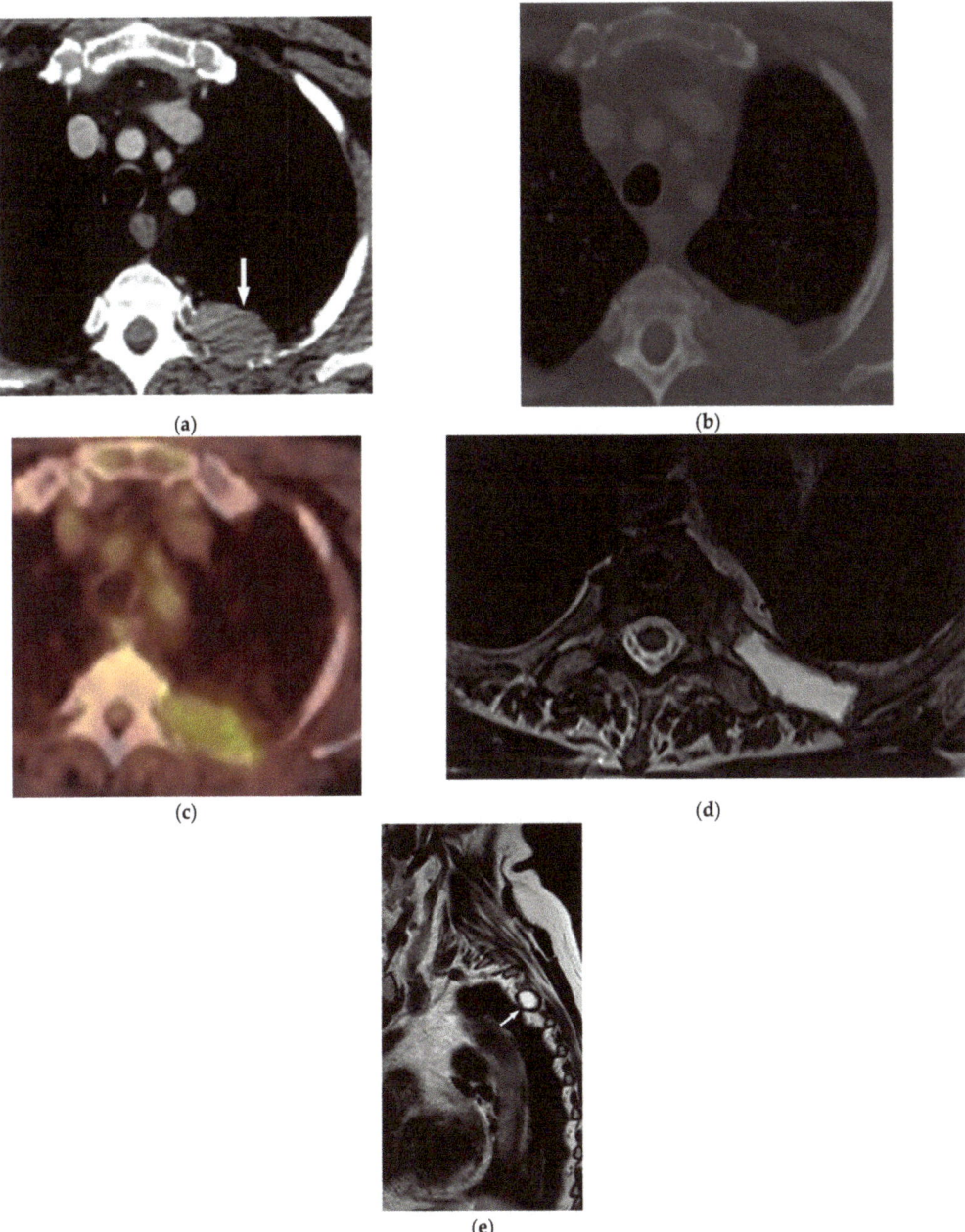

Figure 6. A 63-year-old woman with incidentally detected mass at the left posteromedial chest wall. Axial chest CT with mediastinal (**a**) and bone (**b**) window show a well-defined expansile mass (arrow) with the destruction of the adjacent rib. There is no internal calcification. No neural foraminal extension was seen (not shown). (**c**) T2W images of another patient with the same pathology show mildly expansile marrow replacing lesions at proximal posterior rib with high T2 signal intensity without cortical disruption or soft tissue mass. Increased metabolic activity is present on 18F-FDG PET/CT (**d**) Axial and (**e**) sagittal (arrow).

7. Benign Bone Tumors

Radiologic characteristics of benign bone tumors are summarized in Table 2.

7.1. Aneurysmal Bone Cyst

An aneurysmal bone cyst (ABC) is an uncommon benign bone tumor that consists of multiple blood-filled cysts, which can present as a primary tumor or as secondary changes of other bone tumors [1,16,27]. The most common location of chest wall ABCs is vertebral bodies with extension through adjacent soft tissue structures [27].

ABC's imaging appearance on radiography and CT is a well-defined expansile osteolytic lesion with thin marginal sclerosis, typical fluid-fluid level, and internal septation [1]. T1-weighted hyperintensity might be found secondary to the subacute timeline of internal hemorrhage (Figure 7) [16,27].

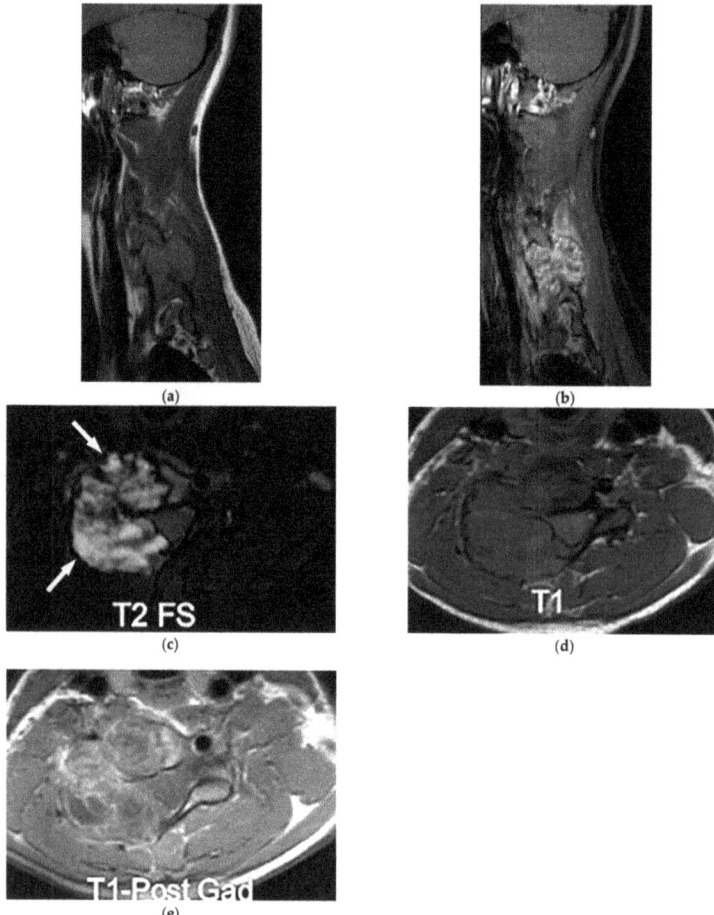

Figure 7. A 14-year-old boy with neck stiffness and scoliosis. The sagittal pre- and post-contrast T1WFS (**a,b**) demonstrate hypointense destructive spine lesion with low signal rim and heterogeneous enhancement of solid component. Axial images (**c–e**) show an expansile multiloculated mass (arrow) with the destruction of the vertebral body, spinous process, and lamina of the cervical spine. Fluid-fluid level and variable signal intensity caused by various-aged hemorrhage also were seen on T2WFs. It extends through the right lateral recess with canal stenosis. Slight hyperintensity on T1W is secondary to intratumoral hemorrhage. After injection of contrast, septal enhancements are seen.

7.2. Fibrous Dysplasia

Fibrous dysplasia (FD) is a developmental bone lesion caused by immature bone and marrow fibrous tissue replacement. It affects patients during the first and second decades of life. Rib is the most commonly affected site [1,16].

Fibrous dysplasia presents as a well-defined intramedullary osteolytic lesion with fusiform bony expansion and endosteal scalloping with preservation of cortical contour (Figure 8a). Increased trabeculation, thickened cortex, and "Ground glass" appearance caused by amorphous woven bone formation are other imaging findings (Figure 8c). FD has typical low intensity on T1-weighted and variable low to high intensity on T2-weighted MRI sequences depending on varying amounts of fibrous tissue (Figure 8b) [16,28]. FD metabolic activity on 18F-FDG PET/CT ranges from normal to intense, and it depends on the number of proliferating fibroblasts [29].

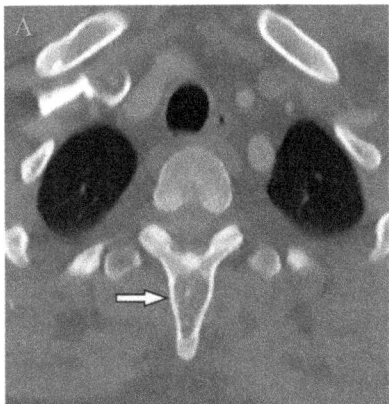
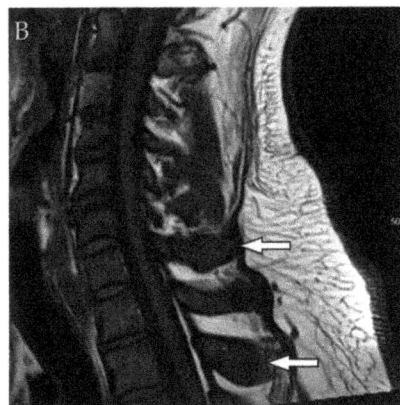
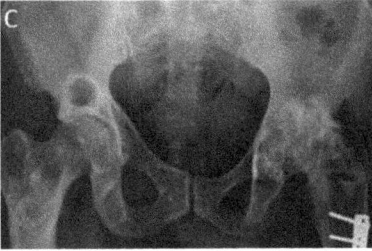

Figure 8. A 24-year-old man with multiple bone lesions. (**A**) The axial non-contrast CT in bone window demonstrates expansile lytic bone lesion with intact cortex within the spinous process of thoracic vertebrae (arrow); no periosteal reaction, cortical disruption, or soft tissue mass was found. (**B**) Sagittal T1W image shows expansile bone lesions with hyposignal intensity and intact cortex within the spinous process of multiple cervical spines (arrow). (**C**) Frontal image of pelvis shows bilateral expansile lytic bone lesions with bubbly appearance and typical shepherd's crook deformity in the left side.

7.3. Giant Cell Tumor

Chest wall giant cell tumor (GCT) originates from the subchondral region of tubular or flat bones, e.g., clavicle, ribs, sternum, and vertebrae. It usually affects patients during the third or fourth decade of age, with a female predilection. Thoracic vertebrae is the most common location for spinal GCT after sacrum [8,30].

On CT, GCTs manifest as osteolytic lesions, bone expansion with cortical thinning, heterogeneous soft-tissue attenuation, and area of hemorrhage or necrosis with no internal calcification (Figure 9a,b) [30]. MRI typically reveals low to intermediate intensity on both T1-weighted and T2-weighted sequences, representing an abundant amount of hemosiderin and collagen deposition. Fluid-level occurrence is less frequent than in ABC (Figure 9c,d) [8,31]. 18F-FDG PET/CT may cause misdiagnosis of the GCT as a high-grade osseous sarcoma [30].

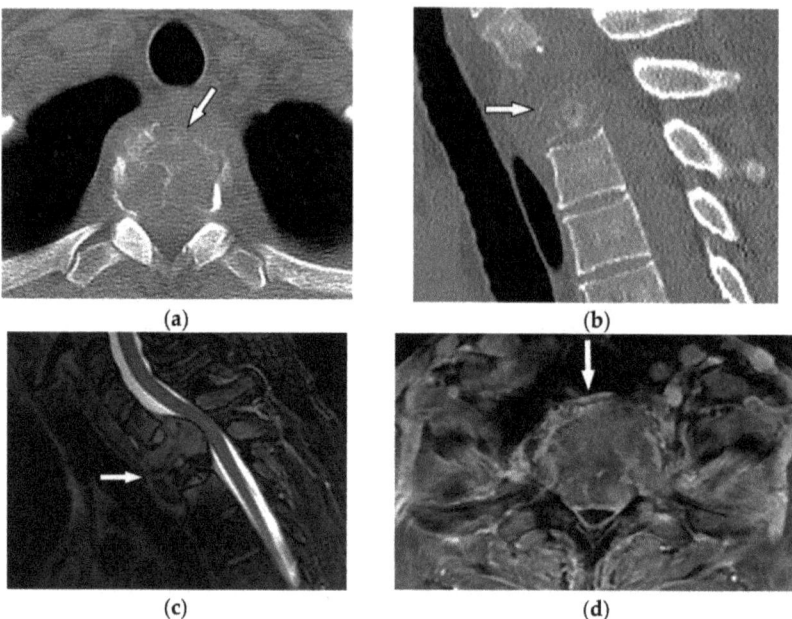

Figure 9. A 52-year-old man with bilateral leg weakness and paresthesia. The axial non-contrast CT in bone window demonstrates expansile osteolytic bone lesion with destruction and collapse of the vertebral body with pressure effect over the spinal cord and paravertebral soft tissue; the edge of vertebral body cortex disappeared (arrow) (**a**,**b**). Sagittal T2W shows heterogeneous iso signal mass with the collapse of the T2 vertebral body with compression of the dura and spinal cord (arrow); anterior soft tissue mass is also shown. The Intervertebral disc was intact. The visible internal hypointense lines are caused by thickened trabecular or hemosiderin deposition (**c**). T1W after injection of gadolinium shows heterogeneous marked enhancement of the tumor (arrow) (**d**).

7.4. Enchondroma

Enchondroma is the most common benign rib neoplasm after fibrous dysplasia, accounting for 15–20% of benign rib tumors. It typically arises from the costochondral or costovertebral junction due to its cartilaginous nature [32].

CT reveals focally expansile well-demarcated osteolytic lesion with or without cortical bulging. MRI helps depict enchondroma, especially when matrix calcification is vague on CT. Enchondroma has pronounced hypointensity on T1-weighted images as opposed to adjacent hypersignal fatty bone marrow. Hyaline cartilaginous content [rich in water] results in hyperintensity on T2-weighted images, and internal calcification foci produce hypointensity on all sequences [8,32].

7.5. Chondromyxoid Fibroma

Chondromyxoid fibroma is a rare benign cartilaginous tumor that contains various proportions of fibrous, myxomatous, and chondroid components [1,6]. It infrequently occurs within the chest wall from the scapula, spine, or ribs [33].

Cortical expansion with lobulated border, abundant peripheral sclerosis, and rarely internal calcification are the main radiologic appearances of chondromyxoid fibroma on radiograph and CT [3,33]. Cortical expansion with lobulated border, abundant peripheral sclerosis, and rarely internal calcification are the main radiologic appearances of chondromyxoid fibroma on radiograph and CT [3,33]. On MRI, varying degrees of signal intensity can be identified. Isointensity on T1-weighted and intermediate to high intensity on T2-weighted images have been reported. Peripheral hypointense rim seen on both T1-weighted and T2-weighted images reflects the sclerotic rim. The absence of diffusion restriction and diffuse moderate to intense contrast enhancement is noticeable (Figure 10) [3,33]. The absence of diffusion restriction and diffuse moderate to intense contrast enhancement is noticeable (Figure 10) [3,33].

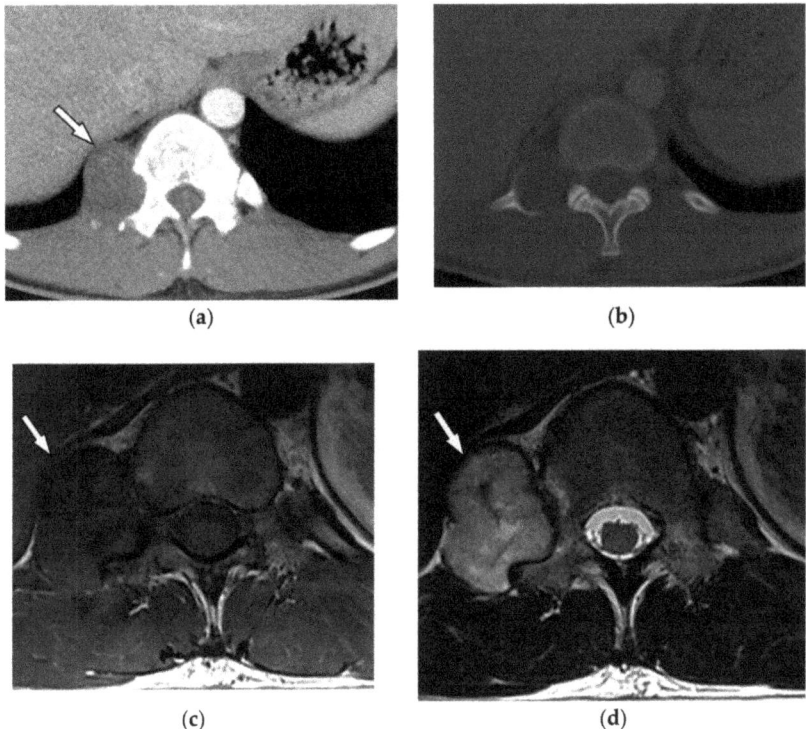

Figure 10. A 26-year-old man with right chest pain. The axial contrast-enhanced CT in soft tissue (**a**) and bone window (**b**) demonstrate well-defined oval eccentric lytic bone lesion within the posteromedial aspect of the chest wall on the right side (arrow) without intracanal extension or periosteal reaction; adjacent focal vertebral body scalloping is also shown. (**c,d**) Axial T1W and T2W show low signal intensity in T1W and intermediate to high intensity in T2W with the peripheral hypointense rim due to the sclerotic rim (arrow).

7.6. Chondroblastoma

Chondroblastoma is a rare, relatively benign bone neoplasm with a characteristic intercellular cartilaginous matrix and internal foci of calcification. It is usually found in the epi-metaphyseal regions of long bones. However, few cases of rib involvement have been reported [1,34]. It is frequently associated with cortical destruction and periosteal bone formation resembling malignant bone tumors [1,34,35].

The main radiologic appearance of chondroblastoma on radiograph and CT is an oval or round well-circumscribed lesion with internal matrix mineralization [1,34]. It appears homogenously hypointense on T1-weighted and heterogeneous on T2-weighted MRI sequences [36].

7.7. Paget's Disease of the Rib

Paget's disease is a chronic bone disorder characterized by abnormal osseous remodeling with three phases: lytic, mixed lytic and blastic, and sclerotic. It occurs in patients older than 40 years old with a male predilection. Rib involvement happens approximately in 1–4% of cases [35].

Imaging findings vary among different stages of the disease. The initial lytic active phase display osteolysis with no marginal sclerosis. While late blastic phase reveals cortical thickening and trabecular coarsening with bony enlargement. CT scan is useful in better delineation of the classic Paget's disease triad: osseous expansion, cortical thickening, and trabecular coarsening (Figure 11) [35,37]. Fat-like signal intensity is the most common pattern of the Paget disease seen on MRI, indicating long-lasting disease. Other stage-specific MRI findings are explained in Table 2 [35,37]. The relationship between 18-F FDG uptake and Paget's disease activity is still controversial, but a mild and diffuse pattern of FDG uptake is beneficial to differentiate it from bone metastasis [38].

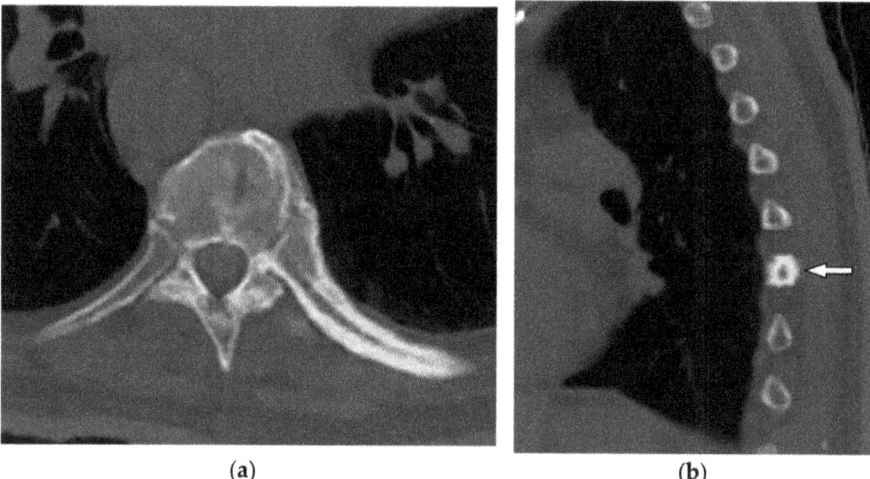

(a) (b)

Figure 11. A 53-year-old woman with localized chest wall tenderness. The axial non-contrast CT in the bone window (**a**) and sagittal (**b**) images show enlarged vertebral body associated with trabecular coarsening, osseous expansion, and thickened cortex of right eighth rib (arrow).

8. Spondylodiskitis

Spondylodiskitis is an infectious process that initially affects the anterior portion of the vertebral bodies and then spreads to the adjacent intervertebral disk via medullary spaces [39]. Staphylococcus aureus is the most common cause of pyogenic spondylodiskitis, which commonly presents as a single-level lumbar involvement of two vertebral bodies and intervertebral disk. Tuberculosis spondylodiskitis, the most common non-pyogenic spine infection, more commonly involves the thoracic spine [39,40].

8.1. Pyogenic Spondylodiskitis

Pyogenic spondylodiskitis presents with loss of vertebral end plate definition and marrow edema. It displays hypointensity on T1-weighted images and hyperintensity on T2-weighted and STIR images. Various types of disk post-contrast enhancement (e.g., homogenous, patchy, and peripheral) may be detected [39]. Abscess or phlegmons demonstrate heterogeneous mixed signal intensity on both T1-weighted and T2-weighted images, with probable spinal cord compression. Rim-like or diffuse post-contrast enhancement are usually seen within these soft tissues. Diffusion weighted imaging (DWI) is valuable for differentiating the abscess from other paravertebral lesions (Figure 12) [39,41].

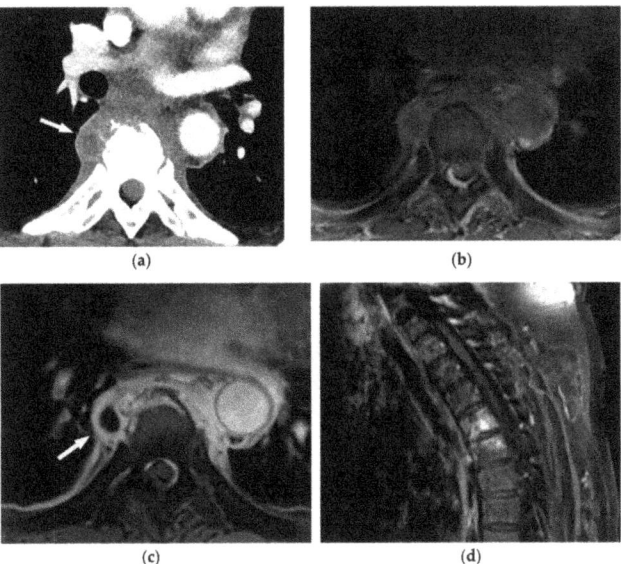

Figure 12. A 71-year-old man with back pain and fever. The contrast-enhanced CT in axial plane (**a**) demonstrates para-spinal soft tissue mass (arrow) with adjacent vertebral body cortical destruction. Axial pre-contrast (**b**) and post-contrast T1WFS (**c**) images at the level of T6-T7 show hypo to isointense paravertebral soft tissue mass with peripheral rim enhancement (arrow) after injection of gadolinium suggestive for paravertebral abscess formation. Sagittal STIR (**d**) image shows adjacent subchondral bone marrow edema as hypersignal intensity. Posterior elements are spared with normal signal intensity. Aspiration was performed and culture was compatible for brucellosis.

8.2. Tuberculosis Spondylodiskitis

Tuberculosis spondylodiskitis has a more gradual and chronic clinical course, which leads to multi-level involvement and paravertebral cold abscess formation with well-circumscribed thin wall. Subligamentous spread of infection to adjacent vertebral levels, relative preservation of intervertebral disk, and kyphotic angulation (gibbous deformity) are other imaging findings. CT scan is more sensitive in delineating calcification within paravertebral cold abscess, end plate erosion, and bony fragment visualization (Figure 13) [39,42].

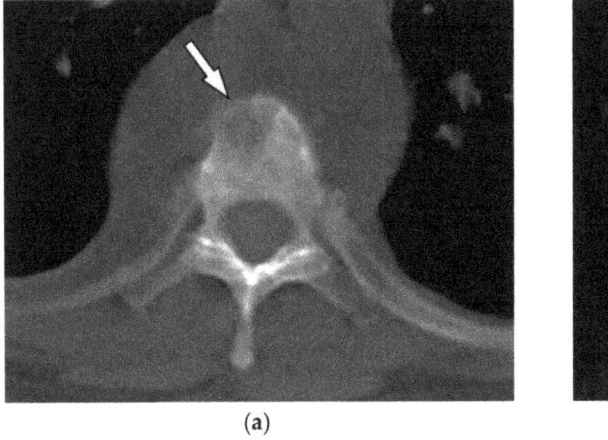 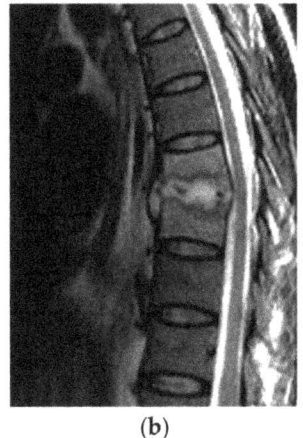

Figure 13. *Cont.*

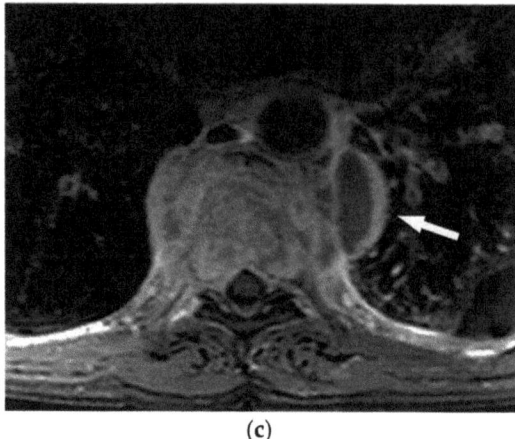

(c)

Figure 13. A 65-year-old man with fever, weight loss, and night sweeting. The non-contrast-enhanced CT (bone window) in axial plane (**a**) shows paraspinal soft tissue mass with erosion of right lateral aspect of adjacent vertebral body. Sagittal T2W image of another patient with the same pathology (**b**) shows hypersignal intensity within T8-T9 vertebral bodies with also intervertebral disc destruction and narrowing of spinal canal pushing the spinal cord posteriorly. Axial T1WFS + C (**c**) identified the enhancing paraspinal mass with peripheral rim enhancement (arrow) in its left posteromedial side, which is suggestive of abscess formation. Culture of aspirated pus under guide of CT was compatible with tuberculosis infection.

9. Soft-Tissue Tumors and Tumor-Like Lesions

9.1. Primary Neurogenic Lesions

Neurogenic tumors of the chest wall can arise from the intercostal nerve, spinal nerve roots, and even from the distal branch of the brachial plexus. They consist of benign and malignant groups, including Neurofibroma, Schwannoma, and malignant peripheral nerve sheet tumors (Table 3).

9.1.1. Schwannoma

Schwannoma is an encapsulated slow-growing peripheral nerve sheet neoplasm typically occurring in patients between 20–50 years old [6,16]. Chest wall schwannomas arise from spinal nerve roots with a dumbbell shape appearance and extend through the course of intercostal nerves, paravertebral region, or spinal canal [7,43].

Schwannoma presents a well-defined homogenous mass on CT scan with attenuation similar or less than muscle. The "Fat-split" sign caused by adjacent surrounding fat is indicative of its non-infiltrating growing pattern. It also shows remarkable post-contrast enhancement except for areas of necrosis or cystic changes (Figure 14). On MR images, it has intensity equal to or slightly more than muscle on T1-weighted and marked hyperintensity on T2-weighted images. Scalloping or bony erosions might be the only radiographic manifestations reflecting its benign nature [6,7,16,43].

9.1.2. Neurofibroma

Neurofibroma is another slow-growing peripheral nerve sheet neoplasm that affects patients in their 20s to 30s with equal male and female prevalence. Localized Neurofibroma, which includes approximately 90% of cases, is not typically associated with neurofibromatosis type 1 (NF1). However, the majority of cases with plexiform type have underlying NF1 [7,16].

The main CT findings are well-circumscribed mass with smooth margin, soft tissue attenuation, possible internal calcifications, and adjacent rib erosion. Neural foraminal widening secondary to tumor extension can be accurately identified on multidetector CT (Figure 15). "Target sign" appears on both T2-weighted and gadolinium-enhanced MR images. It is related to the peripheral abundant stromal matrix surrounding the high cellular center, presenting as hyperintense rim and hypointense center, respectively (Figures 16 and 17) [7,16,43].

Table 3. Imaging manifestations of posteromedial chest wall soft-tissue tumors.

Tumor Type	Imaging Findings	
	CT	MRI
Primary Neurogenic Tumors		
Schwannoma	Well-defined mass with homogenous attenuation, "fat-split" sign, internal calcification in long-standing schwannomas, postcontrast enhancement except for areas of necrosis.	T1W: iso or slightly hyperintense; T2W: significantly hyperintense
Neurofibroma	Well-circumscribed mass with smooth margin and soft tissue attenuation, possible internal calcifications, rib erosion, neural foramina widening because of tumor extension along with the spinal nerve roots.	T2W, T1WFS + C: so-called "target sign" appearance: hyperintense rim and hypointense center
Neuroblastoma [7,16,43]	Ill-defined paravertebral soft tissue mass with heterogeneous attenuation with internal calcification in at least 30% of cases (spotty calcification).	T1W: hyposignal T2W: hyperintense T1WFS + C: heterogeneous enhancement Calcification has a signal void in all sequences
Ganglioneuroma [7,16,43]	Homogenous or heterogeneous attenuation with internal calcification in 25% of cases.	T1W, T2W: intermediate signal with the curvilinear or nodular low signal band making the whorled appearance
Lipomatosis Tumors		
Lipoma	Homogenous similar attenuation to macroscopic fat with approximate HU: −100.	T1W, T2W: signal intensity identical to subcutaneous fat T1WFS + C: no enhancement (mild enhancement can be visible for septa < 2 mm thickness)
Liposarcoma	A heterogeneous mass mixture of fat and soft tissue: higher attenuation than normal fat (hypercellularity), necrosis, and calcification in myxoid subtype. Attenuation similar to fat in well-differentiated subtype. Thick septa, enhancing solid component.	T1W: variable hyperintense (myxoid liposarcoma), hypointense (well-differentiated), and intermixed hyper and hypointense (dedifferentiated subtype) T2W: hyperintense (myxoid liposarcoma and dedifferentiated subtype) T1WFS + C: variable enhancement
Others		
Rhabdomyosarcoma	Invasive, destructive homogenous mass with no mineralization and rapid growth with adjacent soft tissue and bone invasion.	T1W: isointense T2W: hyperintense with hypointense areas reflecting area of necrosis (alveolar and pleomorphic subtypes) T1WFS + C: homogenous or ring-like enhancement
Mesothelioma	Circumferential pleural thickening, bony or cartilaginous differentiation, unilateral pleural effusion, interlobular septal thickening, tumoral extension, thoracic and extrathoracic metastasis.	T1W: unilateral hyperintense pleural effusion, iso to slightly hyperintense pleural thickening T2W: moderately hyperintense T1WFS + C: typical enhancement is expected
Extramedullary Plasmacytoma	Soft tissue masses with nonspecific imaging manifestations. Larger lesions show aggressive behavior such as infiltration, destruction, and encasement.	T1W: isointense T2W: iso to hyperintense T1WFS + C: variable enhancement (from mild to marked enhancement)

T1W = T1-weighted, T2W = T2-weighted, FS = fat saturated, C = contrast; DWI = Diffusion weighted imaging.

9.1.3. Neuroblastoma

Thoracic Neuroblastoma is a non-encapsulated tumor that arises from extra-adrenal sympathetic ganglia. The mediastinum is the second most common tumor location after the abdomen that has a better prognosis than other sites.

Neuroblastoma appears as an ill-defined paravertebral soft tissue mass on a CT scan with heterogeneous attenuation caused by hemorrhage, necrosis, or cystic degeneration. Internal calcification is seen at least in 30% of cases [7,16]. MRI shows irregular margin with possible local invasion to the spinal canal, presenting T1-hypointensity and

T2-hyperintensity with heterogeneous enhancement. Calcification has a signal void in all sequences (Figures 18 and 19). It is reported that tumors with higher metabolic activity on 18F-FDG PET/CT have lower overall survival [44,45]. Metaiodobenzylguanidine labeled as 123I (MIBG) is highly sensitive for detecting catecholamine-producing tumors like neuroblastoma [7,16].

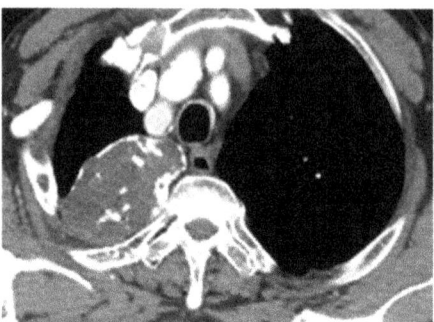

Figure 14. A 39-year-old woman with right vague chest pain. The contrast-enhanced axial CT demonstrates right-sided well-defined posterior mediastinal paraspinal mass with foci of calcifications within it. The round configuration is typical for peripheral nerve tumors. The attenuation is equal to chest wall muscles. Histopathological examination confirms Schwannoma.

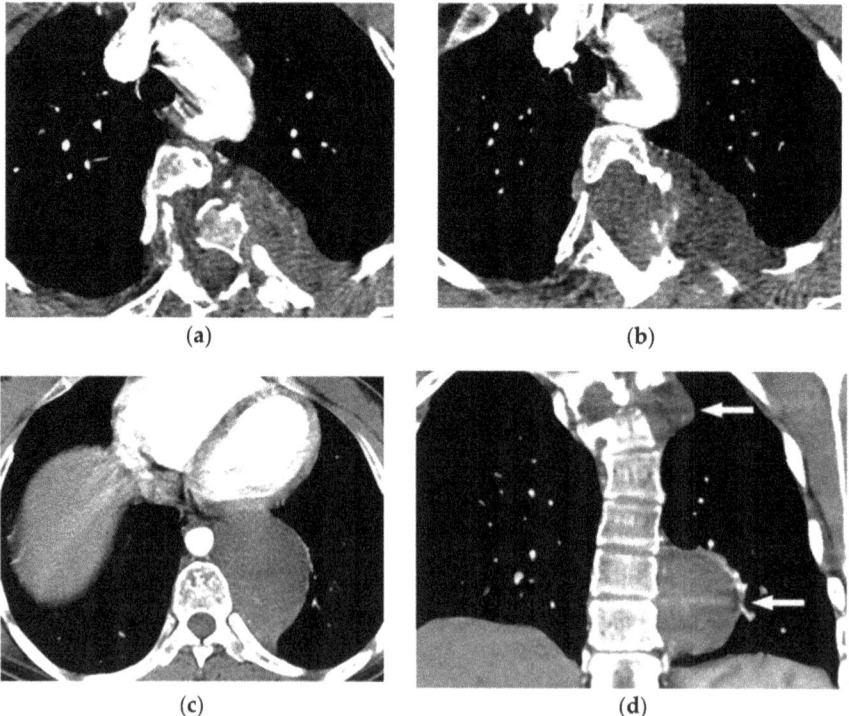

Figure 15. A 27-year-old male with scoliosis. Contrast-enhanced CT in the axial plane (soft tissue window) shows vertebral anomaly and dural ectasia. Left-sided well-defined lobular mass with the widening of adjacent neural foramen with intra- and extraspinal extension are offered (**a**–**c**), coronal CT (**d**) shows scoliosis in upper thoracic vertebrae, associated with two well-defined homogenous masses (arrow) with similar appearance in upper and lower posterior mediastinum.

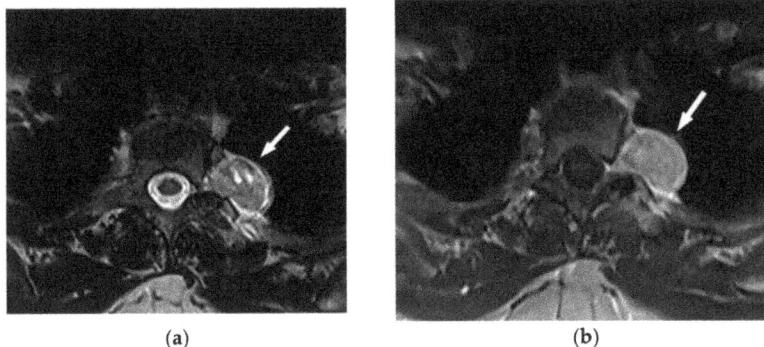

Figure 16. A 31-year-old woman with incidental findings. The axial T2W (**a**) and T1WFS + C (**b**) images show a sharply marginated lobular mass with heterogeneous peripheral hyper signal intensity in T2W, and internal hyper intensity of cystic changes, extending through the right-sided neural foramina (arrow). It has heterogeneous enhancement after contrast administration (**b**); no adjacent vertebral body scalloping was found.

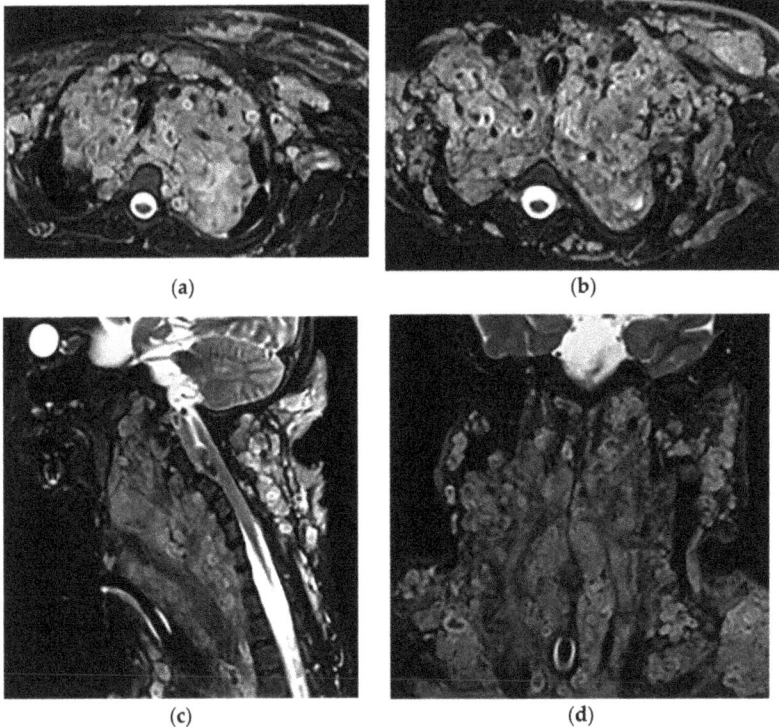

Figure 17. A 34-year-old man, with a case of neurofibromatosis type 1. The axial T2W images (**a**,**b**) show multiple confluent infiltrative paraspinal masses within the neck and upper thorax along the course of sympathetic chain and nerves with high signal intensity and central focus of hypointensity (target sign) surrounding the mediastinal vessels that are typical for plexiform Neurofibroma. Sagittal T2W (**c**) and coronal (**d**) images show the extensive infiltrative nature of this lesion with multi-compartment involvement and extension to pharyngeal space and pressure effect over cervical and thoracic vertebrae.

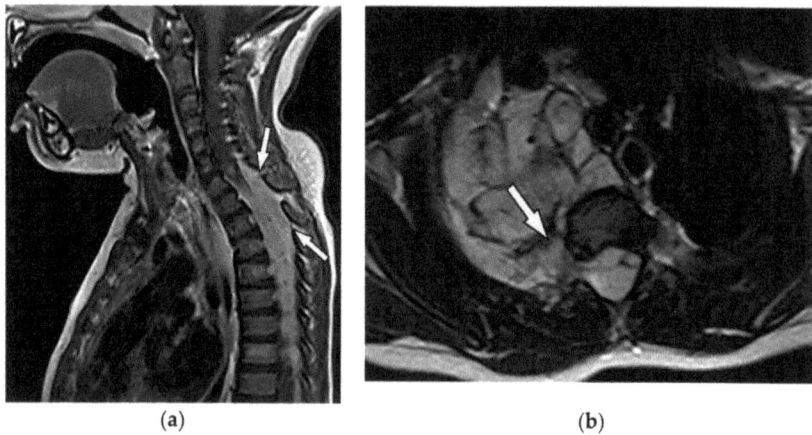

Figure 18. A 6-year-old boy with posterior mediastinal mass with histopathological confirmation for Neuroblastoma. Axial (**a**) T2W shows an ill-defined lobulated group (arrow) with heterogeneous and hyper-intense signal intensity and area of a signal void within the posterior mediastinum. It has intracanal extension via right-sided neural foramina and extradural components at multiple levels. It displaced the spinal cord anteriorly, as shown in sagittal T1W after gadolinium administration (arrow) (**b**).

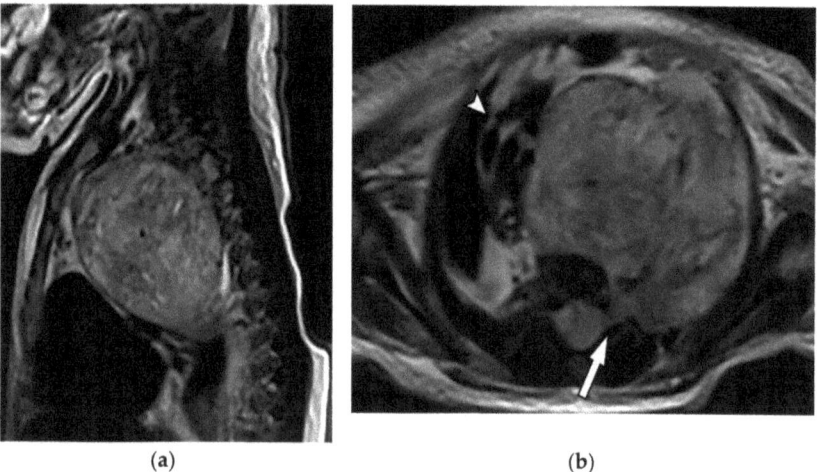

Figure 19. A 4-year-old girl with the opsomyoclonus-myoclonus syndrome. Sagittal (**a**) and axial (**b**) T2W images show large lobulated paraspinal masses (arrowhead) crossing the midline within the posterior superior mediastinum. It shows heterogeneous and hyperintense signal intensity with internal foci of the signal void caused by calcification. It extends through the spinal canal via neural foramina (arrow). Right anterolateral displacement of mediastinal great vessels is also identified.

9.1.4. Ganglioneuroma

Ganglioneuromas are differentiated slow-growing neurogenic tumors originating from sympathetic ganglia that affect young patients. They appear as a paravertebral oval mass with a smooth border and vertical orientation following the sympathetic chain direction. Posterior mediastinum is the most common site of involvement of thoracic ganglioneuroma.

It has homogenous or heterogeneous attenuation on CT images with probable internal calcification (speckled, fine, or coarse). MR imaging displays lesions with intermediate signal intensity on both T1-weighted and T2-weighted images with curvilinear or nodular low signal bands, which form the whorled appearance (Figure 20) [7,16,43].

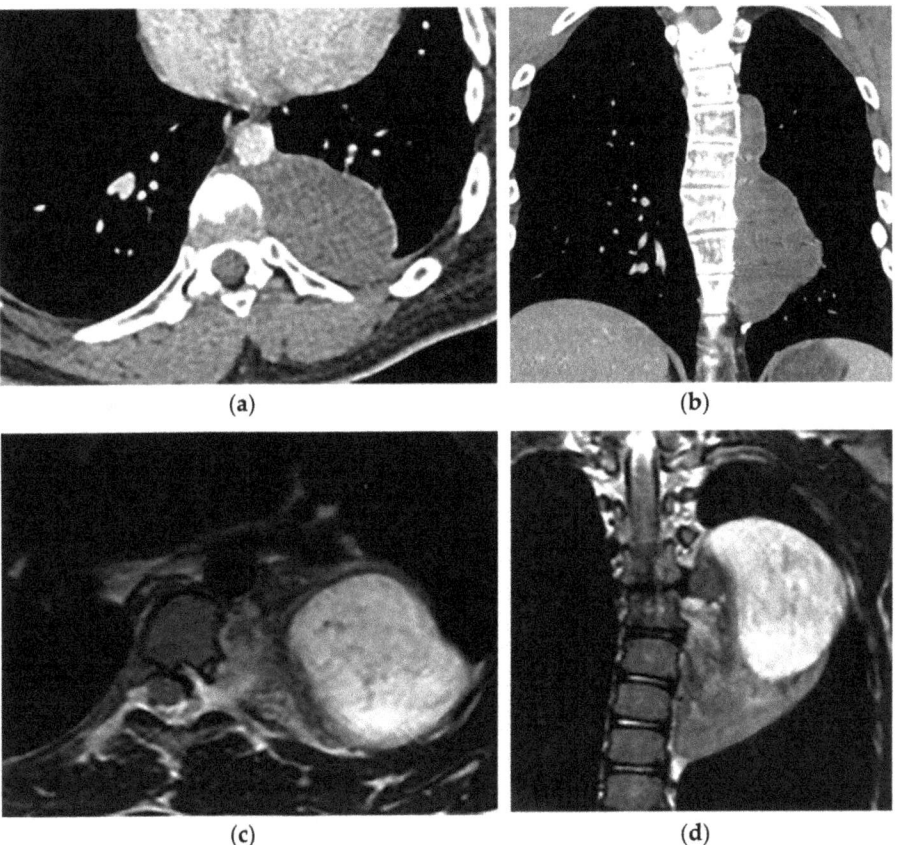

Figure 20. A 26-year-old man with incidental findings. The CT in axial and coronal views (**a**,**b**) shows a well-defined lobulated posterior mediastinal mass with homogenous attenuation and no significant enhancement after injection of contrast extending about five vertebral bodies length in the right posterior mediastinum with close contact to vertebral bodies, but with no vertebral erosion. Axial (**c**) and coronal T2W (**d**) of another patient with the same pathology show well-defined elliptical posterior mediastinal mass with heterogeneously high signal intensity intermixed with internal patchy and linear hypointensity. It also erodes the left lateral aspect of the vertebral body but with no intradural extension. Vertical orientation is typical for sympathetic chain tumors.

9.2. Lateral Meningocele

Lateral thoracic Meningocele is a rare condition defined as herniation of meninges through the vertebral column defect or enlarged neural foramina. It can be unilateral or bilateral and is usually associated with neurofibromatosis type 1 (Table 4). It is most common during the 4th to 5th decades of age, with female predominance [46].

Lateral Meningocele presents as a well-circumscribed paravertebral mass with similar attenuation to CSF. CT myelography reveals ipsilateral neural foramina enlargement communicating with subarachnoid space. This is a key differentiation feature from Neurofibroma [45]. On MR imaging, lateral Meningocele has T1-hypointensity and T2-hyperintensity with no post-contrast enhancement identical to CSF (Figure 21) [25,46].

Table 4. Imaging manifestations of posteromedial chest wall soft-tissue tumor-like lesions.

Tumor Type	Imaging Findings	
	CT	MRI
Neurogenic		
Lateral Meningocele	Well-circumscribed paravertebral mass with attenuation similar to CSF. CT myelography: ipsilateral neural foramina enlargement communicating with subarachnoid space.	T1W: hypointense T2W: hyperintense (similar intensity to CSF) T1WFS + C: lack of enhancement
Pseudomeningocele	Differentiated from Meningocele by lack of dura wrapping.	T1W: hypointense T2W: hyperintense (similar intensity to CSF) T1WFS + C: lack of enhancement [47]
Others		
Extramedullary hematopoiesis	Heterogeneous mass with internal foci of fat with lack of calcification.	T1W, T2W: heterogeneous with internal foci of hyperintensity in old lesions (representative of fat), the intermediate intensity with subtle or no enhancement in active lesions
Asbestos-related pleural plaques	Calcified or non-calcified focal pleural thickening, "Comet tail" appearance usually seen in lower lobes [48].	T1W: hypo to isointense T2W: hypointense (due to fibrosis or calcification) [49]
Empyema necessitance	Connection of pleural collection to extrapleural mass, soft tissue inflammation, rib destruction with periosteal reaction, and fluid collection.	T1W: hypointense effusion and fluid collection T2W: hyperintense effusion, increased thickness of extrapleural fat, and chest wall muscles with hyperintense on T2WFS T1WFS + C: pleural and septal enhancement

T1W = T1-weighted, T2W = T2-weighted, FS = fat saturated, C = contrast; DWI = Diffusion weighted imaging.

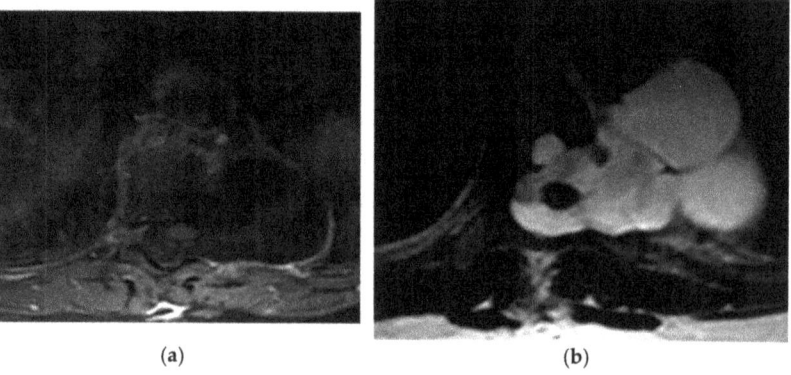

(a) (b)

Figure 21. A 21-year-old man with Neurofibromatosis type 1. The axial T1FS (a) and T2W (b) show lateral expansion of CSF-filled sac through T6-T7 level with scalloping of the adjacent vertebral body. It has similar signal intensity to CSF in both T1W and T2W sequences and hypo and hypersignal intensity, respectively. No entrapped fat or neural elements were seen. Slightly anterior spinal cord displacement was also identified, which is compatible with lateral Meningocele.

9.3. Pseudomeningocele

Pseudomeningocele or meningeal pseudocyst is an abnormal extradural CSF collection that communicates with the brain and spinal canal. It can be congenital (thoracolumbar), traumatic (cervical), or iatrogenic (laminectomy of the lumbar spine). Congenital Pseudomeningocele can be seen in Marfan syndrome or NF1 [25].

The Pseudomeningocele can be differentiated from Meningocele by lack of dura wrapping the collection. The absence of nerve roots within the CSF collection helps in identifying the brachial plexus Pseudomeningocele. On MR imaging, it has similar intensity to CSF with a lack of post-contrast enhancement (Figure 22) [25,47]. The Pseudomeningocele can be differentiated from Meningocele by lack of dura wrapping the collection. The absence of nerve roots within the CSF collection helps in identifying the brachial plexus Pseudomeningocele. On MR imaging, it has similar intensity to CSF with a lack of post-contrast enhancement (Figure 22) [25,47].

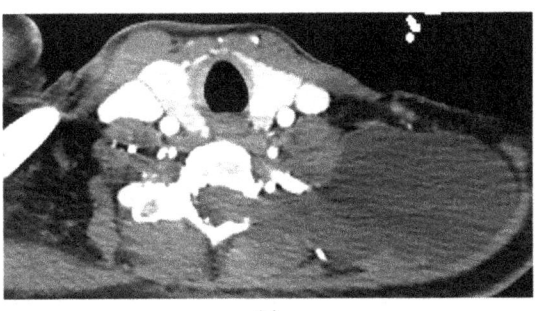
(a)

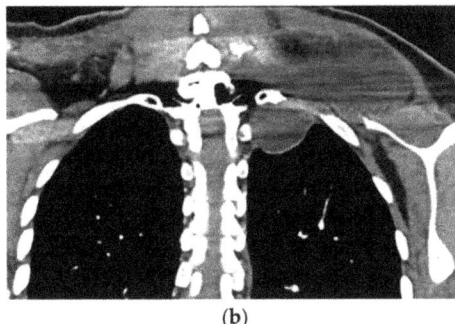
(b)

Figure 22. A 38-year-old man with a history of a remote motor vehicle collision. The axial (**a**) and coronal (**b**) contrast-enhanced CT show abnormal well-defined extraspinal fluid collection at the level C6-T1, which extends through the left neural foramina (lateral recess), communicating with CSF space. There is no edema, solid component, or abnormal enhancement within the mentioned collection or adjacent muscles. Regarding the history of trauma, a Pseudomeningocele diagnosis was made and was confirmed in MRI (not shown).

10. Lipomatosis Tumors

Radiologic characteristics of lipomatosis tumors are summarized in Table 3.

10.1. Lipoma

Chest wall fatty tumors are relatively common, and lipoma is the most frequent. It is a well-defined mesenchymal tumor arising from adipose tissue usually seen in patients between 50–70 years old. Most chest wall lipomas are located deeply, involve intramuscular or intermuscular layers, and show larger size with less distinct borders than superficial ones [1,8,16,50].

On multidetector CT scan, lipomas are homogenous and have similar attenuation to macroscopic fat with approximate -100 HU radiodensity (Figure 23); other non-adipose components such as calcification and septa might also be seen. On MR imaging, signal intensity is identical to subcutaneous fat on T1-weighted and T2-weighted images. It typically does not enhance gadolinium-enhanced MR images except for septa with less than 2 mm thickness [8,16,50,51].

10.2. Liposarcoma

Liposarcoma consists of lipoblasts with various differentiations. Well-differentiated type is the most common subtype with near 50–75% internal fat component. The less frequent subtypes are dedifferentiated, myxoid, pleomorphic, and mixed subtypes. Chest wall involvement is not common [1,2,8].

On multidetector CT, liposarcoma has higher attenuation than normal fat secondary to a mixture of fat and malignant cells. Necrosis and calcification are uncommon in well-differentiated subtypes in contrast to the myxoid subtype (Figure 24). On MR imaging, Myxoid Liposarcoma has hyperintensity on both T1-weighted and T2-weighted images. Dedifferentiated subtype should be suspected when an area of T2-hyperintensity and T1-hypointensity are identified within preexisting well-differentiated liposarcoma [16,50]. Septal thickening of 2 mm or more, older age, larger size, and nodular non-adipose components are features that help to categorize liposarcoma over lipoma [16,50]. 18F-FDG metabolic activity can predict the liposarcoma grading, although there are some overlapping features [1].

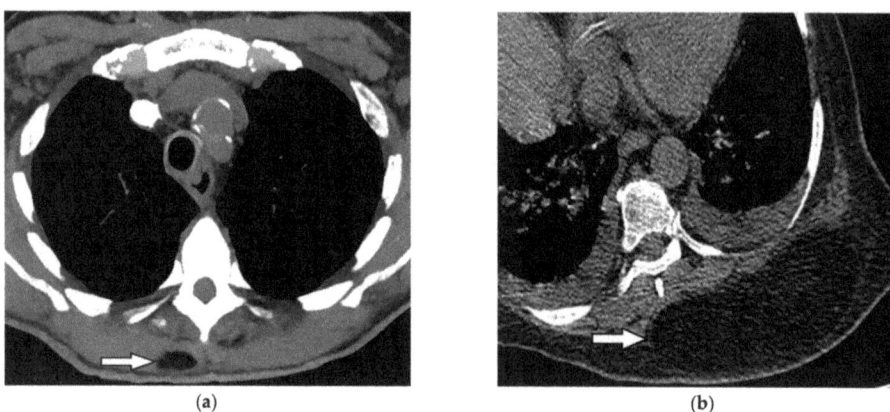

Figure 23. A 34-year-old man, with a case of SVC thrombosis with incidental finding. (**a**) Non-contrast-enhanced CT in axial plane demonstrates well-circumscribed lesion in the right posteromedial aspect of the chest wall with similar attenuation to subcutaneous fat with no internal septa. Multiple collaterals are also shown in the anterior aspect of the chest wall, maybe formed due to underlying SVC occlusion. (**b**) Axial plane CT of another patient shows large posteromedial chest wall mass with attenuation similar to adjacent subcutaneous fat compatible with lipoma.

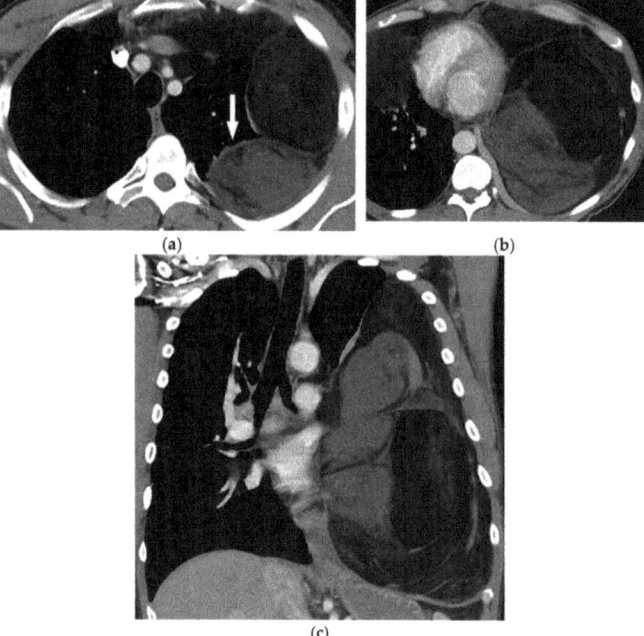

Figure 24. A 58-year-old man with dyspnea. (**a,b**) Axial contrast-enhanced CT shows a large heterogeneous mass with enhancing non-adipose solid components (arrow). The mass has extensive fat attenuation that is intermixed with soft tissue density. (**c**) Coronal image better characterizes the craniocaudal extension of the mass, which also shows a large inhomogeneous fat-containing lesion with an internal enhancing solid component.

11. Pleural Diseases

11.1. Empyema Necessitance

Empyema necessitance is a chronic pleural space infection that can affect both immunocompromised and immunocompetent people. Empyema leakage to chest wall soft tissues manifests as an extrapleural collection of empyema. Its usual location is the anterior aspect of the chest wall. Mycobacterium Tuberculosis is the most prevalent pathogen, with Nocardia Asteroides, Actinomyces Israelii, Staphylococcus, Aspergillosis, and Blastomycosis spp. being less common [1,8,52,53].

On CT, a communication between the pleural and extrapleural collection is a pathognomonic finding of empyema necessitans (Figure 25). A peripheral rim of soft tissue inflammation and thickening, draining sinus tracts, and rib destruction with periosteal reaction are other radiologic findings. MRI is extremely helpful in detecting vertebral and spinal canal involvement if the posteromedial part of the chest wall is affected (Table 4) [54].

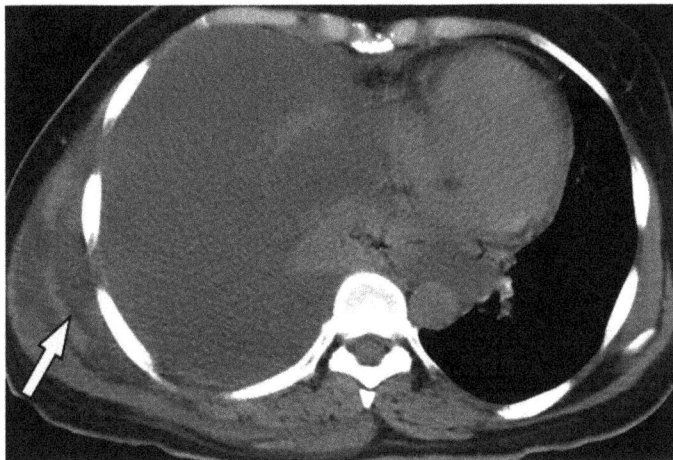

Figure 25. A 46-year-old man with high-grade fever and chills. The axial contrast-enhanced CT shows significant right-sided pleural effusion with the near complete collapse of the right lung resulting in a shift of the heart and mediastinum to the left side. There is pleural thickening and enhancement. There is an extrapleural component within the adjacent chest wall with rim enhancement (arrow). Aspiration was performed under the guidance of ultrasonography, and diagnosis of empyema necessitans was made as a complication of Actinomyces Israelii.

11.2. Asbestos-Related Pleural Diseases

Asbestos-induced conditions include non-neoplastic and neoplastic pleural and lung diseases ranging from pleural effusion, thickening, plaques to malignant mesothelioma, and lung cancer. Pleural plaques are the most common disease [48,49,55].

Paravertebral and anterior plaques are better delineated on CT scans than radiography (Figure 26). On MRI, pleural plaques are hypo to isointense to skeletal muscle on T1-weighted, and hypointense on T2-weighted images. These findings are representative of fibrosis and internal calcification (Table 4) [48,49,55].

11.3. Mesothelioma

Malignant mesothelioma is the most common primary tumor of the pleura, which is related to prior asbestos exposure with a relatively poor prognosis [56].

Multidetector CT effectively reveals the primary tumoral extension, lymphadenopathy, and extrathoracic metastasis (Figures 27 and 28) [56]. Another CT finding is circumferential pleural thickening (most common finding) with extension along the fissures. Large or punctate osseous or cartilaginous differentiation is more in favor of malignant mesothelioma rather than linear calcification that usually occurs within asbestosis plaques. Dynamic contrast-enhanced computed tomography (DCE CT) enables measuring intratumoral capillary permeability and blood flow, which are beneficial in evaluating treatment response [56–58].

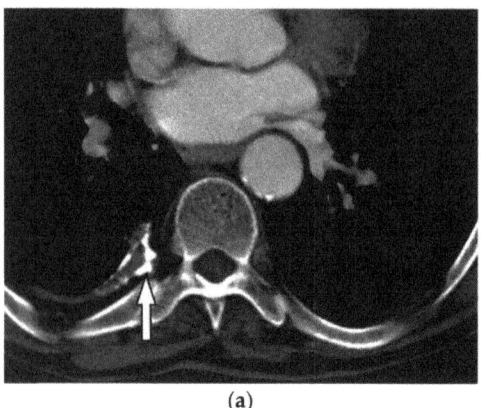
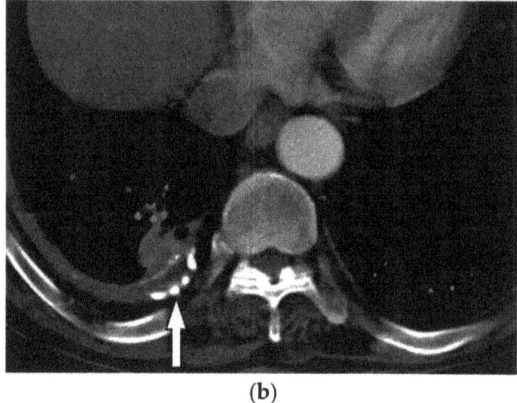

Figure 26. A 78-year-old man with dyspnea. The axial contrast-enhanced CT (**a**,**b**) demonstrates right-sided calcified pleural plaque (arrow) and small pleural effusion due to previous asbestosis exposure. Adjacent round atelectasis is also shown.

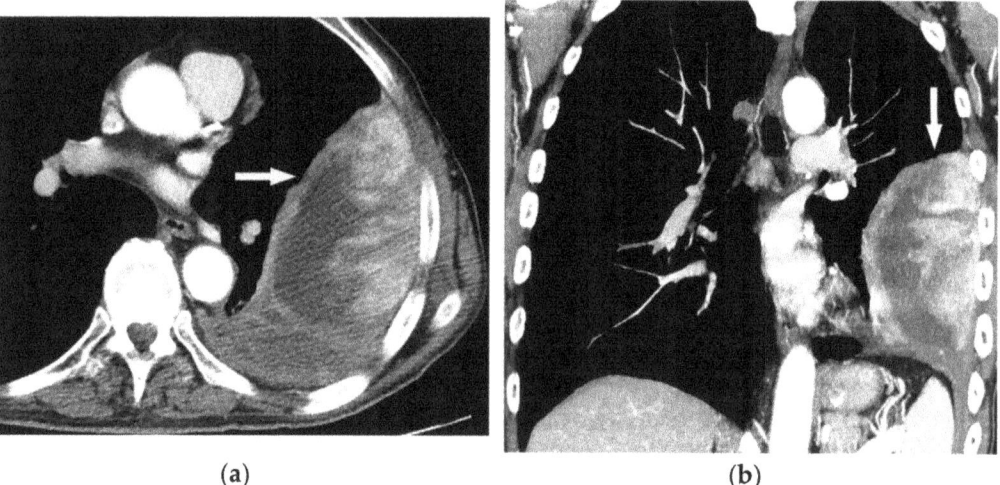

Figure 27. A 67-year-old man with dyspnea and chest pain. Contrast-enhanced CT in axial (**a**) and coronal (**b**) planes demonstrate left-sided localized enhancing pleural mass (arrow) with internal areas of necrosis that extend to the posteromedial aspect of the chest wall. Involvement of diaphragmatic pleura and elevation of left hemidiaphragm are also identified.

MR imaging and 18F-FDG PET/CT are useful in further evaluation of chest wall, diaphragm, and mediastinal invasion [56–59]. Malignant mesothelioma appears as unilateral hyperintense pleural effusion and pleural thickening with iso to slight hyperintensity to chest wall muscles on T1-weighted and moderate hyperintensity on T2-weighted images. Post-contrast enhancement is expected (Table 3). It is believed that higher metabolic activity on 18F-FDG PET/CT is associated with poor prognosis and shorter survival time [25,56–58].

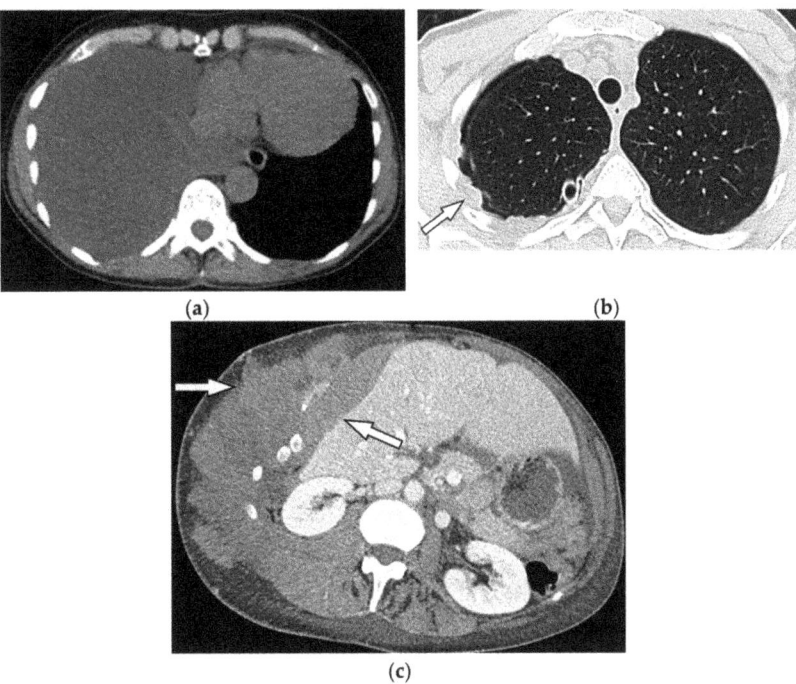

Figure 28. A 70-year-old man with dyspnea. The non-contrast CT in the axial plane demonstrates right-sided large pleural effusion, near complete collapse of the right lung (**a**) after the chest tube insertion; thick circumferential nodular pleural thickening of parietal pleura was shown (arrow) (**b**). Contrast-enhanced CT of the upper abdomen shows the extension of mesothelioma through the abdominal cavity and wall with indentation over adjacent liver parenchyma (arrow) (**c**).

12. Other Soft Tissue Lesions

12.1. Rhabdomyosarcoma

Rhabdomyosarcoma is a high-grade sarcoma that mostly affects children and usually appears before 40. Chest wall rhabdomyosarcomas are uncommon tumors with poor prognosis and usually manifest as rapidly growing mass with adjacent bone invasion and nerve compression [1,16].

CT scan demonstrates homogenous mass with no mineralized matrix invading adjacent bone and soft tissue structures (Figure 29) [16]. MRI is the modality of choice for better delineation of tissue characterization, tumor extension, and medullary involvement. It is isointense to muscle on T1-weighted and hyperintense on T2-weighted images. Typical homogenous or ring-like enhancements are expected. Non-enhanced areas of hypointensity are reflective of necrosis (Table 3) [1,16,60]. 18F-FDG PET/CT is valuable in the primary staging, restaging, prognosis, and therapeutic assessment [61].

12.2. Extramedullary Hematopoiesis

Extramedullary hematopoiesis is a compensatory marrow hyperplasia in conditions with insufficient red blood cell production. Paraspinal areas are less frequently involved than lymph nodes, spleen, and liver. It typically arises from posterior ribs in the lower thoracic and upper lumbar area as unilateral or bilateral masses with no adjacent rib destruction [62].

On CT, it presents as a heterogeneous mass with internal foci of fat and no calcification. Lesions with hematopoietic activity demonstrate heterogeneous intermediate intensity on both T1-weighted and T2-weighted sequences with subtle or no enhancement. However, lesions with no hematopoietic activity might show foci of hyperintensity on both T1-weighted and T2-weighted images due to fat component or hypointensity on both T1-weighted and T2-weighted images secondary to iron deposition (Table 4) (Figure 30) [62,63].

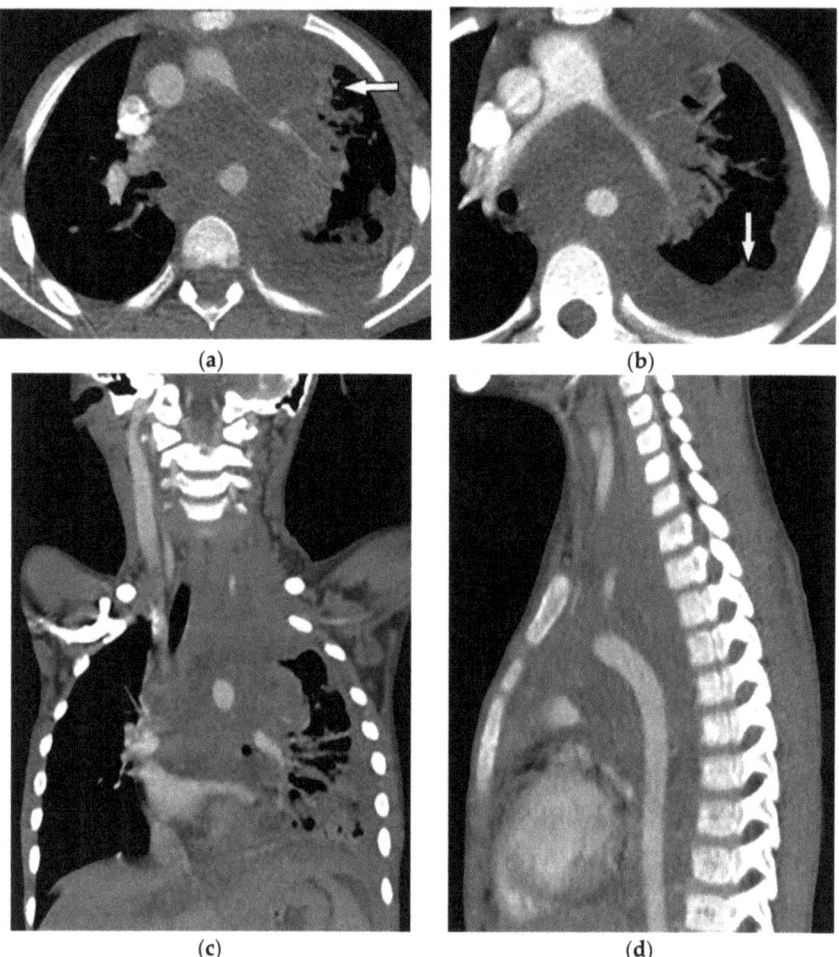

Figure 29. A 5-year-old girl with dyspnea. The axial contrast-enhanced CT in soft tissue window was obtained at the level of the main pulmonary artery (**a,b**), showing a large infiltrative soft tissue mass (arrow) with irregular border and slight enhancement encasing great mediastinal vessels. Left-sided pleural effusion was also identified. Coronal (**c**) and sagittal (**d**) CT better delineate the extension of the tumor and demonstrates infiltrative soft tissue mass within the superior, mid, and posterior mediastinum extending to the thoracic inlet and neck.

12.3. Extramedullary Plasmacytoma

Extramedullary plasmacytoma accounts for less than 3% of all plasma cell neoplasms and can occur in any location. It presents as soft tissue masses with nonspecific imaging manifestations [64].

Larger lesions show aggressive behavior such as infiltration and destruction of adjacent soft tissue and encasement of vascular structures. It typically presents as isointense compared to muscle on T1-weighted images and iso to hyperintensity on T2-weighted images [64,65].

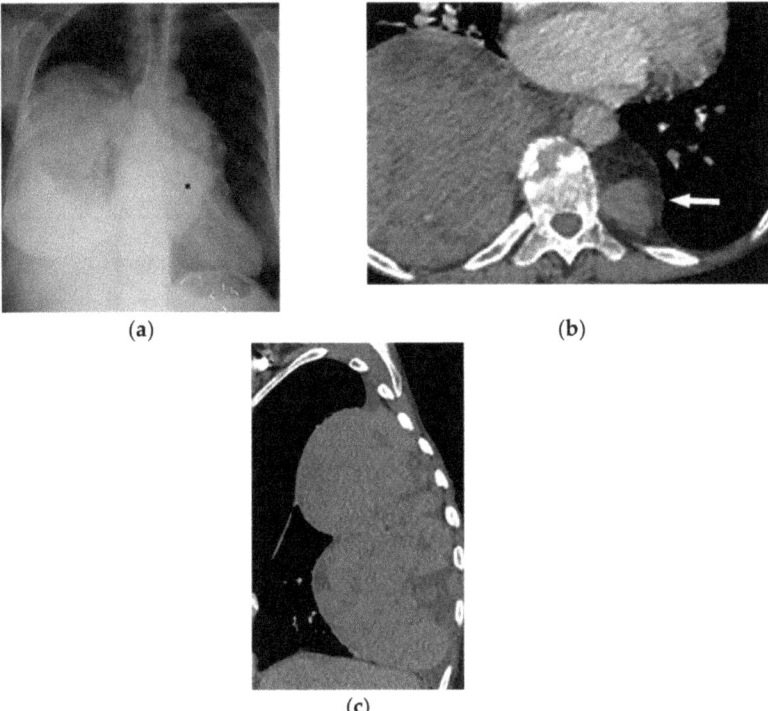

Figure 30. A 42-year-old woman with beta-thalassemia major presented with progressive dyspnea. PA radiograph (**a**) shows right basilar mass with meniscus sign and mass-like density over the mediastinum (asterisk). Surgical clips in LUQ of the abdomen from the previous splenectomy are noted. Axial CT with intravenous contrast (**b**) shows large heterogeneous well-defined soft tissue mass with some areas of internal hypo-density and no internal calcification in the right posteromedial chest wall; another similar appearing smaller lesion is detectable on the left side (arrow). Sagittal CT of the chest (**c**) along the long axis of the lesion demonstrates the craniocaudal extension of the lobulated retro-mediastinal mass. Biopsy confirmed the diagnosis of EMH.

13. Conclusions

Chest wall neoplasms are a group of heterogeneous lesions, and the posteromedial chest wall is a source of different pathologies due to its complex anatomy. Many of these pathologies can be differentiated by imaging. A comprehensive systematic approach with varying imaging modalities is needed to identify the correct diagnosis or limit the differential diagnosis and determine the appropriate further investigation. This article illustrates the various posteromedial chest wall pathologies and their imaging features. Ill-defined border, heterogeneous enhancement, and local invasion are more suggestive of a malignant lesion. In contrast, well-defined borders and the absence of local invasion or distant metastasis favor benign nature. The pattern of mineralization helps in the differentiation of osseous/cartilaginous neoplasm from other neoplasms. We also explored key imaging features as well as strengths and limitations of each imaging modality. Therefore, the familiarity of radiologists with the imaging features of posteromedial chest wall lesions is crucial and can avoid unnecessary invasive procedures. Future investigation is required using quantitative novel imaging modalities to increase the diagnostic accuracy of radiology. Furthermore, improvement in deep learning and radiomics may increase patients' benefit from reduced need for biopsy and individualized treatment options.

Author Contributions: Conceptualization, M.C., B.M. and D.Y.; methodology, S.H. and B.M.; software, M.S. and F.S.Z.; validation, D.Y., M.C., B.M. and H.C.; investigation, S.H. and P.K.; resources, M.S. and F.S.Z.; data curation, S.H.; writing—original draft preparation, S.H., P.K., M.S. and F.S.Z.; writing—review and editing, M.C., H.C. and B.M.; visualization, P.K., M.S. and F.S.Z.; supervision, M.C., H.C., D.Y. and B.M.; project administration, S.H. All authors have read and agreed to the published version of the manuscript.

Funding: This research received no external funding.

Conflicts of Interest: The authors declare no relevant conflict of interest.

Abbreviations

MRI = Magnetic resonance imaging, CT = Computed tomography, 18F-FDG = Fluorine 18 fluorodeoxyglucose, PET/CT = Positron emission tomography/computed tomography, GCT = Giant cell tumor, MM = Multiple myeloma, SBP = Solitary plasmacytoma of the bone, ABC = Aneurysmal bone cyst, FD = Fibrous dysplasia, DCE = Dynamic contrast-enhanced.

References

1. Carter, B.W.; Benveniste, M.F.; Betancourt, S.L.; De Groot, P.M.; Lichtenberger, J.P., III; Amini, B.; Abbott, G.F. Imaging evaluation of malignant chest wall neoplasms. *Radiographics* **2016**, *36*, 1285–1306. [CrossRef] [PubMed]
2. Mullan, C.P.; Madan, R.; Trotman-Dickenson, B.; Qian, X.; Jacobson, F.L.; Hunsaker, A. Radiology of chest wall masses. *Am. J. Roentgenol.* **2011**, *197*, W460–W470. [CrossRef] [PubMed]
3. Tateishi, U.; Gladish, G.; Kusumoto, M.; Hasegawa, T.; Yokoyama, R.; Tsuchiya, R.; Moriyama, N. Chest wall tumors: Radiologic findings and pathologic correlation: Part 1. Benign tumors. *Radiographics* **2003**, *23*, 1477–1490. [CrossRef] [PubMed]
4. Bueno, J.; Lichtenberger, J.P.; Rauch, G.; Carter, B.W. MR imaging of primary chest wall neoplasms. *Top. Magn. Reson. Imaging* **2018**, *27*, 83–93. [CrossRef]
5. Clemens, M.W.; Evans, K.K.; Mardini, S.; Arnold, P.G. *Introduction to Chest Wall Reconstruction: Anatomy and Physiology of the Chest and Indications for Chest Wall Reconstruction*; Seminars in Plastic Surgery Thieme Medical Publishers: New York, NY, USA, 2011; pp. 5–15.
6. Imperato, M.C.; Monti, R.; Cappabianca, S.; Caranci, F.; Conforti, R. Thoracic Boundary Pathology: Radiological Investigation and Review. *J. Radiol. Clin. Imaging* **2021**, *4*, 141–158. [CrossRef]
7. Pavlus, J.D.; Carter, B.W.; Tolley, M.D.; Keung, E.S.; Khorashadi, L.; Lichtenberger, J.P., 3rd. Imaging of thoracic neurogenic tumors. *Am. J. Roentgenol.* **2016**, *207*, 552–561. [CrossRef]
8. Nam, S.J.; Kim, S.; Lim, B.J.; Yoon, C.-S.; Kim, T.H.; Suh, J.-S.; Ha, D.H.; Kwon, J.W.; Yoon, Y.C.; Chung, H.W. Imaging of primary chest wall tumors with radiologic-pathologic correlation. *Radiographics* **2011**, *31*, 749–770. [CrossRef]
9. Maheshwarappa, R.P.; Rajdev, M.; Nagpal, P.; Gholamrezanezhad, A.; Soni, N.; Gupta, A. Multimodality imaging of the extrapleural space lesions. *Clin. Imaging* **2021**, *79*, 64–84. [CrossRef]
10. Jaiswal, L.S.; Neupane, D. Benign rib tumors: A case series from tertiary care Centre of Nepal and review of literature. *J. Surg. Case Rep.* **2021**, *2021*, rjab518. [CrossRef]
11. Aboughalia, H.A.; Ngo, A.-V.; Menashe, S.J.; Kim, H.H.; Iyer, R.S. Pediatric rib pathologies: Clinicoimaging scenarios and approach to diagnosis. *Pediatr. Radiol.* **2021**, *51*, 1783–1797. [CrossRef]
12. Graeber, G.M.; Nazim, M. The anatomy of the ribs and the sternum and their relationship to chest wall structure and function. *Thorac. Surg. Clin.* **2007**, *17*, 473–489. [CrossRef]
13. Taralli, S.; Giancipoli, R.G.; Caldarella, C.; Scolozzi, V.; Ricciardi, S.; Cardillo, G.; Calcagni, M.L. The Prognostic Value of 18F-FDG PET Imaging at Staging in Patients with Malignant Pleural Mesothelioma: A Literature Review. *J. Clin. Med.* **2022**, *11*, 33. [CrossRef]
14. Chassagnon, G.; Vakalopoulou, M.; Paragios, N.; Revel, M.-P. Artificial intelligence applications for thoracic imaging. *Eur. J. Radiol.* **2020**, *123*, 108774. [CrossRef]
15. Fischer, A.M.; Yacoub, B.; Savage, R.H.; Martinez, J.D.; Wichmann, J.L.; Sahbaee, P.; Grbic, S.; Varga-Szemes, A.; Schoepf, U.J. Machine learning/deep neuronal network: Routine application in chest computed tomography and workflow considerations. *J. Thorac. Imaging* **2020**, *35*, S21–S27. [CrossRef]
16. Tateishi, U.; Gladish, G.W.; Kusumoto, M.; Hasegawa, T.; Yokoyama, R.; Tsuchiya, R.; Moriyama, N. Chest wall tumors: Radiologic findings and pathologic correlation: Part 2. Malignant tumors. *Radiographics* **2003**, *23*, 1491–1508. [CrossRef]
17. Gladish, G.W.; Sabloff, B.M.; Munden, R.F.; Truong, M.T.; Erasmus, J.J.; Chasen, M.H. Primary thoracic sarcomas. *Radiographics* **2002**, *22*, 621–637. [CrossRef] [PubMed]
18. Zhang, J.; Dong, A.; Cui, Y.; Wang, Y. FDG PET/CT in a case of primary pulmonary Ewing sarcoma. *Clin. Nucl. Med.* **2019**, *44*, 666–668. [CrossRef]

19. Guimarães, J.B.; Rigo, L.; Lewin, F.; Emerick, A. The importance of PET/CT in the evaluation of patients with Ewing tumors. *Radiol. Bras.* **2015**, *48*, 175–180. [CrossRef]
20. Jesus-Garcia, R.; Osawa, A.; Filippi, R.Z.; Viola, D.C.; Korukian, M.; de Carvalho Campos Neto, G.; Wagner, J. Is PET-CT an accurate method for the differential diagnosis between chondroma and chondrosarcoma? *SpringerPlus* **2016**, *5*, 236. [CrossRef]
21. Ormond Filho, A.G.; Carneiro, B.C.; Pastore, D.; Silva, I.P.; Yamashita, S.R.; Consolo, F.D.; Hungria, V.T.M.; Sandes, A.F.; Rizzatti, E.G.; Nico, M.A.C. Whole-Body Imaging of Multiple Myeloma: Diagnostic Criteria. *Radiographics* **2019**, *39*, 1077–1097. [CrossRef] [PubMed]
22. Hanrahan, C.J.; Christensen, C.R.; Crim, J.R. Current concepts in the evaluation of multiple myeloma with MR imaging and FDG PET/CT. *Radiographics* **2010**, *30*, 127–142. [CrossRef]
23. Singal, R.; Dalal, U.; Dalal, A.K.; Attri, A.K.; Gupta, S.; Raina, R. Solitary plasmacytoma of the rib: A rare case. *Lung India* **2011**, *28*, 309–311. [CrossRef] [PubMed]
24. Kayhan, S.; Yilmaz, M.A. Solitary Plasmacytoma of the Chest Wall. *J. Clin. Anal. Med.* **2015**, *6*, 496–498.
25. Haaga, J.R.; Boll, D. *Computed Tomography & Magnetic Resonance Imaging of The Whole Body E-Book*; Elsevier Health Sciences: Amsterdam, The Netherlands, 2016.
26. Albano, D.; Bosio, G.; Treglia, G.; Giubbini, R.; Bertagna, F. 18F-FDG PET/CT in solitary plasmacytoma: Metabolic behavior and progression to multiple myeloma. *Eur. J. Nucl. Med. Mol. Imaging* **2018**, *45*, 77–84. [CrossRef]
27. Song, W.; Suurmeijer, A.J.H.; Bollen, S.M.; Cleton-Jansen, A.M.; Bovée, J.; Kroon, H.M. Soft tissue aneurysmal bone cyst: Six new cases with imaging details, molecular pathology, and review of the literature. *Skelet. Radiol.* **2019**, *48*, 1059–1067. [CrossRef]
28. Aras, M.; Ones, T.; Dane, F.; Nosheri, O.; Inanir, S.; Erdil, T.Y.; Turoglu, H.T. False Positive FDG PET/CT Resulting from Fibrous Dysplasia of the Bone in the Work-Up of a Patient with Bladder Cancer: Case Report and Review of the Literature. *Iran. J. Radiol.* **2012**, *10*, 41–44. [CrossRef]
29. Fitzpatrick, K.A.; Taljanovic, M.S.; Speer, D.P.; Graham, A.R.; Jacobson, J.A.; Barnes, G.R.; Hunter, T.B. Imaging findings of fibrous dysplasia with histopathologic and intraoperative correlation. *AJR Am. J. Roentgenol.* **2004**, *182*, 1389–1398. [CrossRef]
30. Muheremu, A.; Ma, Y.; Huang, Z.; Shan, H.; Li, Y.; Niu, X. Diagnosing giant cell tumor of the bone using positron emission tomography/computed tomography: A retrospective study of 20 patients from a single center. *Oncol. Lett.* **2017**, *14*, 1985–1988. [CrossRef]
31. Chakarun, C.J.; Forrester, D.M.; Gottsegen, C.J.; Patel, D.B.; White, E.A.; Matcuk, G.R., Jr. Giant cell tumor of bone: Review, mimics, and new developments in treatment. *Radiographics* **2013**, *33*, 197–211. [CrossRef]
32. Zarqane, H.; Viala, P.; Dallaudière, B.; Vernhet, H.; Cyteval, C.; Larbi, A. Tumors of the rib. *Diagn. Interv. Imaging* **2013**, *94*, 1095–1108. [CrossRef]
33. Yamamoto, A.; Takada, K.; Motoi, T.; Imamura, T.; Furui, S. Chondromyxoid fibroma of the rib with prominent exophytic configuration. *Jpn. J. Radiol.* **2012**, *30*, 81–85. [CrossRef] [PubMed]
34. Brandolini, J.; Bertolaccini, L.; Pardolesi, A.; Salvi, M.; Valli, M.; Solli, P. Chondroblastoma of the rib in a 47-year-old man: A case report with a systematic review of literature. *J. Thorac. Dis.* **2017**, *9*, E907–E911. [CrossRef] [PubMed]
35. Levine, B.D.; Motamedi, K.; Chow, K.; Gold, R.H.; Seeger, L.L. CT of rib lesions. *AJR Am. J. Roentgenol.* **2009**, *193*, 5–13. [CrossRef] [PubMed]
36. Kaim, A.H.; Hügli, R.; Bonél, H.M.; Jundt, G. Chondroblastoma and clear cell chondrosarcoma: Radiological and MRI characteristics with histopathological correlation. *Skelet. Radiol.* **2002**, *31*, 88–95. [CrossRef]
37. Theodorou, D.J.; Theodorou, S.J.; Kakitsubata, Y. Imaging of Paget disease of bone and its musculoskeletal complications: Review. *AJR Am. J. Roentgenol.* **2011**, *196* (Suppl. 6), S64–S75. [CrossRef]
38. Park, E.T.; Kim, S.E. Radiography, Bone Scan, and F-18 FDG PET/CT Imaging Findings in a Patient with Paget's Disease. *Nucl. Med. Mol. Imaging* **2010**, *44*, 87–89. [CrossRef]
39. Hong, S.H.; Choi, J.-Y.; Lee, J.W.; Kim, N.R.; Choi, J.-A.; Kang, H.S. MR Imaging Assessment of the Spine: Infection or an Imitation? *Radiographics* **2009**, *29*, 599–612. [CrossRef]
40. Ramadani, N.; Dedushi, K.; Kabashi, S.; Mucaj, S. Radiologic Diagnosis of Spondylodiscitis, Role of Magnetic Resonance. *Acta Inf. Med.* **2017**, *25*, 54–57. [CrossRef]
41. Kumar, Y.; Gupta, N.; Chhabra, A.; Fukuda, T.; Soni, N.; Hayashi, D. Magnetic resonance imaging of bacterial and tuberculous spondylodiscitis with associated complications and non-infectious spinal pathology mimicking infections: A pictorial review. *BMC Musculoskelet. Disord.* **2017**, *18*, 244. [CrossRef]
42. Yeom, J.A.; Lee, I.S.; Suh, H.B.; Song, Y.S.; Song, J.W. Magnetic Resonance Imaging Findings of Early Spondylodiscitis: Interpretive Challenges and Atypical Findings. *Korean J. Radiol.* **2016**, *17*, 565–580. [CrossRef]
43. Rha, S.E.; Byun, J.Y.; Jung, S.E.; Chun, H.J.; Lee, H.G.; Lee, J.M. Neurogenic tumors in the abdomen: Tumor types and imaging characteristics. *Radiographics* **2003**, *23*, 29–43. [CrossRef]
44. Kumar, R.; Dhull, V.; Sharma, P.; Agarwala, S.; Bakhshi, S.; Bal, C.; Bhatnagar, V.; Malhotra, A. Utility of 18F-FDG PET-CT in pediatric neuroblastoma: Comparison with 131I-MIBG scintigraphy. *J. Nucl. Med.* **2013**, *54* (Suppl. 2), 199.
45. Amr, M. Predictive value of FDG PET/CT in pediatric Neuroblastoma patients. *Egypt. J. Nucl. Med.* **2014**, *10*, 46–59. [CrossRef]
46. Kumar, B.E.P.; Hegde, K.V.; Kumari, G.L.; Agrawal, A. Bilateral multiple level lateral meningocoele. *J. Clin. Imaging Sci.* **2013**, *3*, 1. [CrossRef]

47. Teplick, J.G.; Peyster, R.G.; Teplick, S.K.; Goodman, L.R.; Haskin, M.E. CT identification of postlaminectomy pseudomeningocele. *Am. J. Neuroradiol.* **1983**, *4*, 179–182. [CrossRef]
48. Elboga, U.; Yılmaz, M.; Uyar, M.; Çelen, Y.Z.; Bakır, K.; Dikensoy, Ö. The role of FDG PET-CT in differential diagnosis of pleural pathologies. *Rev. Española Med. Nucl. Imagen Mol.* **2012**, *31*, 187–191. [CrossRef]
49. Kusaka, Y.; Hering, K.G.; Parker, J.E. *International Classification of HRCT for Occupational and Environmental Respiratory Diseases*; Springer: Berlin, Germany, 2005.
50. Gaerte, S.C.; Meyer, C.A.; Winer-Muram, H.T.; Tarver, R.D.; Conces, D.J., Jr. Fat-containing lesions of the chest. *Radiographics* **2002**, *22*, S61–S78. [CrossRef]
51. Baffour, F.I.; Wenger, D.E.; Broski, S.M. 18F-FDG PET/CT imaging features of lipomatous tumors. *Am. J. Nucl. Med. Mol. Imaging* **2020**, *10*, 74.
52. Yauba, M.S.; Ahmed, H.; Imoudu, I.A.; Yusuf, M.O.; Makarfi, H.U. Empyema necessitans complicating pleural effusion associated with proteus species infection: A diagnostic dilemma. *Case Rep. Pediatr.* **2015**, *2015*, 108174.
53. Kellie, S.P.; Shaib, F.; Forster, D.; Mehta, J.P. Empyema Necessitatis. *Chest* **2010**, *138*, 39A. [CrossRef]
54. Babamahmoodi, F.; Davoodi, L.; Sheikholeslami, R.; Ahangarkani, F. Tuberculous Empyema Necessitatis in a 40-Year-Old Immunocompetent Male. *Case Rep. Infect. Dis.* **2016**, *2016*, 4187108. [CrossRef] [PubMed]
55. Roach, H.D.; Davies, G.J.; Attanoos, R.; Crane, M.; Adams, H.; Phillips, S. Asbestos: When the dust settles an imaging review of asbestos-related disease. *Radiographics* **2002**, *22*, S167–S184. [CrossRef] [PubMed]
56. Nickell, L.T., Jr.; Lichtenberger, J.P., 3rd; Khorashadi, L.; Abbott, G.F.; Carter, B.W. Multimodality imaging for characterization, classification, and staging of malignant pleural mesothelioma. *Radiographics* **2014**, *34*, 1692–1706. [CrossRef] [PubMed]
57. Tyszko, S.M.; Marano, G.D.; Tallaksen, R.J.; Gyure, K.A. Best cases from the AFIP: Malignant mesothelioma. *Radiographics* **2007**, *27*, 259–264. [CrossRef]
58. Wang, Z.J.; Reddy, G.P.; Gotway, M.B.; Higgins, C.B.; Jablons, D.M.; Ramaswamy, M.; Hawkins, R.A.; Webb, W.R. Malignant pleural mesothelioma: Evaluation with CT, MR imaging, and PET. *Radiographics* **2004**, *24*, 105–119. [CrossRef]
59. Yildirim, H.; Metintas, M.; Entok, E.; Ak, G.; Ak, I.; Dundar, E.; Erginel, S. Clinical value of fluorodeoxyglucose-positron emission tomography/computed tomography in differentiation of malignant mesothelioma from asbestos-related benign pleural disease: An observational pilot study. *J. Thorac. Oncol.* **2009**, *4*, 1480–1484. [CrossRef]
60. Saboo, S.S.; Krajewski, K.M.; Zukotynski, K.; Howard, S.; Jagannathan, J.P.; Hornick, J.L.; Ramaiya, N. Imaging features of primary and secondary adult rhabdomyosarcoma. *AJR. Am. J. Roentgenol.* **2012**, *199*, W694–W703. [CrossRef]
61. Dong, Y.; Zhang, X.; Wang, S.; Chen, S.; Ma, G. 18F-FDG PET/CT is useful in initial staging, restaging for pediatric rhabdomyosarcoma. *Q. J. Nucl. Med. Mol. Imaging* **2017**, *61*, 438–446. [CrossRef] [PubMed]
62. Georgiades, C.S.; Neyman, E.G.; Francis, I.R.; Sneider, M.B.; Fishman, E.K. Typical and atypical presentations of extramedullary hemopoiesis. *AJR Am. J. Roentgenol.* **2002**, *179*, 1239–1243. [CrossRef]
63. Roberts, A.S.; Shetty, A.S.; Mellnick, V.M.; Pickhardt, P.J.; Bhalla, S.; Menias, C.O. Extramedullary haematopoiesis: Radiological imaging features. *Clin. Radiol.* **2016**, *71*, 807–814. [CrossRef]
64. Ooi, G.C.; Chim, J.C.; Au, W.Y.; Khong, P.L. Radiologic manifestations of primary solitary extramedullary and multiple solitary plasmacytomas. *AJR Am. J. Roentgenol.* **2006**, *186*, 821–827. [CrossRef] [PubMed]
65. Daghighi, M.H.; Poureisa, M.; Shimia, M.; Mazaheri-Khamene, R.; Daghighi, S. Extramedullary plasmacytoma presenting as a solitary mass in the intracranial posterior fossa. *Iran. J. Radiol.* **2012**, *9*, 223–226. [CrossRef] [PubMed]

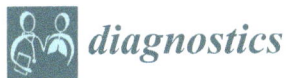

Review

Radiographic Findings of Inflammatory Arthritis and Mimics in the Hands

Fatemeh Ezzati [1] and Parham Pezeshk [2,*]

1. Division of Rheumatic Disease, Department of Internal Medicine, UT Southwestern Medical Center, Dallas, TX 75390, USA
2. Division of Musculoskeletal Radiology, Department of Radiology, UT Southwestern Medical Center, Dallas, TX 75390, USA
* Correspondence: parham.pezeshk@utsouthwestern.edu

Abstract: Clinical presentation could be challenging in patients with arthralgia, and imaging plays an important role in the evaluation of these patients to make the diagnosis or narrow the differential diagnosis. Radiography of the hands is a commonly available imaging modality that can provide crucial information with regard to the pattern and pathology of the involved joints. It is important that radiologists and rheumatologists are familiar with the imaging findings of different rheumatic diseases to make the diagnosis in the early stages of disease to initiate treatment.

Keywords: imaging; radiographs; inflammatory arthritis

1. Introduction

Hand radiographs are frequently ordered as the first imaging modality in the assessment of patients presenting with peripheral arthritis. They can provide invaluable information about the bones, joints, mineralization, soft tissues and the distribution of abnormalities. Given the wide spectrum of rheumatic diseases, it might be challenging to make the diagnosis solely based on the clinical findings and imaging plays an important role in narrowing the differential diagnosis. Having the knowledge of the common radiographic manifestations of inflammatory arthritis is of paramount importance for clinicians and radiologists to diagnose the underlying disease in early stages of disease in order to start treatment. The purpose of the article is to review the key radiographic findings of common rheumatic diseases in the hands.

2. Radiographic Views

The standard radiographic views of the hands for evaluation of rheumatic disease include a posteroanterior (PA), an oblique, and a lateral view. Norgaard view (aka. ball-catcher view) can be obtained as an alternative to oblique views to evaluate the joints in an oblique angle [1]. The PA view is useful to assess soft tissues, alignment, mineralization, erosions and joint spaces. The oblique or Norgaard views are more sensitive for evaluation of erosions in the corners of the joints that may be obscured on the PA and lateral views (Figure 1). In Norgaard view, the patient is asked to position the hands similar to holding a ball with the palms facing up. This maneuver flexes the joints and exposes the corners of the joints to the X-ray beams.

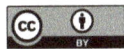

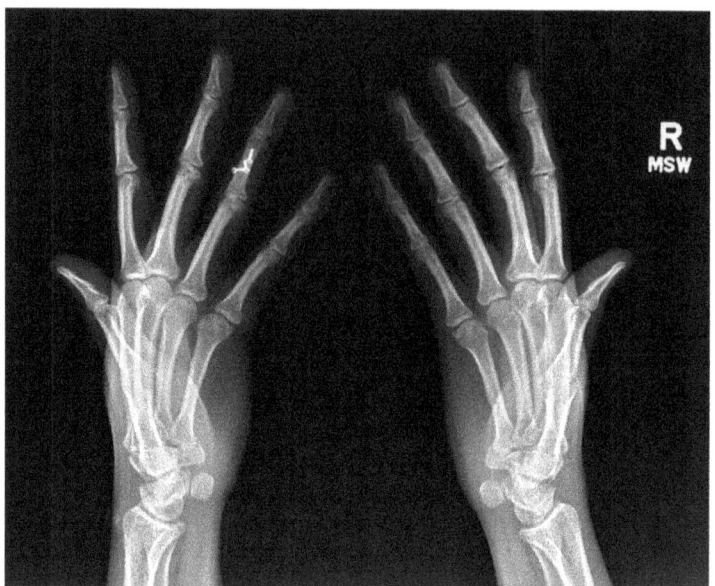

Figure 1. Norgaard (ball-catcher) view.

3. Interpretation of the Hand Radiographs

To ensure a thorough assessment of hand radiographs, the mnemonics of "ABCDES" can be followed. In evaluating the alignment (A), attention should be paid to subluxation, dislocation, angulation and deviation of the joints. Bones (B) should be evaluated for trabecular pattern, destruction, and osseous lesions. Joint spaces should be evaluated for cartilage loss (C) and joint space narrowing, and bones need to be assessed for bone density and demineralization (D). The evaluation of erosions (E) as well as their pattern and distribution is also an important step in the assessment of patients with inflammatory arthritis. Soft tissue (S) swelling and calcifications can add crucial information to narrow the differential diagnosis. Upon gathering all the information, the clinician will have a better insight into the nature of underlying disease in the light of clinical findings. Radiographs of the hands can be used for evaluation of new patients as well as monitoring the progression of known disease.

The purpose of this note is to review the main radiographic findings of common rheumatic diseases and their mimics in the hands. Table 1 summarizes the radiographic findings that will be discussed in further details.

Table 1. Summary of imaging findings of different arthritis in the hand radiography.

Disease	Rheumatoid Arthritis	Psoriasis	Erosive OA	CPPD	Gout	SLE
Joints	MCP > IP DIP unusual	IP > MCP	IP > MCP (mostly DIP)	MCP Radiocarpal	Any	Typically MCPs
Osteopenia	Juxta-articular then diffuse	No		Not primarily	No	Juxta-articular
Erosions	Marginal	Marginal and then central	Central	Not dominant	Well-defined with sclerotic margins	Typically absent
Periostitis	No periostitis	Periostitis				

Table 1. Cont.

Disease	Rheumatoid Arthritis	Psoriasis	Erosive OA	CPPD	Gout	SLE
Distribution	Polyarticular	2/3 asymmetric and mono-oligoarticular	Polyarticular Bilateral Usually symmetric	MCP Radiocarpal	Asymmetrical polyarticular	Polyarticular
Hallmarks		Sausage-digits Micky-mouse Pencil-in-cup. No osteophyte formation	Gull-wing (not specific, also can be seen in RA and PsA)	More prominent cysts Wrong distribution for primary OA Elbow and shoulders involved Chondrocalcinosis involving the triangular fibrocartilage complex (TFCC), scapholunate and lunotriquetral ligaments	Punched out erosions with overhanging edges	Reducible deformity and subluxations Non-erosive

4. Rheumatoid Arthritis

Rheumatoid arthritis (RA) is a daily disease seen in rheumatology clinics. It predominantly involves the appendicular skeleton. The axial skeleton is mostly spared except for the cervical spine where instability can occur and can be carefully assessed with cervical spine radiographs in flexion and extension. Radiographs may show erosion at the C1-C2 level with destruction of the transverse ligament that can result in atlantoaxial subluxation [2].

In the early stage of the disease, synovitis and inflammation of the joints result in fusiform and symmetric juxta-articular soft tissue swelling. Due to hyperemia of the synovium and soft tissues in the setting of inflammation, bone resorption and peri-articular demineralization develops. The bare areas of the bones, where no covering cartilage exists, are exposed to the inflamed synovium and can be eroded [3,4]. These marginal erosions are the first erosive changes seen through the course of the disease and happen before joint space loss. Early erosive changes are appreciated as subtle loss and discontinuity in the cortex in the metacarpal heads as well as the radial base of the proximal phalanges at the metacarpophalangeal joints [4]. In the wrist, erosive changes are typically seen in the ulnar styloid, waists of the scaphoid and hamate, as well as the fifth carpometacarpal joint (Figure 2). As the cartilage destruction continues, symmetric and uniform loss of joint spaces develops and the underlying bone becomes exposed and eroded, which manifests as subchondral erosions. In contrast to osteoarthritis, the joint space loss in the RA is symmetric and mechanical reactive bony changes such as osteophytosis, sclerosis, or cystic changes are not appreciated as the initial manifestations until a later stage of the disease when secondary osteoarthritis develops. Rheumatoid arthritis does not typically involve the distal interphalangeal joints (DIPs) [5] and other possibilities should be entertained when DIP joints are involved (Figures 3 and 4). Radiographs have low sensitivity in detection of bone erosions in the early stage of rheumatoid arthritis and some studies suggest that such findings do not predict the development of inflammatory arthritis in at-risk individuals with positive CCP (cyclic citrullinated peptide) [6]. Ultrasound and MRI with contrast are more sensitive imaging modalities to assess inflammation in the early phase when radiographs are normal.

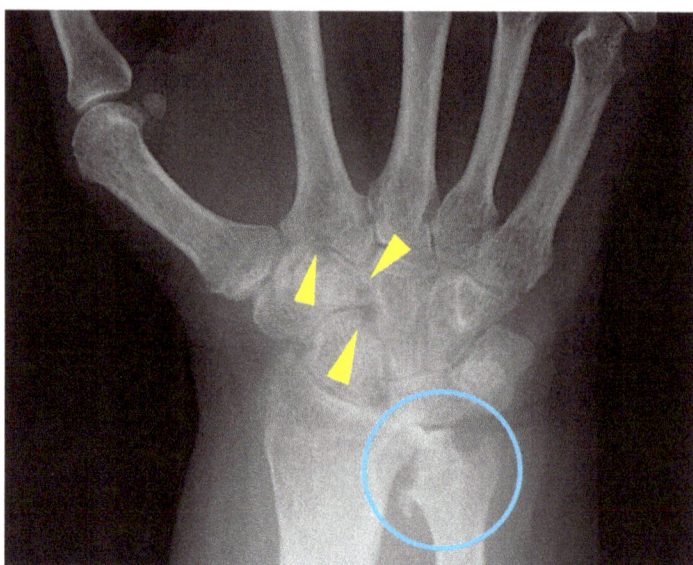

Figure 2. 57-year-old female with rheumatoid arthritis. Moderate demineralization with scattered erosions in the carpal bones (yellow arrowheads) as well as distal radius and ulna (blue circle) are noted.

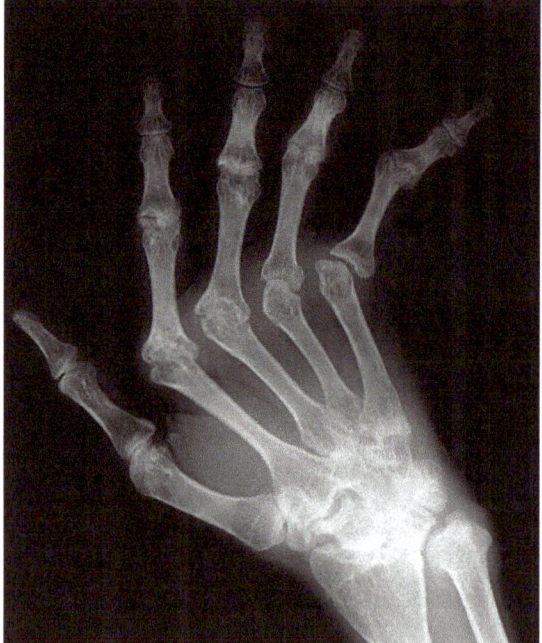

Figure 3. 60-year-old female with long-standing rheumatoid arthritis. Hand radiographs shows erosive changes in the PIP and MCP joints as well as the wrist. Ulnar subluxation of the fingers at MCP joints is also present. Note the distal interphalangeal joints are spared.

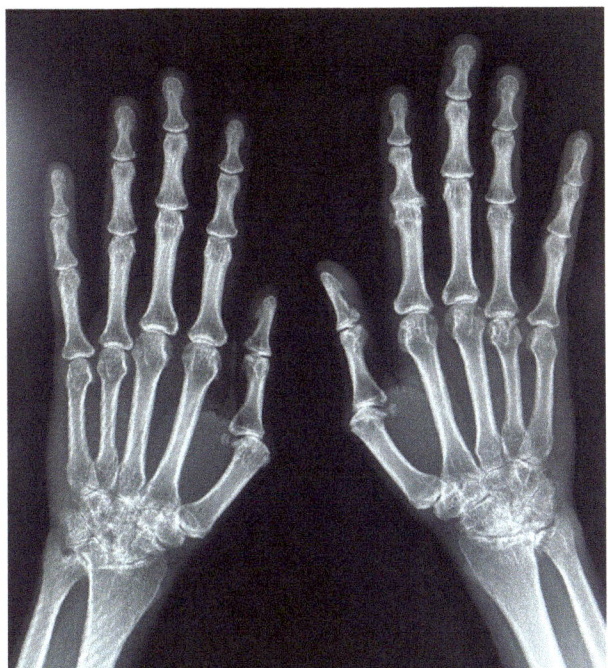

Figure 4. Frontal view of the hand in a 40-year-old female with rheumatoid arthritis. Severe pancarpal joint space loss is present as well as juxta-articular demineralization. Distal interphalangeal joints are spared.

Scoring radiographic findings in rheumatoid arthritis is used as an outcome measure to help estimate the progress of disease. Findings such as erosions, joint-space narrowing, demineralization, malalignment, soft tissue swelling, subluxation, ankylosis and cysts are used in different methods of scoring. The most commonly used scoring methods include van der Heijde-modified Sharp, Simple Erosion Narrowing Score (SENS) [7].

Inflammation of the tendons and ligaments around the joints of the hands results in malalignment and deformity of the joints. These deformities include subluxation of the MCP joints with ulnar and palmar subluxation of the proximal phalanges as well as boutonniere and swan-neck deformities of the distal phalanges. In the later stages of the disease, diffuse demineralization and ankylosis of the joints can also occur. Deformity of the hand can eventually present as arthritis mutilans (Figure 5).

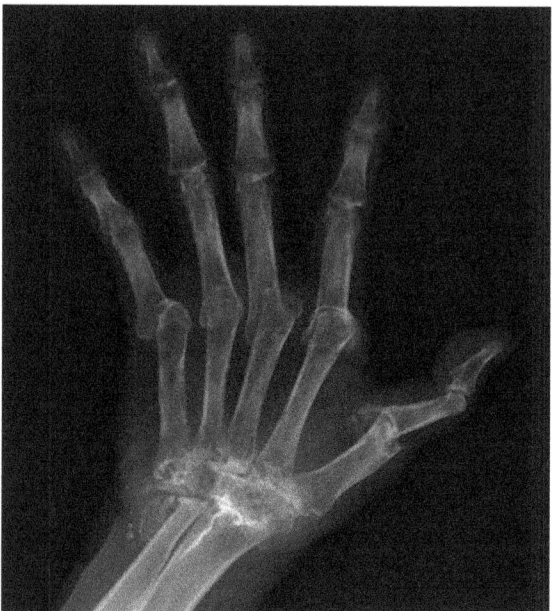

Figure 5. 59-year-old female rheumatoid arthritis. Hand radiograph shows extensive erosive changes and osseous loss in the wrist and metacarpophalangeal joints with telescoping and ulnar deviation at the MCP joints. Severe demineralization is also present. Findings represent arthritis mutilans which also can be seen in psoriatic arthritis.

5. Psoriatic Arthritis (PsA)

Psoriasis arthritis coincide or develop after skin changes. In 15% of cases, arthritis can precede skin changes by 2 years [8] and imaging can play an important role in diagnosis in this timeframe. Hands are the most commonly involved joints in psoriatic arthritis and interphalangeal joints are the predominantly affected [9]. Fusiform periarticular soft tissue swelling can be seen and in approximately 25% of the patients soft-tissue swelling extends beyond the joints and diffusely involves the entire digit resulting in dactylitis that is commonly known as hot-dog or sausage-digits (Figure 6). PsA mainly involves the distal and proximal interphalangeal joints [9]. Normal mineralization is usually maintained through the course of the disease, although early transient juxta-articular demineralization can be seen. Initially, marginal erosions develop which over time progress to central erosions with "pencil-in-cup" deformity. Arthritis mutilans occurs in about 5% of the patients and manifests as destruction of the joints and clinical "telescoping" of the joints where fingers can be pulled back to normal length. Acro-osteolysis is often a prominent feature of psoriatic arthritis [10]. Bony proliferation is the main finding in psoriatic arthritis, which, along with DIP involvement, differentiates it from the rheumatoid arthritis. Erosions in psoriasis are predominantly marginal, which can help differentiate it from central erosion in erosive osteoarthritis (Figures 6 and 7). Marginal erosions with periostitis result in a mouse-ear appearance known as the "Mickey mouse" sign.

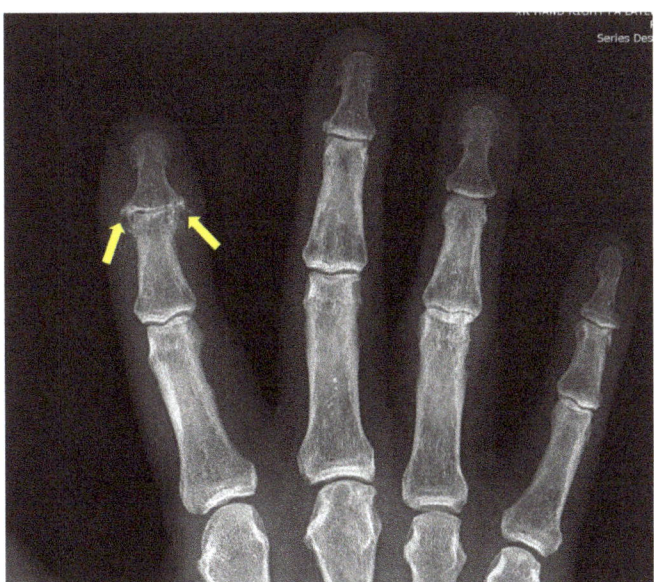

Figure 6. 79-year-old male with psoriatic arthritis. Hand radiographs demonstrate diffuse soft-tissue swelling in the index finger (sausage finger). Small marginal erosions are present in the DIP joint along with mild fluffy periosteal reaction.

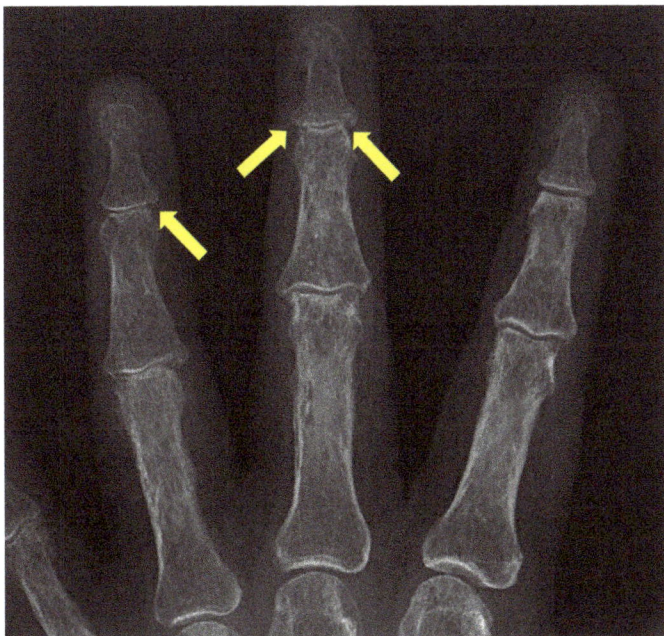

Figure 7. 59-year-old female with psoriatic arthritis. Hand radiographs show marginal erosions in the distal interphalangeal joints of the index and middle fingers (yellow arrows). Mild periosteal reaction is seen at the middle finger DIP joints.

6. Erosive Osteoarthritis

Erosive osteoarthritis (EOA) is a type of osteoarthritis with a strong inflammatory component. It occurs most commonly in females over the age of 60 and usually involves the interphalangeal joints in the hands. Radiographic findings typically include a combination of bony proliferation and erosions [11]. Distal interphalangeal joints are mostly affected and metacarpal (MCP) joints are usually spared. The hallmark of EOA is central erosions in the interphalangeal joints that result in gull-wing or seagull appearance [12] (Figures 8 and 9). The first carpometacarpal joint is also frequently involved. In later stages, ankylosis of the joints might occur as well [13]. The main differential diagnosis of EOA includes classic osteoarthritis, rheumatoid arthritis, and psoriatic arthritis. Joint erosions and interphalangeal ankylosis are absent in classic osteoarthritis. While osteophyte formation is a consistent phenomenon in EOA, it develops secondary to degenerative changes in RA and PsA and is almost never seen as a primary feature in these two entities [11]. Unlike EOA, the DIP joints are spared in adult-onset RA; however, DIPs may be involved in juvenile idiopathic arthritis. In addition, RA demonstrates juxta-articular demineralization, a feature that is usually absent in EOA. Both EOA and PsA involve the DIP joints, but the erosions of PsA are marginal simiar to RA rather than central in EOA. PsA involves the joints asymmetrically unlike EOA, which almost invariably has a symmetric distribution [14]. PsA demonstrates additional features such as skin lesions, sacroiliitis, and enthesophytes followed by fluffy periostitis and sometimes bone erosions [15]. The DIP erosions in PsA has a "mouse-ear" appearance rather a "gull-wing" configuration of EOA [14]. Acro-osteolysis, pencil-in-cup deformity, and arthritis mutilans are absent in EOA [11].

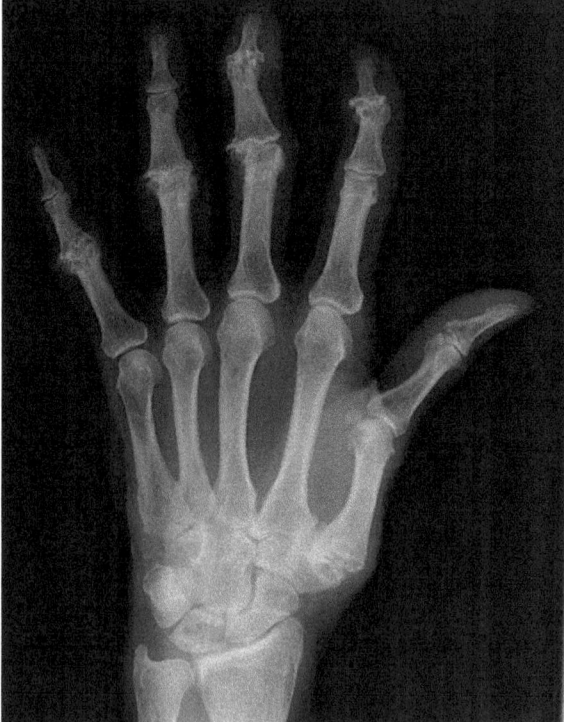

Figure 8. 76-year-old female with erosive arthritis. Severe osteoarthritis of most of the distal and proximal interphalangeal joints with central erosions and seagull appearance.

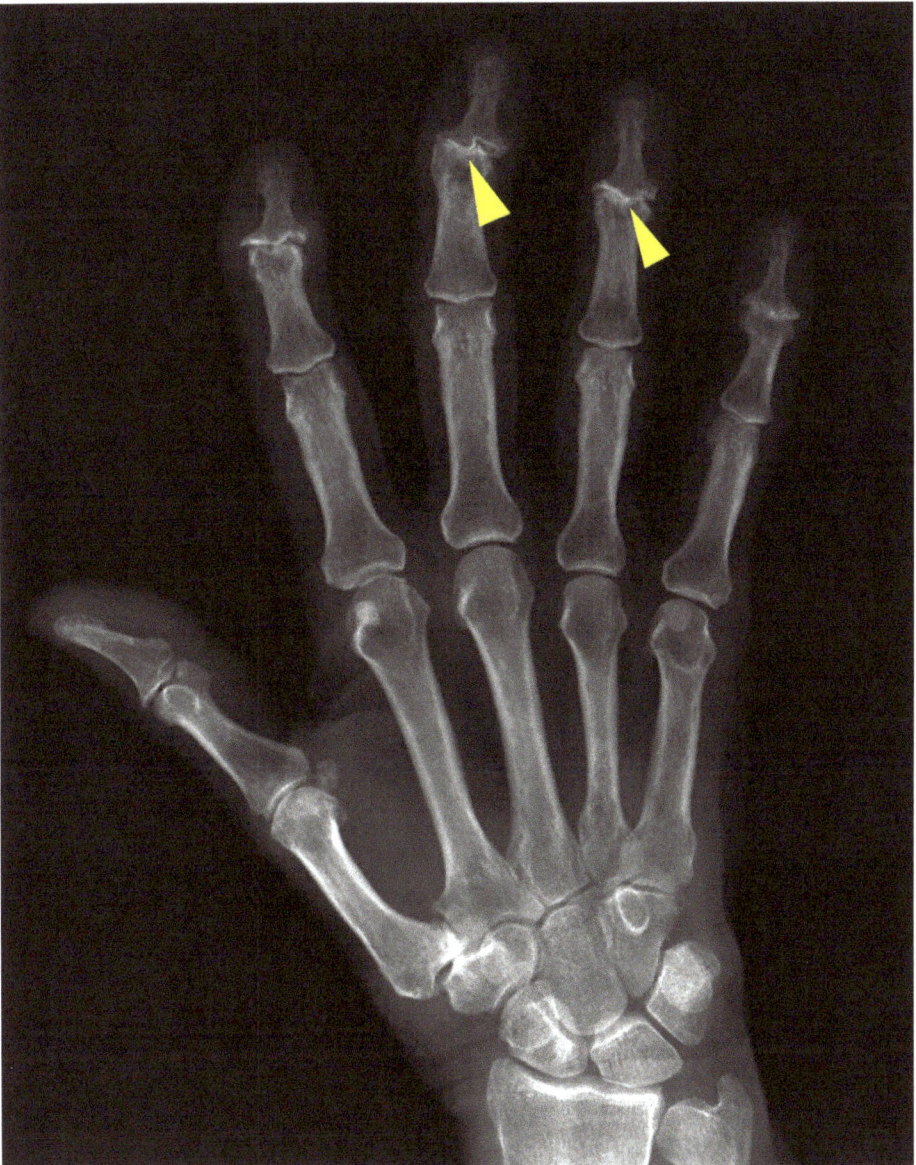

Figure 9. 50-year-old female with erosive arthritis. Severe osteoarthritis of DIP joints with central erosions and seagull appearance (yellow arrowheads).

7. Calcium Pyrophosphate Dehydrate Arthropathy (CPPD)

Calcium pyrophosphate dihydrate (CPPD) crystal deposition disease, also known as pseudogout, is the most common crystal arthropathy and is typically seen in the middle-aged and elderly population. Chondrocalcinosis is the deposition of CPPD crystals in the cartilage. CPPD arthropathy can present clinically as acute and chronic arthritis or destructive arthropathy [16]. It can be primary or secondary and the secondary form is the consequence of metabolic diseases such as hyperparathyroidism and hemochromatosis [17]. Chondrocalcinosis most frequently involve the knees, symphysis pubis and wrists.

Two main radiographic manifestations of CPPD include calcifications and arthropathy [17]. In the hands and wrists, chondrocalcinosis is mostly seen in the triangular fibrocartilage and cartilage adjacent to scaphoid, lunate and metacarpophalangeal joints. Bone mineralization is normal; however, it can be seen due to other etiologies such as aging. Joint-space loss is noted with subchondral new bone formation. CPPD arthropathy resembles osteoarthritis but in an atypical distribution. Common radiographic findings in CPPD include joint-space narrowing, subchondral cyst formation and osteophyte formation. Subchondral cysts are more significant than in primary osteoarthritis and could be the dominant picture in radiography. In the hands, CPPD arthropathy is usually confined to the metacarpophalangeal (MCP) joints, mostly involving 1st to 3rd MCPs, and spares interphalangeal (IP) joints. Beak-like osseous projections, also known as "hook osteophytes" could be seen in the 2nd and 3rd metacarpal head (Figure 10). In the wrist, CPPD arthropathy most commonly affects the radiocarpal joint and ligaments, including the lunotriquetral ligament, scapholunate ligament and triagnulat fibrocartilage complex (TFCC). Involvement and rupture of the scapholunate ligament may result in scapholunate advance collapse (SLAC) wrist [18].

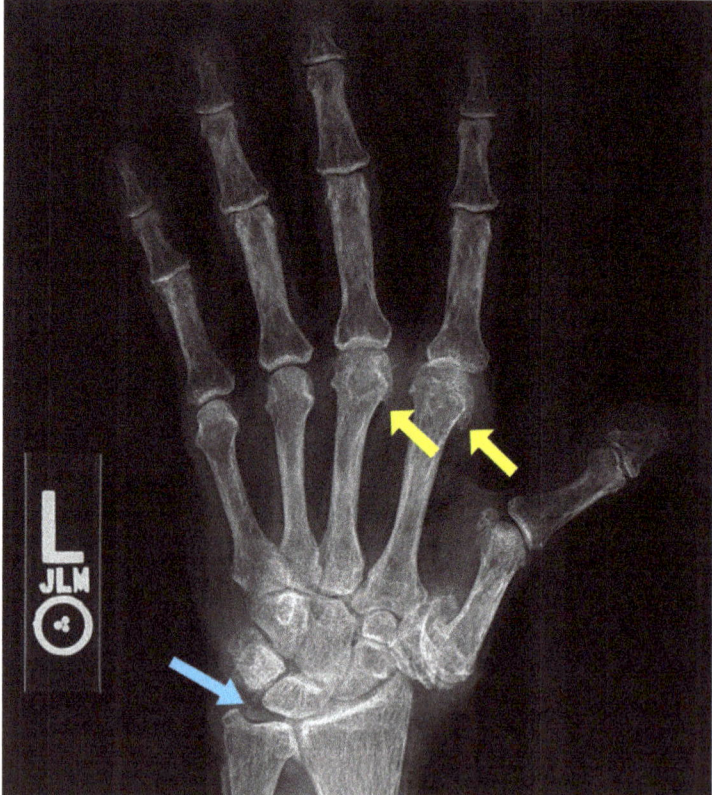

Figure 10. 80-year-old male with CPPD arthropathy. Severe first carpometacarpal osteoarthritis, chondrocalcinosis (blue arrow), degenerative changes and hook osteophytes in the second and third metacarpals (yellow arrows) are findings to lead to the diagnosis.

The distribution of degenerative changes in CPPD is different from the primary osteoarthritis and the "wrong" distribution of degenerative changes should raise the possibility of CPPD arthropathy [19]. In addition, cysts are more prominent in CPPD than in osteoarthritis and shoulder and elbow joints are involved unlike osteoarthritis (Figures 10 and 11).

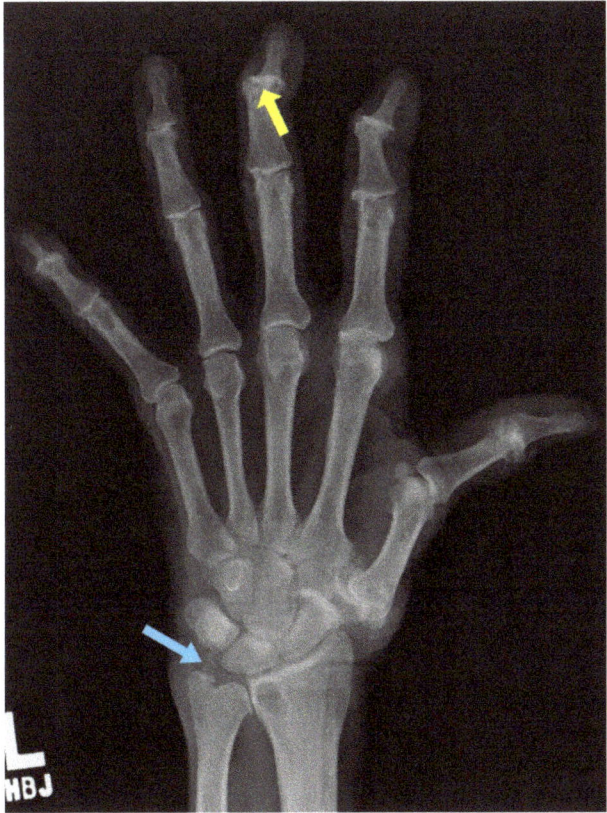

Figure 11. 82 year-old-female with hand pain. Chondrocalcinosis (blue arrow). Severe osteoarthritis of the first carpometacarpal and sever joint space narrowing in the second MCP with a small hook osteophyte. Severe osteoarthritis of the DIP joints with central erosions predominantly seen in the middle finger DIP joint. Patient has findings of CPPD arthtopahy and erosive osteoarthritis.

8. Gout

Gout results from the deposition of monosodium urate crystals, affects males more frequently than the females and is the most common cause of inflammatory arthritis in men older than 60 years [20]. The prevalence of gout increases in postmenopausal females after the protective effect of estrogen begins to fade away. In primary gout, the uric acid level increases due to inborn error of metabolism. In secondary gout, the level of the uric acid increases by either increased production or decreased excretion due to various diseases.

The deposition of monosodium urate crystals occurs in tissues with poor blood supply such as cartilage and tendon sheaths and the radiographic findings depends on the location of the tophus. Urate crystals are not radio-opaque; however, depending on the degree of secondary calcium deposition in the tophi, calcifications can be seen with various densities. It takes an average of 7–10 years for radiographic findings of gout to appear, so in this timeframe radiographs are mostly normal or show nonspecific joint effusion or juxta-articular soft tissue swelling [17]. Serum concentration of uric acid can be normal at the time of an acute flare in up to one-third of the patients [21], therefore a normal serum uric acid level does not exclude the diagnosis.

The imaging findings of gout in hand radiography include an asymmetrical polyarticular distribution, juxta-articluar eccentric and lobulated soft tissue masses due to tophus deposition, normal mineralization, well-defined erosions with sclerotic margins (punched-out lesions) and overhanging margins (Figure 12). There is preference of joint involvement in the hands, and erosions can be intra-articular or juxta-articular. As synovitis is not the primary pathophysiology in gout, cartilage damage and joint-space loss are not the primary findings till secondary osteoarthritis develops in the later stages. Extensive erosions from the long-standing soft-tissue tophi can mimic a "mouse or rat bite" appearance [22]. Gouty arthritis can mimic other arthritides and can happen anywhere in the musculoskeletal system so a high index of suspicion should be maintained if the imaging findings are not typical for other types of arthritis.

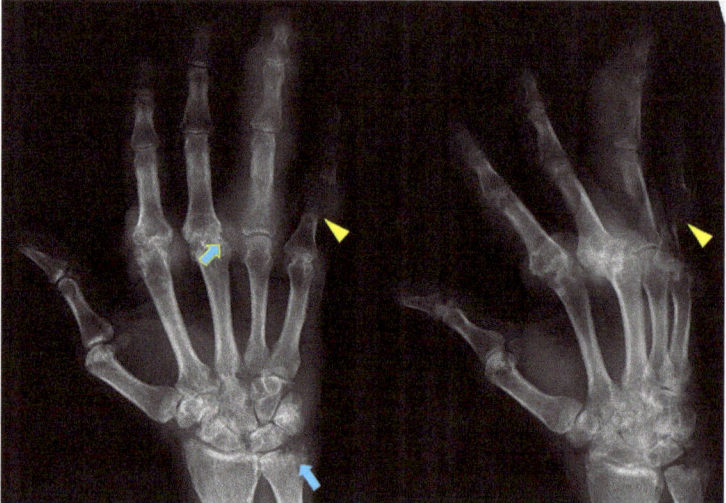

Figure 12. 52-year-old male with gout. Mass-like soft tissue densities representing tophi in the second and third MCP joints as well as the ring and fifth fingers with underlying erosive changes and osseous destruction. Sclerosis at the margins of some of the erosions are noted giving the "punched-out" appearance (blue arrows). Overhanging edge is seen in the fifth finger at the margin of the erosion (yellow arrowhead).

9. Systemic Lupus Erythematous (SLE)

SLE is a systemic autoimmune disease characterized by inflammation of multiple organs. Articular manifestations range from mild and self-limiting arthralgia to persistent arthritis, which can be deforming (i.e., Jaccoud's arthropathy) and/or erosive (i.e., Rhupus; an entity considered by some clinicians as an overlap syndrome between rheumatoid arthritis and SLE) [23]. The most frequent imaging finding in the hand radiographs is deformity and subluxation without erosions (Figure 13). Except for Rhupus, SLE is considered traditionally as non-erosive [23,24]. Deformities are reducible and alignment improves when the patients' hands are supported on the radiographic cassette [8]. Other features on radiographs include peri-articular soft-tissue swelling and juxta-articular demineralization. Soft-tissue calcifications are uncommon.

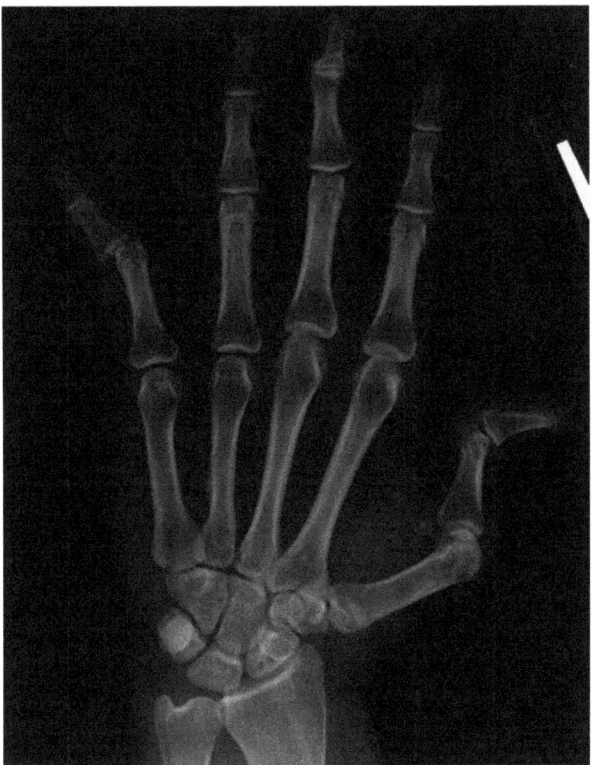

Figure 13. 42-year-old female with SLE. Frontal hand radiograph with Boutonnière deformity of the thumb and ulnar subluxation of the fifth finger PIP joint. Note the absence of erosions.

Jaccoud arthropathy is a non-erosive and deformity arthropathy of the metacarpophalangeal (MCP) and proximal interphalangeal joints, wrists and knees. Hand deformities present as ulnar deviation and subluxation of the MCP similar to RA; however, the deformities are due to ligament laxity and muscle imbalance rather than joint involvement [25].

10. Osteoarthritis (OA)

Osteoarthtritis is the most common arthopathy. In primary osteoarthritis, the change in the dynamics and mechanics of a joint results in cartilage loss and bony reactive changes. In secondary osteoarthritis, the cartilage is lost due to the other pathologies such as infection, inflammatory arthritis, gout, CPPD, trauma and hemophilia. Following the loss of cartilage and joint space, the articulating bones come into closer contact and undergo reactive bony changes such as marginal osteophytosis, subchondral cystic changes and sclerosis. Cartilage pieces can be released into the joint space and continue to grow and ossify over time to form osteochondral bodies as joint fluid provides nutrients to the chondrocytes.

Radiography remains the gold-standard imaging modality to evaluate osteoarthritis [12]. The findings of primary OA in the hands include normal mineralization, osteophyte and cyst formation, and asymmetrical joint space loss. Primary OA involves the distal and proximal interphalangeal joints (DIPs and PIPs) and relatively spares the metacarpophalangeal joints (MCPs). Peri-articular soft-tissue swelling along with osteophyte formation can develop in the PIP and DIP joints, which are known as Bouchard and Heberden nodes, respectively.

11. Systemic Sclerosis

Systemic sclerosis, also known as scleroderma, is a multisystem disorder with skin thickening and vasculitis. Acro-osteolysis (osseous loss of the distal phalanges of the hands and feet) and soft-tissue calcifications are the main radiographic findings. Acro-osteolysis is seen in approximately 40–80% of the cases and manifests as resorption of the tufts, penciling, and resorption of the entire distal phalanx [8]. Other main differential diagnoses of acro-osteolysis include hyperparathyroidism, psoriatic arthritis, and thermal injuries. Arthritis is uncommon in early stages of the disease and might develop later on as erosions and cartilage loss. Digital soft-tissue calcification is seen in 10–30% of patients with systemic sclerosis [8] (Figures 14 and 15).

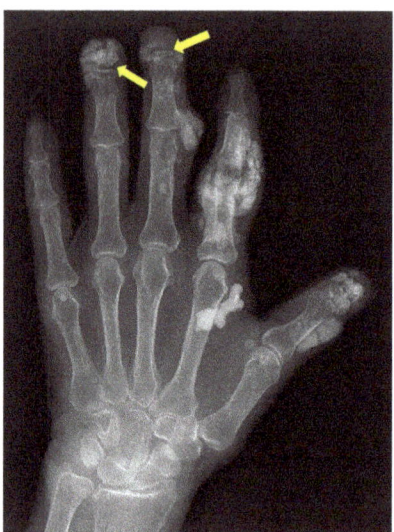

Figure 14. 75-year-old female with scleroderma. There is partial osseous loss of the distal tufts of the middle and ring fingers, known as acro-osteolysis (yellow arrows). Soft-tissue calcifications are noted in the thumb, index, middle and ring fingers.

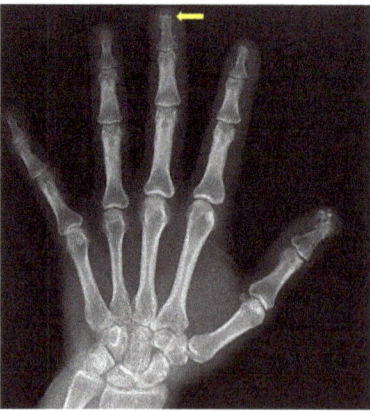

Figure 15. 43-year-old female with scleroderma. Early acro-osteolysis at the tip of the middle finger distal tuft (yellow finger). Foci of soft-tissue calcifications in the thumb, index and middle fingers.

Other conditions mimicking inflammatory arthritis:

12. Septic Arthritis

Septic arthritis is an important consideration when only one joint is involved (monoarthritis). Infection of a joint can be the result of direct extension of infection from subjacent soft tissues (e.g., ulcers in diabetes, decubitus ulcer or penetrating injuries) or secondary to hematogenous spread of pathogens. Radiographic findings include soft-tissue swelling and joint effusion in early stages. Joint-space narrowing and erosive changes are appreciated in later stages as the cartilage is destructed due to synovitis and infection. It is important to diagnose septic arthritis in the early stages, as cartilage and joint destruction can result in osteoarthritis in untreated cases. In the cases of chronic septic arthritis, indolent infections such as tuberculosis should be contemplated [26]. Septic arthritis is a diagnosis of exclusion and should be considered in every case of monoarthritis unless proven otherwise (Figure 16).

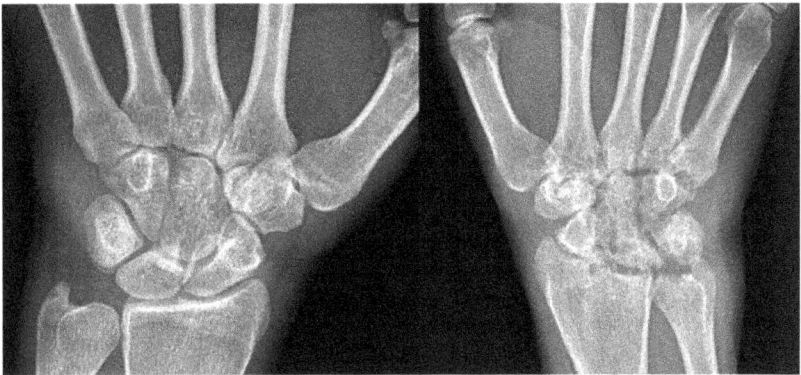

Left   Right

Figure 16. 37-year-old female with septic arthritis of the right wrist. Patient presented with pain and swelling in the right wrist for a few weeks along with fever and chills. Radiographs show erosive changes in the right wrist with soft-tissue swelling. No other joints are involved. Septic arthritis is the diagnosis of exclusion in all patients presenting with monoarthritis and should not be overlooked.

13. Conclusions

Radiography of the hands is a commonly available and cost-effective imaging modality that can provide invaluable information about the pattern of joint involvement and should be the first imaging modality of choice in patients presenting with hand and wrist pain.

Author Contributions: Conceptualization, F.E.; writing—original draft preparation, F.E.; writing—review and editing, F.E. and P.P.; All authors have read and agreed to the published version of the manuscript.

Funding: This research received no external funding.

Institutional Review Board Statement: Not applicable.

Informed Consent Statement: Not applicable.

Conflicts of Interest: The authors declare no conflict of interest.

References

1. Norgaard, F. Earliest Roentgenological Changes in Polyarthritis of the Rheumatoid Type: Rheumatoid Arthritis. *Radiology* **1965**, *85*, 325–329. [CrossRef] [PubMed]
2. Firestein, G.S.; Budd, R.C.; Gabriel, S.E. *Kelley's Textbook of Rheumatology*, 11th ed.; Elsevier: Amsterdam, The Netherlands, 2021.
3. Llopis, E.; Kroon, H.M.; Acosta, J.; Bloem, J.L. Conventional Radiology in Rheumatoid Arthritis. *Radiol. Clin. North Am.* **2017**, *55*, 917–941. [CrossRef] [PubMed]

4. Brower, A.C.; Flemming, D.J. Rheumatoid Arthritis. In *Arthritis in Black and White*; Saunders: Philadelphia, PA, USA, 2012; pp. 170–199.
5. Hant, F.N.; Bolster, M.B.; Monu, J.U. Rheumatoid Arthritis. In *Musculoskeletal Imaging*, 2nd ed.; Saunders: Philadelphia, PA, USA, 2014; pp. 666–674.
6. Di Matteo, A.; Mankia, K.; Nam, J.L.; Cipolletta, E.; Garcia-Montoya, L.; Duquenne, L.; Rowbotham, E.; Emery, P. In anti-CCP+ at-risk individuals, radiographic bone erosions are uncommon and are not associated with the development of clinical arthritis. *Rheumatology* **2021**, *60*, 3156–3164. [CrossRef] [PubMed]
7. Boini, S.; Guillemin, F. Radiographic scoring methods as outcome measures in rheumatoid arthritis: Properties and advantages. *Ann. Rheum. Dis.* **2001**, *60*, 817–827. [PubMed]
8. Manaster, B. *Diagnostic Imaging: Musculoskeletal Non-Traumatic Disease*, 2nd ed.; Elsevier: Amsterdam, The Netherlands, 2016.
9. Brower, A.C.; Flemming, D.J. Psoriatic Arthritis. In *Arthritis in Black and White*, 3rd ed.; Saunders: Philadelphia, PA, USA, 2012.
10. Kemp, S.S.; Dalinka, M.K.; Schumacher, H.R. Acro-osteolysis. Etiologic and radiological considerations. *JAMA* **1986**, *255*, 2058–2061. [CrossRef] [PubMed]
11. Greenspan, A. Erosive osteoarthritis. *Semin. Musculoskelet. Radiol.* **2003**, *7*, 155–159. [PubMed]
12. Guermazi, A.; Hayashi, D.; Eckstein, F.; Hunter, D.J.; Duryea, J.; Roemer, F.W. Imaging of osteoarthritis. *Rheum. Dis. Clin. North Am.* **2013**, *39*, 67–105. [CrossRef] [PubMed]
13. McEwen, C. Osteoarthritis of the fingers with ankylosis. *Arthritis Rheum.* **1968**, *11*, 734–744. [CrossRef] [PubMed]
14. Martel, W.; Stuck, K.J.; Dworin, A.M.; Hylland, R.G. Erosive osteoarthritis and psoriatic arthritis: A radiologic comparison in the hand, wrist, and foot. *AJR Am. J. Roentgenol.* **1980**, *134*, 125–135. [CrossRef] [PubMed]
15. Peterson, C.C., Jr.; Silbiger, M.L. Reiter's syndrome and psoriatic arthritis. Their roentgen spectra and some interesting similarities. *Am. J. Roentgenol. Radium. Ther. Nucl. Med.* **1967**, *101*, 860–871. [CrossRef] [PubMed]
16. Zhang, W.; Doherty, M.; Bardin, T.; Barskova, V.; Guerne, P.A.; Jansen, T.L.; Leeb, B.F.; Perez-Ruiz, F.; Pimentao, J.; Punzi, L.; et al. European League Against Rheumatism recommendations for calcium pyrophosphate deposition. Part I: Terminology and diagnosis. *Ann. Rheum. Dis.* **2011**, *70*, 563–570. [CrossRef] [PubMed]
17. Jacques, T.; Michelin, P.; Badr, S.; Nasuto, M.; Lefebvre, G.; Larkman, N.; Cotten, A. Conventional Radiology in Crystal Arthritis: Gout, Calcium Pyrophosphate Deposition, and Basic Calcium Phosphate Crystals. *Radiol. Clin. North Am.* **2017**, *55*, 967–984. [CrossRef] [PubMed]
18. Kahloune, M.; Libouton, X.; Omoumi, P.; Larbi, A. Osteoarthritis and scapholunate instability in chondrocalcinosis. *Diagn. Interv. Imaging* **2015**, *96*, 115–119. [CrossRef] [PubMed]
19. Brower, A.C.; Flemming, D.J. Calcium Pyrophosphate Dihydrarte Crystal Deposition Disease. In *Arthritis in Black and White*, 3rd ed.; Saunders: Philadelphia, PA, USA, 2012; pp. 309–324.
20. Zhang, W.; Doherty, M.; Pascual, E.; Bardin, T.; Barskova, V.; Conaghan, P.; Gerster, J.; Jacobs, J.; Leeb, B.; Lioté, F.; et al. EULAR evidence based recommendations for gout. Part I: Diagnosis. Report of a task force of the Standing Committee for International Clinical Studies Including Therapeutics (ESCISIT). *Ann. Rheum. Dis.* **2006**, *65*, 1301–1311. [CrossRef] [PubMed]
21. Mikuls, T.R. Gout. In *Rheumatology Secrets*; West, S.G., Ed.; Elsevier: Amsterdam, The Netherlands, 2020; pp. 364–372.
22. Brower, A.C.; Flemming, D.J. Gout. In *Arthritis in Black and White*; Saunders: Philadelphia, PA, USA, 2012; pp. 263–308.
23. Di Matteo, A.; Smerilli, G.; Cipolletta, E.; Salaffi, F.; De Angelis, R.; Di Carlo, M.; Filippucci, E.; Grassi, W. Imaging of Joint and Soft Tissue Involvement in Systemic Lupus Erythematosus. *Curr. Rheumatol. Rep.* **2021**, *23*, 73. [CrossRef] [PubMed]
24. Antonini, L.; Le Mauff, B.; Marcelli, C.; Aouba, A.; de Boysson, H. Rhupus: A systematic literature review. *Autoimmun. Rev.* **2020**, *19*, 102612. [CrossRef] [PubMed]
25. Spina, M.F.; Beretta, L.; Masciocchi, M.; Scorza, R. Clinical and radiological picture of Jaccoud arthropathy in the context of systemic sclerosis. *Ann. Rheum. Dis.* **2008**, *67*, 728–729. [CrossRef] [PubMed]
26. Hogan, J.I.; Hurtado, R.M.; Nelson, S.B. Mycobacterial Musculoskeletal Infections. *Infect. Dis. Clin. North Am.* **2017**, *31*, 369–382. [CrossRef] [PubMed]

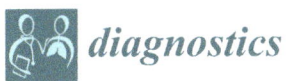

Review

Postoperative Findings of Common Foot and Ankle Surgeries: An Imaging Review

Maryam Soltanolkotabi *, Chris Mallory, Hailey Allen, Brian Y. Chan, Megan K. Mills and Richard L. Leake

Department of Radiology & Imaging Sciences, University of Utah School of Medicine, Salt Lake City, UT 84132, USA; chris.mallory@hsc.utah.edu (C.M.); hailey.allen@hsc.utah.edu (H.A.); brian.chan@hsc.utah.edu (B.Y.C.); megan.mills@hsc.utah.edu (M.K.M.); richard.leake@hsc.utah.edu (R.L.L.)
* Correspondence: maryam.soltanolkotabi@hsc.utah.edu

Abstract: Foot and ankle surgery is increasingly prevalent. Knowledge of the mechanisms underlying common foot and ankle deformities is useful in understanding surgical procedures used to restore normal biomechanics. As surgical techniques evolve, it is important for the radiologist to be familiar with these procedures, their expected postoperative appearance, and potential complications. This article reviews the key imaging findings of a variety of common and important foot and ankle surgical procedures.

Keywords: postoperative foot and ankle; foot and ankle imaging; osteotomy; arthrodesis; articular implants; post-traumatic fixation

1. Introduction

Foot and ankle surgery is increasingly prevalent. In 2000, a total of 548,214 foot and ankle surgeries occurred in the Medicare population. An approximate direct economic burden of USD 11 billion was attributed to these procedures [1]. Additionally, osteoarthritis is a common reason for primary care visits and surgical consultation. The quantity and variety of foot and ankle surgeries has increased over time. Familiarity with these procedures, their expected postoperative imaging findings, and common complications are important for the general radiologist as well as the musculoskeletal subspecialist.

2. Osteotomies

2.1. Hallux Valgus and Metatarsus Primus Varus

Hallux valgus (HV), defined as abnormal fixed abduction of the first metatarsophalangeal (MTP) joint, is the most common form of forefoot malalignment. It is often seen concurrently with metatarsus primus varus (MPV) or abnormal adduction of the first metatarsal related to the other metatarsals. Both HV and MPV can cause foot pain, stiffness, and chronic irritation of the overlying skin.

Foot radiographs are the mainstay for preoperative imaging of HV and MPV. As most foot and ankle deformities have a dynamic biomechanical component, non-weight-bearing radiographs tend to underestimate deformity severity.

Many radiographic measurements have been described to define HV and MPV. Three of the most commonly used measurements include the hallux abductus angle (HAA), the first intermetatarsal angle (IMA), and the metatarsal sesamoid position (MSP) (Figure 1A,B). Normal HAA and IMA are less than 15 and 10 degrees, respectively [2]. The MSP describes the relationship between the longitudinal axis of the first metatarsal and the position of the tibial sesamoid. This is measured on a 7-point scale, with positions 1–3 depicted as normal [3].

As the abduction deformity progresses, the first metatarsal head slides medially in relation to the sesamoids, the medial bony prominence (bunion) increases, and the medial supporting structures attenuate. Many patients do not respond to conservative

management; subsequently, multiple surgical techniques are used to address the underlying malalignment.

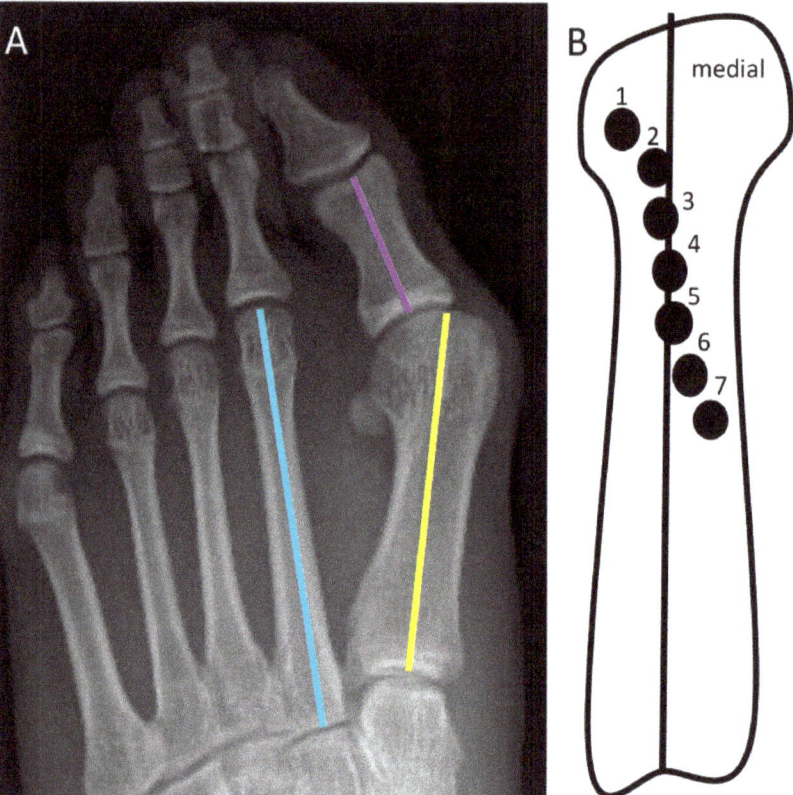

Figure 1. (**A**) Anteroposterior (AP) radiograph of the foot demonstrating the longitudinal axis of the first metatarsal (yellow line), first proximal phalanx (purple line), and second metatarsal (blue line). IMA is the angle between the first and second metatarsal longitudinal axes. HAA is the angle between the first metatarsal and first proximal phalangeal longitudinal axes. (**B**) Schematic of MSP, typically measured on a 7-point scale that increases with progressive medial angulation of the first metatarsal.

The choice of procedure depends on the severity of the deformity. More severe deformities generally require more proximal metatarsal osteotomy or first tarsometatarsal (TMT) arthrodesis. Figure 2 depicts an overview of various techniques used for correction of HV/MPP.

2.2. Akin Osteotomy

The Akin procedure is a medial-wedge osteotomy of the first proximal phalangeal base, typically performed in combination with a first metatarsal osteotomy procedure (Figure 3A,B) [4]. A single screw or cerclage wire are typically used for osteotomy fixation.

2.3. Chevron Osteotomy

Chevron osteotomy, a V-shaped osteotomy of the first-metatarsal head performed in the medial-to-lateral direction, is best for mild deformities [5,6]. Traditionally, the dorsal and plantar osteotomy limbs were equal in size, but more recently, the dorsal limb has been cut longer to accommodate the fixation screw [7]. The distal fragment is then translated laterally and typically fixed with one or two bicortical screws (Figure 3A). Postoperatively, lateral radiographs are important to ensure the screws do not violate the metatarsal–sesamoid articulation and do not protrude into adjacent soft-tissue structures.

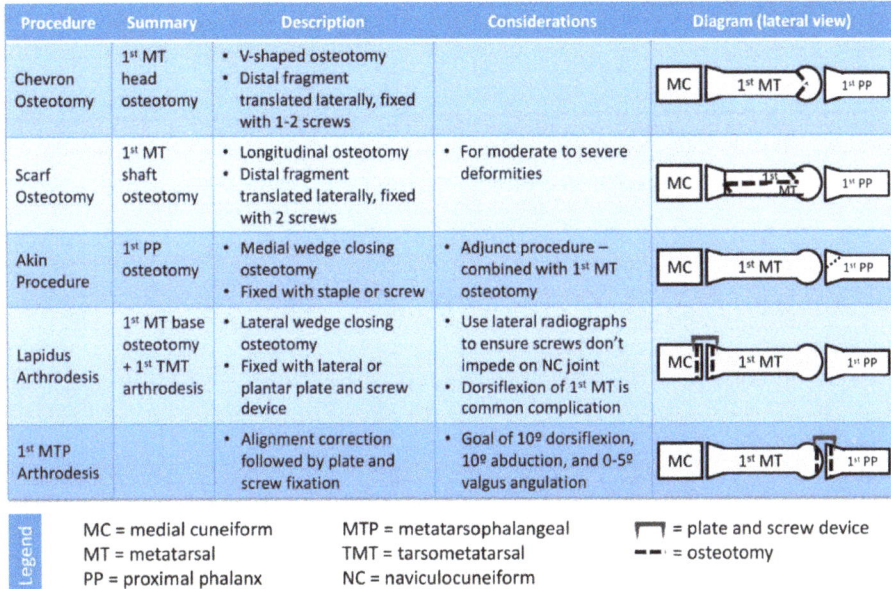

Figure 2. Surgical options for correction of hallux valgus.

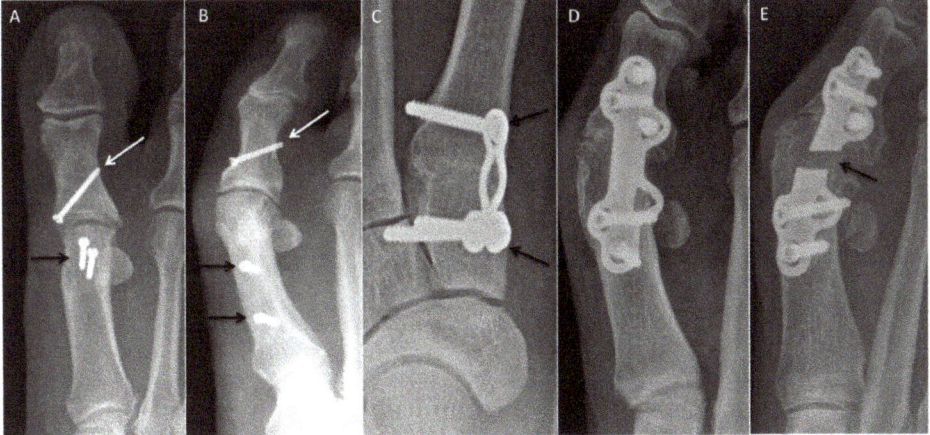

Figure 3. Hallux valgus correction. (**A**) Postoperative AP radiograph demonstrating Chevron (black arrow) and adjunct Akin (white arrow) correction of hallux valgus deformity with first metatarsal head and proximal phalangeal base osteotomies. Two first-metatarsal head screws and one screw in the base of the first proximal phalanx transfix the osteotomy sites. (**B**) Postoperative AP radiograph demonstrating Scarf (black arrows) and adjunct Akin (white arrow) correction of hallux valgus deformity with first-metatarsal shaft and proximal phalangeal base osteotomies. (**C**) Postoperative changes related to Lapidus procedure with first-metatarsal base osteotomy and first TMT arthrodesis (black arrows). (**D**) First MTP arthrodesis for correction of hallux valgus. (**E**) Postoperative complication of first MTP arthrodesis with fractured plate (black arrow).

2.4. Reverdin Osteotomy

The Reverdin osteotomy consists of medial rotation of the articular surface of the first metatarsal head [8]. Radiographs lack sensitivity to depict the exact position of the cartilage-covered metatarsal head. Thus, most surgeons rely on intraoperative findings when making the decision to perform a Reverdin osteotomy.

2.5. Scarf Osteotomy

A longitudinal osteotomy on the first-metatarsal shaft is performed from medial to lateral, often for moderate degrees of hallux valgus [9]. The distal fragment is translated laterally and fixed with two screws (Figure 3B). Lateral postoperative radiographs are especially useful in depiction of screw orientation.

2.6. First-Metatarsal Base Closing Wedge Osteotomy

For severe HV/MPV deformities, procedures at the base of the first metatarsal may be required. One such procedure is the first-metatarsal base-closing-wedge osteotomy, which is a lateral oblique osteotomy fixed with at least one bicortical screw [10].

2.7. Lapidus Arthrodesis

Lapidus arthrodesis is another option for severe deformities, which combines a first-tarsometatarsal arthrodesis and closing-wedge osteotomy of the first-metatarsal base (Figure 3C) [11]. A potential complication is excursion of the screws into the naviculo-cuneiform joint; this is best appreciated on lateral radiographs.

2.8. First Metatarsophalangeal Arthrodesis

Arthrodesis is an option for patients with severe HV/MPV deformities and first MTP osteoarthritis (Figure 3D,E). Joint instability, as can be seen in patients with rheumatoid arthritis, is another indication of arthrodesis. The goal postoperative alignment is approximately 10 degrees of phalangeal abduction (10-degree hallux abductus angle), 10 degrees of dorsiflexion, and 0–5 degrees of valgus.

2.9. Bunionectomy and Bunionettectomy

Resection of the medial and lateral eminences of the condyles of the first and fifth metatarsals—termed bunionectomy and bunionettectomy, respectively—are very common adjunct procedures in the treatment of HV/MPV. They are rarely performed in isolation, as they do not contribute to realignment of the bones. Postoperative radiographic evaluation is mainly performed to assess for complications such as infection or bunion recurrence.

2.10. Second-Metatarsal Shortening

Second-metatarsal shortening is often performed for correction of long-second-toe syndrome and metatarsalgia that has failed conservative treatment. In long-second-toe syndrome, the second toe is longer than the hallux and third toes, resulting in hammertoe deformity, callus formation, ungual lesions, and pain [12]. Surgical options include joint-preserving metatarsal-shortening osteotomy (Weil osteotomy), resection arthroplasty, and arthrodesis [13]. An osteotomy is made from the dorsal aspect of the metatarsal neck, parallel to the plantar surface of the foot. The distal fragment is then translated proximally to achieve the desired shortening (Figure 4A,B). Decreased dislocation rate, pain reduction, and resolution of soft-tissue callus are advantages of the Weil osteotomy. Postoperative improvement in range of motion does not always occur, and postoperative extension contractures and joint stiffness have been reported [14].

2.11. Calcaneal Osteotomy

The calcaneus plays an important role in alignment of the foot during weight-bearing. Calcaneal osteotomies are extra-articular, joint-preserving procedures utilized in the correction of pes planovalgus and pes cavovarus. Not only do calcaneal osteotomies correct alignment through repositioning of the calcaneal tuberosity, but they also change the direction of the pull of the Achilles tendon, transforming it into a corrective force. A variety of calcaneal osteotomies exist and can be broadly divided into translational osteotomies (medializing or lateralizing), closing-wedge osteotomies (Dwyer/modified Dwyer) [15], and rotational osteotomies (Evans or Z-osteotomy) [16]. A major contraindication to these procedures is subtalar osteoarthritis. In the presence of subtalar osteoarthritis, subtalar arthrodesis is preferred.

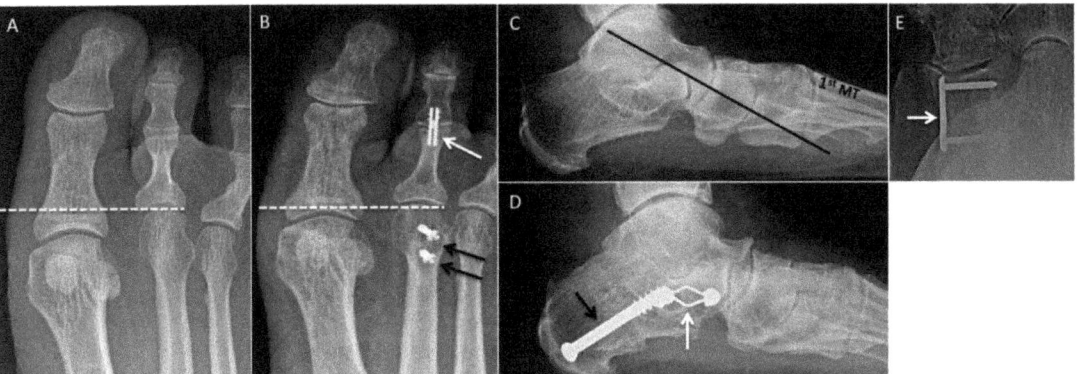

Figure 4. Osteotomies. (**A**) Preoperative AP radiograph demonstrating long-second metatarsal in a patient with plantar pain. (**B**) Postoperative radiograph showing findings of Weil osteotomy with screw fixation (black arrows) with decreased length of the second metatarsal (white dashed lines). Additionally, the patient underwent second PIP arthrodesis (white arrow). (**C**) Preoperative lateral radiograph demonstrating altered tarsometatarsal axis (black line) passing plantar to the first metatarsal. Postoperative lateral (**D**) and AP (**E**) radiographs demonstrating healed medializing calcaneal osteotomy (black arrow) and Evans lengthening osteotomy (white arrows).

2.12. Single-Plane Translational Osteotomy

Single-plane translational osteotomies are simple transverse osteotomies of the posterior calcaneus. The calcaneal tuberosity may be translated medially, laterally, anteriorly, or posteriorly depending on the type of realignment required.

Medializing calcaneal osteotomy is usually performed for correction of pes planovalgus caused by posterior tibialis tendon dysfunction. It reduces strain on the deltoid ligament and other medial support structures. The osteotomy is usually fixed with two retrograde screws or a lateral plate and screw construct. A lateralizing calcaneal osteotomy is utilized for correction of pes cavovarus (Figure 4C,D) [17].

2.13. Closing-Wedge Osteotomy

This procedure, originally described by Dwyer, is performed in cases of mild pes cavovarus, often in the setting of peroneal tendon pathology, and may be performed alongside peroneal tendon repair [15]. An 8–12 mm wedge of bone is resected via a lateral approach osteotomy, theoretically displacing the weight-bearing axis of the hindfoot more laterally. By reducing stress on the repaired peroneal tendons, closing-wedge osteotomies reduce the chance of tendon re-tear. This is a more challenging technique as the osteotomy and tendon repair are often performed through the same incision.

2.14. Rotational Osteotomy

Evans described a lengthening opening-wedge osteotomy of the calcaneal neck to address an overcorrected clubfoot deformity [16]. A wedge-shaped bone allograft is inserted into the osteotomy site, which lengthens the lateral column and rotates the hindfoot and forefoot medially to restore the arch of the foot. This may be performed together with a medial translational osteotomy for correction of severe pes planovalgus. Because the Evans osteotomy accentuates the equinus deformity and leads to varus forefoot alignment, it is commonly performed with a medial cuneiform osteotomy (Cotton osteotomy) to correct forefoot varus. Additionally, a lengthening gastrocnemius/soleus procedure is often performed with the Evans osteotomy to correct ankle equinus (Figure 4E).

Radiographic evaluation of calcaneal osteotomies consists of describing the degree of alignment correction, appropriate healing of the osteotomy and incorporation of graft material if present. Weight-bearing radiographs, including the hindfoot (Saltzman) view, aid the radiologist in describing postoperative alignment [18].

Nonunion or malunion are rare complications associated with calcaneal osteotomies. According to Greenfield et al., this most commonly occurs in patients with systemic comorbidities, including vitamin D deficiency. At-risk patients may receive biologic supplementation in the form of osteoinductive modalities such as bone morphogenetic protein (BMP) at the osteotomy site in hopes of achieving better postoperative outcomes [19].

2.15. Medial Cuneiform Opening-Wedge Osteotomy

Medial cuneiform opening-wedge (Cotton) osteotomy is an adjunct procedure used for correction of the fixed forefoot varus component of adult pes planovalgus. The osteotomy is performed at the midpoint of the medial cuneiform from dorsal to plantar, keeping the plantar cortex intact. A 4–6 mm opening is made in the medial cuneiform to accommodate a wedge-shaped autograft or allograft. In recent years, insertion of trabecular titanium wedges has been proposed in lieu of bone grafts (Figure 5) [20]. The osteotomy is usually fixed with Kirschner wires for 4–6 weeks and the patient is kept non-weight-bearing; permanent screw fixation is usually not required.

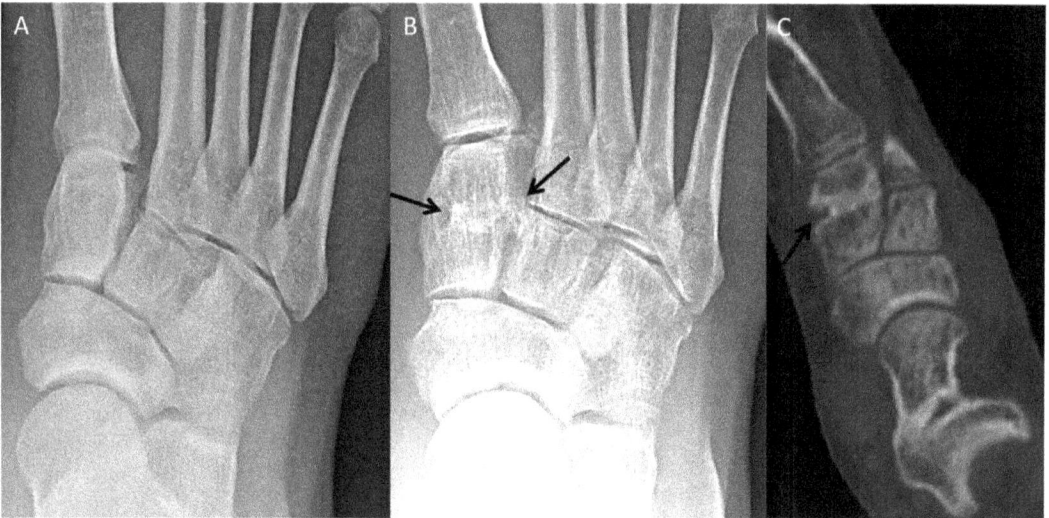

Figure 5. (**A**) Preoperative and (**B**) postoperative AP radiographs, and (**C**) axial CT of the foot demonstrating changes of Cotton osteotomy at the waist of the medial cuneiform with interposition of bone graft material (black arrows).

Postoperative weight-bearing radiographs are utilized to evaluate osteotomy healing and graft incorporation. Meary's (talus-first metatarsal) and Kite's (talus-calcaneal) angles are measured on lateral and anteroposterior radiographs to assess restoration of the plantar arch.

3. Arthrodeses

3.1. Hindfoot

The hindfoot joints include the talonavicular, subtalar, and calcaneocuboid joints. Hindfoot arthrodesis is indicated in symptomatic patients with advanced arthritis or severe hindfoot malalignment (varus or valgus) who have failed conservative management [21,22]. Hindfoot deformity can be painful even in the absence of significant arthritis. In advanced Charcot–Marie–Tooth disease, hindfoot varus can result in symptomatic adult clubfoot. Inflammatory disease such as rheumatoid arthritis can also lead to both deformity and arthritis. Due to the importance of the hindfoot joints in the biomechanics of the foot and ankle, arthrodesis should not be attempted unless other treatment strategies such as tendon transfers, corrective osteotomies, and midfoot arthrodesis have failed.

3.2. Subtalar

Subtalar arthrodesis is performed in the setting of severe arthritis of any etiology (primary, post-traumatic, postseptic, or inflammatory) or in other conditions such as talocalcaneal coalition and acquired pes planus deformity related to posterior tibial tendon dysfunction.

Because of the vital role of this joint in foot and gait biomechanics, anatomic alignment of the fusion is essential with a goal of 5–10 degrees of valgus. Open subtalar arthrodesis is generally preferred for more severe deformities and when additional arthrodeses are planned. Fixation is achieved with two large cannulated screws. One of the screws crosses the joint towards the talar neck. The second screw is placed parallel to the sagittal plane, superior to the first screw into the subchondral bone of the talar dome.

Postoperative radiographs are acquired to assess for degree of fusion, alignment, and possible complications, including hardware failure (Figure 6A–D).

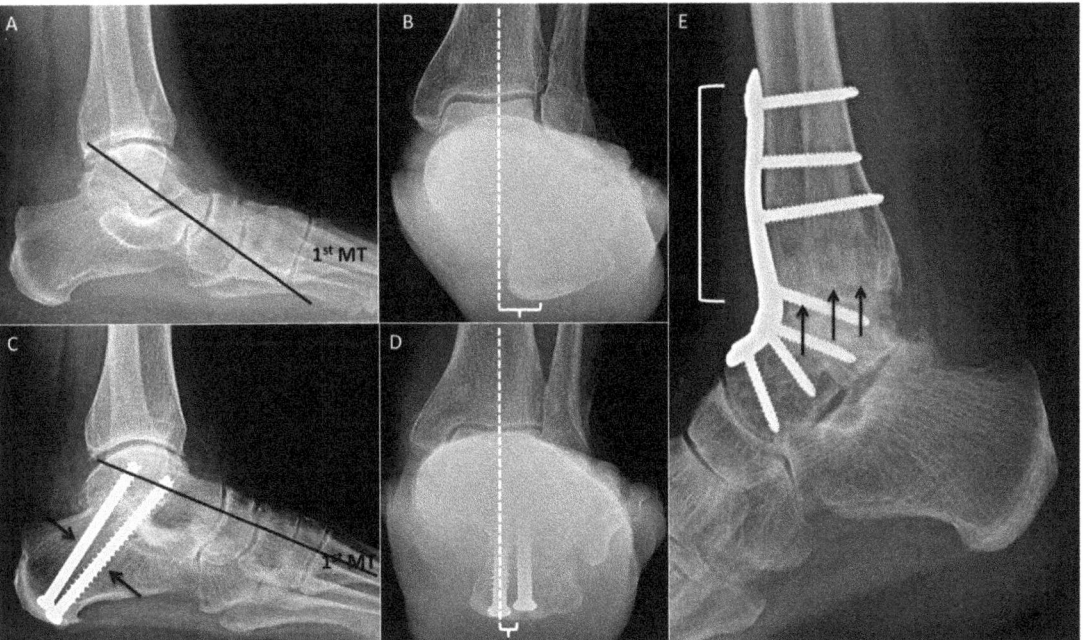

Figure 6. Arthrodeses. (**A,B**) Preoperative weight-bearing radiographs of the hindfoot. (**A**) Weight-bearing lateral radiograph demonstrating the longitudinal axis of the talus (black line) passing plantar

to the first metatarsal (MT), consistent with severe pes planus. There is also mild subtalar osteoarthritis. (**B**) Saltzman view of the hindfoot demonstrating the weight-bearing axis of the tibia (white dashed line) passing far medial to the plantar calcaneus, compatible with hindfoot valgus. (**C,D**) Postoperative weight-bearing radiographs of the hindfoot following subtalar arthrodesis. (**C**) Weight-bearing lateral radiograph demonstrates improved alignment, with the longitudinal axis of the talus (black line) passing through the first MT. Note the talocalcaneal fixation screws (black arrows). (**D**) Saltzman view of the hindfoot demonstrating resolved hindfoot valgus, with the weight-bearing axis of the tibia (white dashed line) passing near the plantar calcaneus. (**E**) Postoperative lateral radiograph demonstrating tibiotalar arthrodesis with plate and multiple screws (white bracket). There is partial ankylosis (black arrows).

3.3. Triple Arthrodesis

Triple arthrodesis involves fusion of the talonavicular (TN), talocalcaneal (TC), and calcaneocuboid (CC) joints (Figure 7). The primary goals of a triple arthrodesis are to relieve pain from arthritic, deformed, or unstable joints. Other goals are the correction of deformity and the creation of a stable, balanced plantigrade foot for ambulation. A variety of techniques exist for this procedure and a combination of screws and plates may be used [23]. Complications include nonunion, hardware failure, malalignment, and adjacent joint arthritis. In the late postoperative period, special attention should be directed to hardware integrity and developing arthritis in the unfused joints.

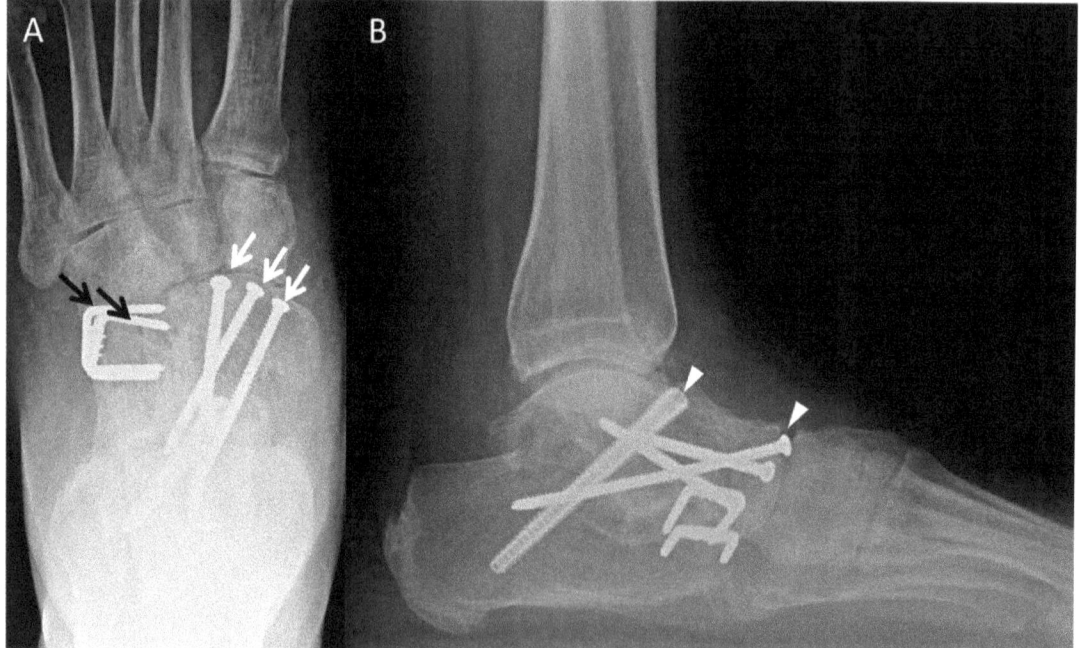

Figure 7. (**A**) AP and (**B**) lateral radiographs of the foot demonstrate hindfoot triple arthrodesis with hardware spanning the subtalar (arrow heads), talonavicular (white arrows) and calcaneocuboid joints (black arrows). The hardware is intact and there is mature ankylosis with decreased conspicuity of the joint space.

3.4. Tibiotalar

The goal of tibiotalar arthrodesis is to solidly fuse the tibia and talus in appropriate alignment, defined as 0–5 degrees of valgus, neutral dorsiflexion, and slight external rotation, in order to obtain pain-free weight-bearing and gait improvement. There is currently no consensus on the best surgical approach for this procedure; hence, a variety of techniques exist. This procedure is performed both open and arthroscopically. The arthroscopic approach is usually selected in patients with minimal-to-no malalignment, whereas the open approach is preferred for patients with moderate-to-severe deformity for better joint visualization and alignment correction. Both internal and external fixation may be used in tibiotalar arthrodesis; successful outcomes have been demonstrated with both methods [24,25].

Various methods of internal fixation have been described, including screws, plates, and retrograde intramedullary nails. Many surgeons prefer to use screws as the primary means of internal fixation because screws are easy to use, have low morbidity, and are less expensive compared to most other methods. However, higher nonunion rates of the ankle joint have been reported with screw fixation, especially in demineralized bone [26]. Plates are advantageous for ankle arthrodesis because they are stiffer constructs than screws and may achieve better union rates; there are also many options available in terms of plate size and shape. However, the extensive dissection needed to place a plate can lead to a higher risk of infection and morbidity [27,28]. A combination of plates and screws may also be used. A recent biomechanical study found that a combination of plates and screws provided significantly greater stiffness than plates or screws alone [28]. Retrograde intramedullary arthrodesis is typically reserved for arthrodesis of both the ankle and subtalar joints.

An osteotomy of the distal fibula is often made proximal to the ankle joint. The resected fibular bone block can be discarded or kept for use as an autologous bone graft later on in the case. The tibiotalar joint is typically fixed using two to three cannulated screws after adequate alignment is obtained. Fusion of lateral malleolus to tibia is then performed using two screws. The fibular bone graft may then be used about the fusion site to facilitate union (Figure 6E).

Radiographs are obtained at regular intervals postoperatively to assess for complications at the fusion site and the adequacy of osseous union. The development of osteoarthritis in adjacent joints should also be monitored.

4. Osseous Resection

4.1. Accessory Navicular Resection

Though the majority of patients with an accessory navicular are asymptomatic, a small fraction of patients may develop pain, which is thought to be related to traction from the posterior tibialis tendon (PTT). A type II accessory navicular (triangular or semicircular ossicle attached to the navicular by a fibrocartilage or hyaline-cartilage synchondrosis) is most likely to become symptomatic [29,30]. Patients are most often managed conservatively, but for refractory cases the accessory navicular may be surgically resected. Surgical techniques can be described with regard to their degree of manipulation of the PTT. In simple excision, the dorsal PTT is lifted away from the ossicle and the plantar PTT is not disturbed. Any dissected PTT is reattached to the navicular proper. In the Kidner procedure the ossicle is resected, the PTT is detached and advanced through a tunnel in the medial navicular and sutured to itself and the navicular periosteum [31,32].

Preoperative radiographs may demonstrate degenerative changes across the synchondrosis associated with a type II accessory navicular. Magnetic resonance imaging (MRI) is superior in detecting bone-marrow edema in the ossicle and/or navicular proper as well as posterior tibial tendinosis. Postoperative radiographs are acquired to confirm complete resection of the ossicle. Postoperative MRI may be obtained as indicated to evaluate the integrity of the PTT (Figure 8).

4.2. Cheilectomy

Cheilectomy (derived from the Greek word, *cheil*, meaning tongue) involves the resection of dorsal osteophytes from the first metatarsal head. Sometimes as much as one-third of the dorsal-metatarsal head bone stock is resected [33]. Typically, cheilectomy is performed for mild-to-moderate first MTP arthritis and results in pain relief and improved range of motion. For severe first MTP arthritis, arthrodesis is preferred. Postoperatively, lateral radiographs are helpful in detecting subtotal resection or osteophyte recurrence.

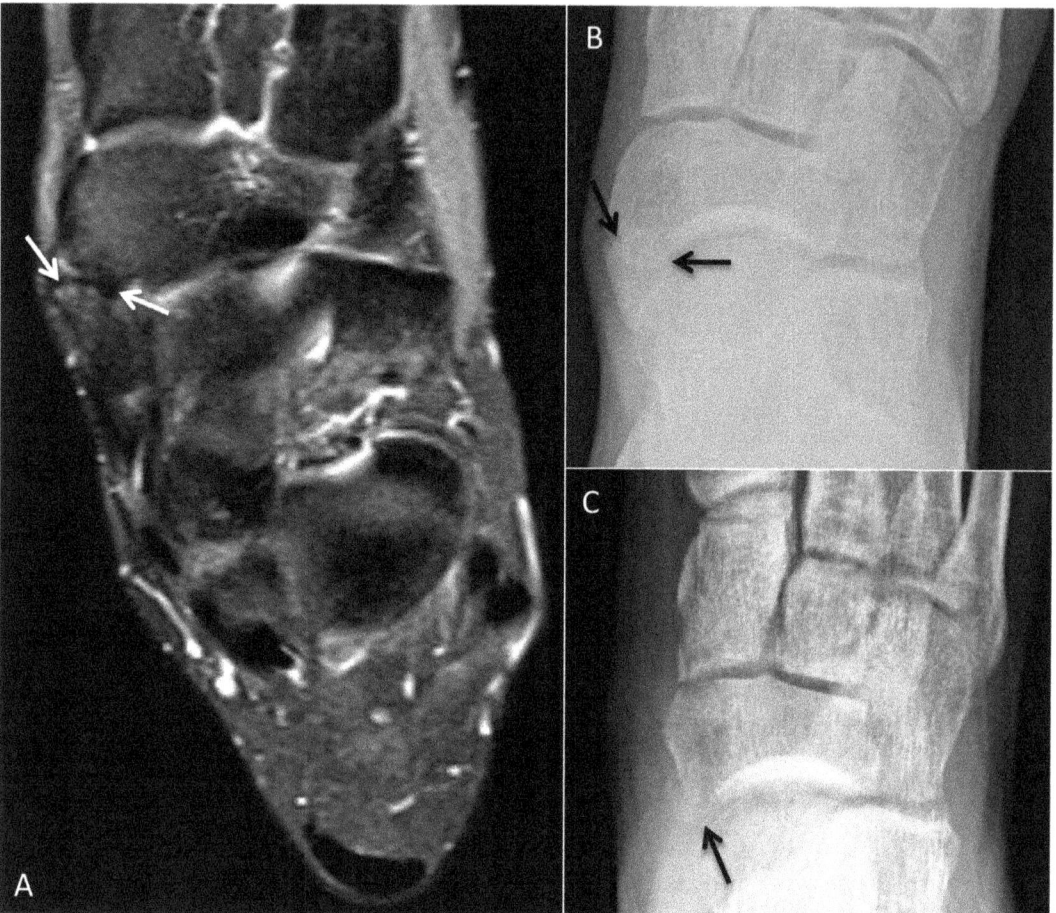

Figure 8. Pre- and postoperative images in a patient with a symptomatic accessory navicular. (**A**) Preoperative axial PD fat-suppressed MR image with mild edema/degenerative changes at the accessory navicular synchondrosis (arrow). (**B**) Preoperative radiograph with type II accessory navicular (arrows). (**C**) Postoperative changes from accessory navicular resection without complication (arrow).

5. Articular Implants

5.1. Polyvinyl Alcohol Hydrogel Hemiarthroplasty/Synthetic Cartilage Implant (SCI)

The goal of polyvinyl alcohol (PVA) hydrogel hemiarthroplasty, commonly known by its trade name Cartiva, is to relieve pain and improve range of motion in patients with first MTP osteoarthritis and/or moderate-to-severe hallux rigidus [33,34]. It can be performed in patients with mild hallux valgus deformities. The implant is made of polyvinyl alcohol, a synthetic polymer with biochemical properties similar to cartilage [35]. A precisely measured cylindrical hole is drilled through the central cartilage and subchondral bone of the metatarsal head and the implant is pressed into place without screws or cement. Cheilectomy is often performed concurrently. The phalangeal side of the joint remains unaltered (Figure 9A).

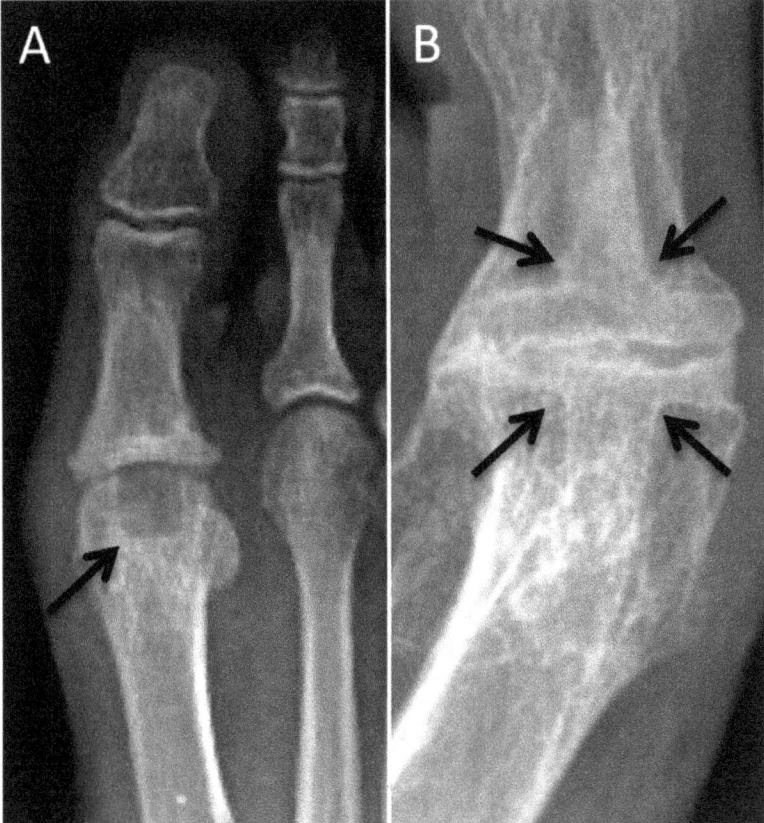

Figure 9. Implants. (**A**) AP radiograph demonstrating postoperative changes related to Cartiva implant (arrow) with geographic rectangular lucency in the first metatarsal head. (**B**) AP radiograph showing silastic implant (arrows) of the first MTP joint. Note flat articular surfaces and triangular shape of stems.

Postoperative radiographs are obtained at regular intervals to assess for complications, including implant displacement, loosening, subsidence, and recurrent osteophyte formation. Radiographically, the implant appears as a geographic rectangular lucency in the first-metatarsal head. Cross-sectional imaging better demonstrates the cylindrical shape of the implant.

5.2. Silastic Implant

Arthroplasty utilizing high-performance silicone implants, termed silastic implants, was originally performed in joints of the hand. In the foot, a single-stem silastic implant for a first MTP hemi-arthroplasty was first used in 1968. The procedure has undergone multiple iterations since that time, with current techniques utilizing double-stem, hinged implants [36]. Indications include severe inflammatory arthritis or osteoarthritis, with or without hallux limitus or hallux rigidus [36–39]. Some authors advocate for the use of this technique in older, less active patients, as this population demonstrates the best clinical outcomes with fewer complications [38]. Prerequisites for silastic-implant placement include intact collateral ligaments and sufficient bone stock. After resection of the articular surface, the medullary cavity is opened, taking care to preserve the collateral ligaments. A trial prosthesis is placed, and the joint is manipulated under fluoroscopy to assess for joint subluxation. The final prosthesis is then inserted with a press-fit technique. The implant acts as a spacer and is not designed to function as a joint replacement. Specific attention must be given to the rebalancing of the soft-tissue structures in an effort to restore the balance of the MTP [36].

Radiographically, silastic implants have increased density relative to the adjacent bone (Figure 9B). The articular surfaces are flat and should closely oppose one another. The component stems are triangular in shape and should be flush with the native bone. Postoperative radiographs should be scrutinized for implant fracture, periprosthetic fracture, and signs of osteolysis or implant loosening [40]. Importantly, the presence of periprosthetic cystic changes and osteolysis may be seen in a large proportion of asymptomatic patients.

5.3. Subtalar Arthroereisis

Patients with flexible flatfoot deformity (hindfoot valgus, talar plantar flexion, and longitudinal arch collapse) who fail conservative management may benefit from surgical intervention [41]. Arthroereisis is a surgical procedure where a bioabsorbable or titanium implant is inserted into the sinus tarsi, expanding the subtalar joint and biomechanically restricting flatfoot deformity [42–44]. The name is derived from the Greek root -ereisis, translated as the action of supporting or lifting up.

Preoperative weight-bearing radiographs demonstrate the degree of flatfoot deformity and the morphology of the subtalar joint, and allow for related presurgical measurements. Intraoperatively, the size of the implant is determined based on the range of motion of the subtalar joint. Intraoperative fluoroscopic or radiographic images are used to assess implant alignment and ensure adequate correction of the deformity. Postoperative radiographs demonstrate the arthroereisis as a radiodense cylindrical implant located between the anterior and posterior subtalar facets near the angle of Gissane (Figure 10). On the lateral radiograph, the tip of the implant should be within the subtalar joint with its long axis parallel to the joint space. On anteroposterior radiographs of the foot, the implant should project over the middle third of the talus. Its lateral margin should align with or be slightly medial to the lateral margin of the calcaneus. Postsurgical weight-bearing radiographs demonstrate the degree of operative correction.

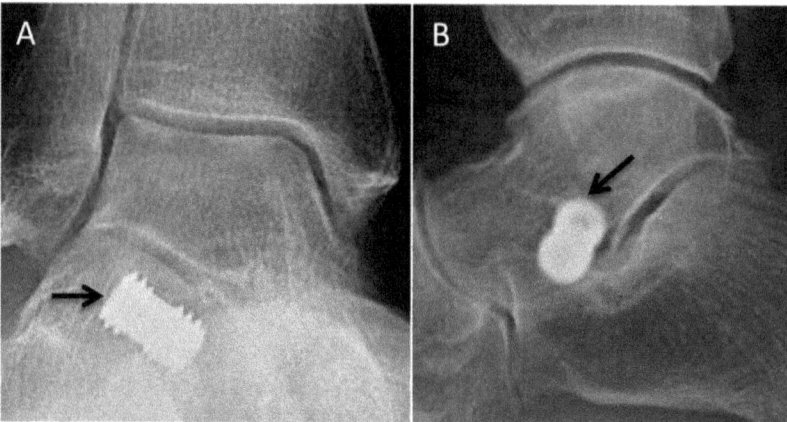

Figure 10. (**A**) AP and (**B**) lateral radiographs demonstrating the arthroereisis screw expanding the subtalar joint (black arrows) positioned between the anterior and posterior subtalar articulations.

Complications such as implant loosening, dislocation, lateral extrusion, and overcorrection of the deformity may be appreciated radiographically (Figure 11) [43]. Subtle implant migration, fractures, and peri-hardware lucency may be better evaluated with CT, whereas MRI may demonstrate postoperative soft-tissue abnormalities or bone-marrow edema [43]. Patients may complain of postoperative pain from sinus tarsi syndrome or accelerated subtalar osteoarthritis, which may be severe enough to require implant removal (Figure 12) [45].

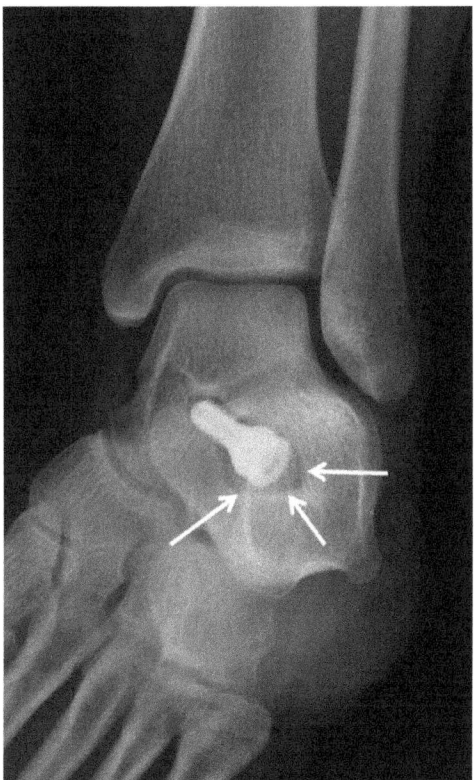

Figure 11. Prior history of subtalar arthroereisis placement. Mortise radiograph of the ankle demonstrates increased lucency surrounding the hardware concerning for loosening (white arrows).

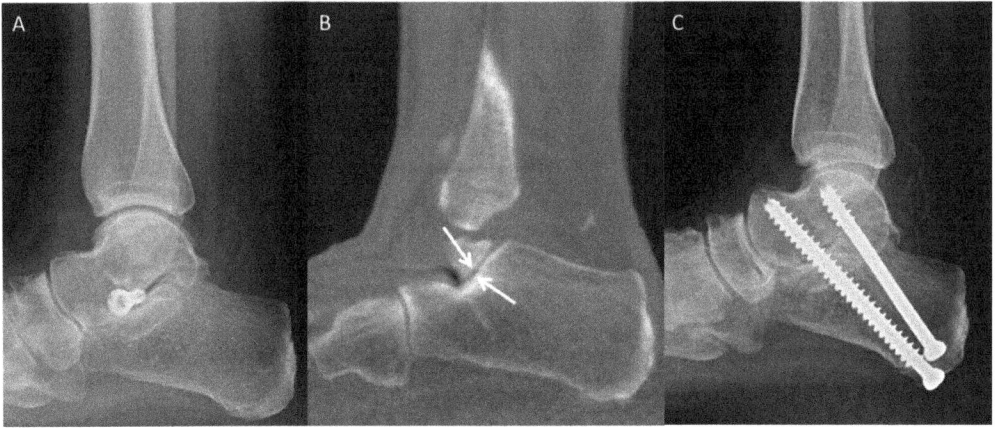

Figure 12. Prior left arthroereisis placement (**A**) developed hindfoot pain. Weight-bearing CT (**B**) demonstrates accelerated posterior subtalar facet degenerative changes (white arrows). Patient underwent implant removal and subsequent subtalar arthrodesis (**C**) with resolution of pain.

5.4. Total Ankle Arthroplasty

Total ankle arthroplasty was developed as an alternative to arthrodesis in patients with end-stage tibiotalar arthrodesis who failed conservative management, with the goals of decreasing pain and restoring ankle alignment while maintaining range of motion. Several generations of these implants exist, with the second and third generations being the most commonly used today. The implants are divided into mobile-bearing and fixed-bearing models based on whether or not the polyethylene spacer is mobile or fixed to the tibial component [46,47].

As with all implants, postoperative evaluation is focused on potential complications, not dissimilar to other arthroplasties, and includes periprosthetic lucency/fracture, osteolysis, and subsidence (Figure 13) [48].

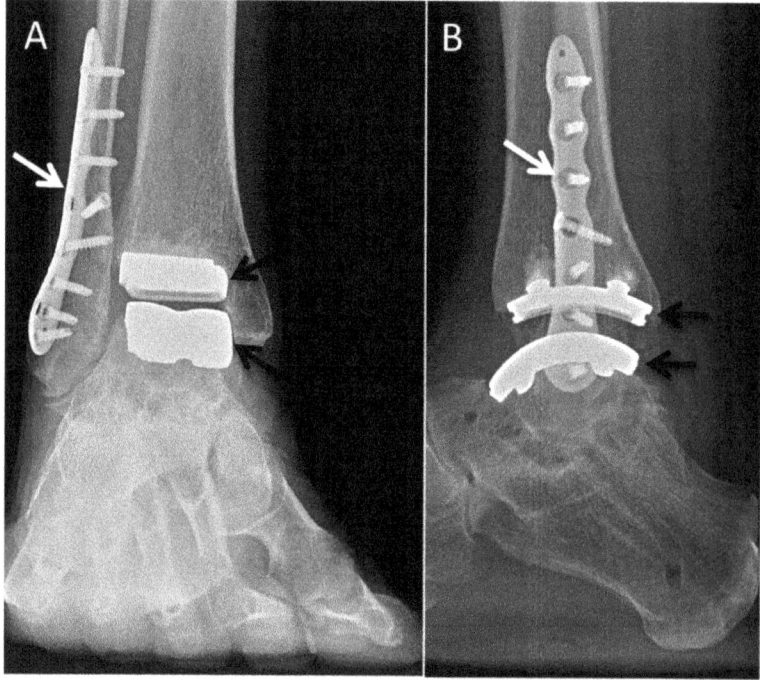

Figure 13. Mobile-bearing total ankle arthroplasty. AP (**A**) and lateral (**B**) radiographs demonstrating well-seated tibial and talar components (black arrows) without abnormal lucency or fracture. Fibular osteotomy (white arrows).

Funding: This review received no external funding.

Institutional Review Board Statement: Not applicable.

Conflicts of Interest: The authors do not have conflict of interest to declare.

References

1. Belatti, D.A.; Phisitkul, P. Economic Burden of Foot and Ankle Surgery in the US Medicare Population. *Foot Ankle Int.* **2014**, *35*, 334–340. [CrossRef] [PubMed]
2. Martin DE, P.J. Introduction and evaluation of hallux abducto valgus. In *McGlamry's Comprehensive Textbook of Foot and Ankle Surgery*; McGlamry, E.D., Banks, A.S., Eds.; Lippincott Williams & Wilkins: Philadelphia, PA, USA, 2001; pp. 481–491. ISBN 978-0-683-30471-8.
3. Ramdass, R.; Meyr, A.J. The Multiplanar Effect of First Metatarsal Osteotomy on Sesamoid Position. *J. Foot Ankle Surg. Off. Publ. Am. Coll. Foot Ankle Surg.* **2010**, *49*, 63–67. [CrossRef]

4. Springer, K.R. The Role of the Akin Osteotomy in the Surgical Management of Hallux Abducto Valgus. *Clin. Podiatr. Med. Surg.* **1989**, *6*, 115–131. [PubMed]
5. Austin, D.W.; Leventen, E.O. A New Osteotomy for Hallux Valgus: A Horizontally Directed "V" Displacement Osteotomy of the Metatarsal Head for Hallux Valgus and Primus Varus. *Clin. Orthop.* **1981**, *157*, 25–30. [CrossRef]
6. Johnson, K.A.; Cofield, R.H.; Morrey, B.F. Chevron Osteotomy for Hallux Valgus. *Clin. Orthop.* **1979**, *142*, 44–47. [CrossRef]
7. Kalish, S.R.; Spector, J.E. The Kalish Osteotomy. A Review and Retrospective Analysis of 265 Cases. *J. Am. Podiatr. Med. Assoc.* **1994**, *84*, 237–242. [CrossRef] [PubMed]
8. Isham, S.A. The Reverdin-Isham Procedure for the Correction of Hallux Abducto Valgus. A Distal Metatarsal Osteotomy Procedure. *Clin. Podiatr. Med. Surg.* **1991**, *8*, 81–94. [PubMed]
9. Weil, L.S. Scarf Osteotomy for Correction of Hallux Valgus. Historical Perspective, Surgical Technique, and Results. *Foot Ankle Clin.* **2000**, *5*, 559–580.
10. Nigro, J.S.; Greger, G.M.; Catanzariti, A.R. Closing Base Wedge Osteotomy. *J. Foot Surg.* **1991**, *30*, 494–505.
11. Hofbauer, M.H.; Grossman, J.P. The Lapidus Procedure. *Clin. Podiatr. Med. Surg.* **1996**, *13*, 485–496.
12. Coughlin, M.J. Lesser Toe Abnormalities. *Instr. Course Lect.* **2003**, *52*, 421–444. [CrossRef] [PubMed]
13. Barouk, L.S. Weil's metatarsal osteotomy in the treatment of metatarsalgia. *Orthopade* **1996**, *25*, 338–344. [CrossRef] [PubMed]
14. Hart, R.; Janecek, M.; Bucek, P. The Weil osteotomy in metatarsalgia. *Z. Orthop. Ihre Grenzgeb.* **2003**, *141*, 590–594. [CrossRef] [PubMed]
15. Dwyer, F.C. Osteotomy of the Calcaneum for Pes Cavus. *J. Bone Jt. Surg. Br.* **1959**, *41*, 80–86. [CrossRef] [PubMed]
16. Evans, D. Calcaneo-Valgus Deformity. *J. Bone Jt. Surg. Br.* **1975**, *57*, 270–278. [CrossRef]
17. Kraus, J.C.; Fischer, M.T.; McCormick, J.J.; Klein, S.E.; Johnson, J.E. Geometry of the Lateral Sliding, Closing Wedge Calcaneal Osteotomy: Review of the Two Methods and Technical Tip to Minimize Shortening. *Foot Ankle Int.* **2014**, *35*, 238–242. [CrossRef] [PubMed]
18. Saltzman, C.L.; el-Khoury, G.Y. The Hindfoot Alignment View. *Foot Ankle Int.* **1995**, *16*, 572–576. [CrossRef]
19. Greenfield, S.; Cohen, B. Calcaneal Osteotomies: Pearls and Pitfalls. *Foot Ankle Clin.* **2017**, *22*, 563–571. [CrossRef]
20. Matthews, M.; Cook, E.A.; Cook, J.; Johnson, L.; Karthas, T.; Collier, B.; Hansen, D.; Manning, E.; McKenna, B.; Basile, P. Long-Term Outcomes of Corrective Osteotomies Using Porous Titanium Wedges for Flexible Flatfoot Deformity Correction. *J. Foot Ankle Surg. Off. Publ. Am. Coll. Foot Ankle Surg.* **2018**, *57*, 924–930. [CrossRef]
21. Wu, B.; Huang, G.; Ding, Z. Application Strategy of Ankle and Hindfoot Arthrodesis. *Zhongguo Xiu Fu Chong Jian Wai Ke Za Zhi Zhongguo Xiufu Chongjian Waike Zazhi Chin. J. Reparative Reconstr. Surg.* **2016**, *30*, 514–517.
22. Wülker, N.; Flamme, C. Hindfoot arthrodesis. *Orthopade* **1996**, *25*, 177–186. [PubMed]
23. Wapner, K.L. Triple Arthrodesis in Adults. *J. Am. Acad. Orthop. Surg.* **1998**, *6*, 188–196. [CrossRef] [PubMed]
24. Wang, L.; Gui, J.; Gao, F.; Yu, Z.; Jiang, Y.; Xu, Y.; Shen, H. Modified Posterior Portals for Hindfoot Arthroscopy. *Arthrosc. J. Arthrosc. Relat. Surg. Off. Publ. Arthrosc. Assoc. N. Am. Int. Arthrosc. Assoc.* **2007**, *23*, 1116–1123. [CrossRef] [PubMed]
25. Stone, J.W. Arthroscopic Ankle Arthrodesis. *Foot Ankle Clin.* **2006**, *11*, 361–368. [CrossRef] [PubMed]
26. Thordarson, D.B.; Markolf, K.; Cracchiolo, A. Stability of an Ankle Arthrodesis Fixed by Cancellous-Bone Screws Compared with That Fixed by an External Fixator. A Biomechanical Study. *J. Bone Jt. Surg. Am.* **1992**, *74*, 1050–1055. [CrossRef]
27. Betz, M.M.; Benninger, E.E.; Favre, P.P.; Wieser, K.K.; Vich, M.M.; Espinosa, N. Primary Stability and Stiffness in Ankle Arthrodes-Crossed Screws versus Anterior Plating. *Foot Ankle Surg. Off. J. Eur. Soc. Foot Ankle Surg.* **2013**, *19*, 168–172. [CrossRef]
28. Clifford, C.; Berg, S.; McCann, K.; Hutchinson, B. A Biomechanical Comparison of Internal Fixation Techniques for Ankle Arthrodesis. *J. Foot Ankle Surg. Off. Publ. Am. Coll. Foot Ankle Surg.* **2015**, *54*, 188–191. [CrossRef]
29. Al-Khudairi, N.; Welck, M.J.; Brandao, B.; Saifuddin, A. The Relationship of MRI Findings and Clinical Features in Symptomatic and Asymptomatic Os Naviculare. *Clin. Radiol.* **2019**, *74*, 80.e1–80.e6. [CrossRef]
30. Chan, B.Y.; Markhardt, B.K.; Williams, K.L.; Kanarek, A.A.; Ross, A.B. Os Conundrum: Identifying Symptomatic Sesamoids and Accessory Ossicles of the Foot. *AJR Am. J. Roentgenol.* **2019**, *213*, 417–426. [CrossRef]
31. Roddy, E.; Menz, H.B. Foot Osteoarthritis: Latest Evidence and Developments. *Ther. Adv. Musculoskelet. Dis.* **2018**, *10*, 91–103. [CrossRef]
32. Cha, S.-M.; Shin, H.-D.; Kim, K.-C.; Lee, J.-K. Simple Excision vs the Kidner Procedure for Type 2 Accessory Navicular Associated with Flatfoot in Pediatric Population. *Foot Ankle Int.* **2013**, *34*, 167–172. [CrossRef] [PubMed]
33. Anderson, M.R.; Ho, B.S.; Baumhauer, J.F. Current Concepts Review: Hallux Rigidus. *Foot Ankle Orthop.* **2018**, *3*, 247301141876446. [CrossRef]
34. Baumhauer, J.F.; Singh, D.; Glazebrook, M.; Blundell, C.; De Vries, G.; Le, I.L.D.; Nielsen, D.; Pedersen, M.E.; Sakellariou, A.; Solan, M.; et al. Prospective, Randomized, Multi-Centered Clinical Trial Assessing Safety and Efficacy of a Synthetic Cartilage Implant Versus First Metatarsophalangeal Arthrodesis in Advanced Hallux Rigidus. *Foot Ankle Int.* **2016**, *37*, 457–469. [CrossRef]
35. Younger, A.S.E.; Baumhauer, J.F. Polyvinyl Alcohol Hydrogel Hemiarthroplasty of the Great Toe: Technique and Indications. *Tech. Foot Ankle Surg.* **2013**, *12*, 164–169. [CrossRef]
36. Lemon, B.; Pupp, G.R. Long-Term Efficacy of Total SILASTIC Implants: A Subjective Analysis. *J. Foot Ankle Surg. Off. Publ. Am. Coll. Foot Ankle Surg.* **1997**, *36*, 341–346; discussion 396–397. [CrossRef]
37. Sullivan, M.R. Hallux Rigidus: MTP Implant Arthroplasty. *Foot Ankle Clin.* **2009**, *14*, 33–42. [CrossRef] [PubMed]

38. Morgan, S.; Ng, A.; Clough, T. The Long-Term Outcome of Silastic Implant Arthroplasty of the First Metatarsophalangeal Joint: A Retrospective Analysis of One Hundred and Eight Feet. *Int. Orthop.* **2012**, *36*, 1865–1869. [CrossRef]
39. Brage, M.E.; Ball, S.T. Surgical Options for Salvage of End-Stage Hallux Rigidus. *Foot Ankle Clin.* **2002**, *7*, 49–73. [CrossRef]
40. Manaster, B.J. Diagnostic Imaging. In *Musculoskeletal: Non-Traumatic Disease*; Elsevier: Philadelphia, PA, USA, 2016; ISBN 978-0-323-39252-5.
41. Nelson, S.C.; Haycock, D.M.; Little, E.R. Flexible Flatfoot Treatment with Arthroereisis: Radiographic Improvement and Child Health Survey Analysis. *J. Foot Ankle Surg. Off. Publ. Am. Coll. Foot Ankle Surg.* **2004**, *43*, 144–155. [CrossRef]
42. Metcalfe, S.A.; Bowling, F.L.; Reeves, N.D. Subtalar Joint Arthroereisis in the Management of Pediatric Flexible Flatfoot: A Critical Review of the Literature. *Foot Ankle Int.* **2011**, *32*, 1127–1139. [CrossRef]
43. Nevalainen, M.T.; Roedl, J.B.; Zoga, A.C.; Morrison, W.B. Imaging Findings of Arthroereisis in Planovalgus Feet. *Radiol. Case Rep.* **2016**, *11*, 398–404. [CrossRef] [PubMed]
44. LiMarzi, G.M.; Scherer, K.F.; Richardson, M.L.; Warden, D.R.; Wasyliw, C.W.; Porrino, J.A.; Pettis, C.R.; Lewis, G.; Mason, C.C.; Bancroft, L.W. CT and MR Imaging of the Postoperative Ankle and Foot. *RadioGraphics* **2016**, *36*, 1828–1848. [CrossRef] [PubMed]
45. Dimmick, S.; Chhabra, A.; Grujic, L.; Linklater, J.M. Acquired Flat Foot Deformity: Postoperative Imaging. In *Seminars in Musculoskeletal Radiology*; Thieme Medical Publishers: New York, NY, USA, 2012; Volume 16, pp. 217–232. [CrossRef]
46. Haddad, S.L.; Coetzee, J.C.; Estok, R.; Fahrbach, K.; Banel, D.; Nalysnyk, L. Intermediate and Long-Term Outcomes of Total Ankle Arthroplasty and Ankle Arthrodesis. A Systematic Review of the Literature. *J. Bone Jt. Surg. Am.* **2007**, *89*, 1899–1905. [CrossRef]
47. Kim, H.J.; Suh, D.H.; Yang, J.H.; Lee, J.W.; Kim, H.J.; Ahn, H.S.; Han, S.W.; Choi, G.W. Total Ankle Arthroplasty versus Ankle Arthrodesis for the Treatment of End-Stage Ankle Arthritis: A Meta-Analysis of Comparative Studies. *Int. Orthop.* **2017**, *41*, 101–109. [CrossRef] [PubMed]
48. Hanna, R.S.; Haddad, S.L.; Lazarus, M.L. Evaluation of Periprosthetic Lucency after Total Ankle Arthroplasty: Helical CT versus Conventional Radiography. *Foot Ankle Int.* **2007**, *28*, 921–926. [CrossRef] [PubMed]

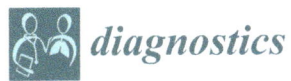

Article

Short-Term and Long-Term Changes of Nasal Soft Tissue after Rapid Maxillary Expansion (RME) with Tooth-Borne and Bone-Borne Devices. A CBCT Retrospective Study.

Pietro Venezia [1], Ludovica Nucci [2], Serena Moschitto [1], Alessia Malgioglio [1], Gaetano Isola [1], Vincenzo Ronsivalle [1], Valeria Venticinque [1], Rosalia Leonardi [1], Manuel O. Lagraverè [3] and Antonino Lo Giudice [1,*]

[1] Department of Medical-Surgical Specialties, Section of Orthodontics, School of Dentistry, University of Catania, Policlinico Universitario "G. Rodolico-San Marco", Via Santa Sofia 78, 95123 Catania, Italy; pierovenezia@gmail.com (P.V.); serenamoschitto@gmail.com (S.M.); ale.malgioglio@gmail.com (A.M.); gaetano.isola@unict.it (G.I.); vincenzo.ronsivalle@hotmail.it (V.R.); valeria251996@gmail.com (V.V.); rleonard@unict.it (R.L.)

[2] Multidisciplinary Department of Medical-Surgical and Dental Specialties, University of Campania "Luigi Vanvitelli", Via Luigi de Crecchio 6, 80138 Naples, Italy; ludortho@gmail.com

[3] Orthodontic Graduate Program, University of Alberta, Edmonton, AB T6G 2B7, Canada; manuel@ualberta.ca

* Correspondence: antonino.logiudice@unict.it

Abstract: The objective of the study was to assess the changes in nasal soft tissues after RME was performed with tooth-borne (TB) and bone-borne (BB) appliances. Methods. This study included 40 subjects with a diagnosis of posterior cross-bite who received tooth-borne RME (TB, average age: 11.75 ± 1.13 years) or bone-borne RME (BB, average age: 12.68 ± 1.31 years). Cone-beam computed tomography (CBCT) was taken before treatment (T0), after a 6-month retention period (T1), and one year after retention (T2). Specific linear measurements of the skeletal components and of the soft-tissue region of the nose were performed. All data were statistically analyzed. Results. Concerning skeletal measurements, the BB group showed a greater skeletal expansion of the anterior and posterior region of the nose compared to the TB group ($p < 0.05$) immediately after RME. Both TB and BB RME induce a small increment (>1 mm) of the alar base and alar width, without significant differences between the two expansion methods ($p > 0.05$). A high correlation was found between skeletal and soft-tissue expansion in the TB group; instead, a weaker correlation was found in the BB group. Conclusion. A similar slight increment of the alar width and alar base width was found in both TB and BB groups. However, the clinical relevance of these differences, in terms of facial appearance, remains questionable.

Keywords: rapid maxillary expansion; bone-borne RME; tooth-borne RME; orthodontic; facial aesthetics

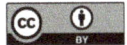

1. Introduction

Rapid maxillary expansion (RME) is the treatment of choice for the correction of transverse maxillary deficiency [1]. RME consists of the separation of the mid-palatal suture, obtained by applying orthopaedic forces through intra-oral devices [2]. The most common design of RME devices is a tooth-borne (TB) expander [3]. Since the TB expander is directly anchored to the teeth, generally the upper first molars, the forces generated by the activation of the appliance can determine undesirable effects on the dentition and alveolar structures [4]. In this regard, common side-effects in TB-RME have been described, such as dental tipping, root resorption, marginal bone loss and reduction in buccal bone thickness [5–7], and to moderate these side effects, it has been proposed to support palatal expanders with temporary skeletal anchorage devices (TADs) [8,9]. The skeletal effects and pattern of expansion of TB-RME-RME have been widely documented in the literature [10];

also, recent evidence has suggested that bone-borne (BB) expander could generate greater skeletal expansion compared to TB expander [8].

The effects of RME are not limited to the maxilla but can be extended to the circummaxillary structure as well as several other adjacent structures in the face and the cranium [11,12]. In particular, it can also influence the anatomy and the physiology of the nasal structures [13]. Previous studies [14,15] showed that RME enlarges the dimension of the nasal cavity (about one-third of appliance expansion) and increases its volume by displacing the nasal lateral walls apart. These changes could explain the improvement of nasal breathing and the reduction in nasal airway resistance often recorded in treated subjects [16].

Conversely, the effect of RME on nasal soft tissue has not been deeply investigated, and the few studies available are mostly related to the evaluation of post-treatment changes of surgically assisted RME in adult subjects [17,18]. In this regard, it would be interesting to understand if certain dimensional changes of nasal soft tissue should be expected after RME even in growing subjects, considering that treatment results, including nasal proportions, influence patients' aesthetic appearance [19]. This aspect is of great clinical relevance considering that transverse skeletal maxillary deficiency is one of the most common skeletal deformities of the craniofacial region among youngsters [20]. In this respect, the aim of the present study was to assess the soft tissue changes of the nose after RME was performed on growing subjects and to evaluate if these changes are different between TB and BB maxillary expanders. For this purpose, we analysed the 3D rendered facial models obtained from cone-beam computed tomography (CBCT) scans of the included subjects. Since BB-RME has shown greater skeletal effects compared to TB-RME [8], we assumed that RME supported by skeletal anchorage (BB-RME) might determine greater soft tissue nasal changes compared to TB-RME, and this assumption was the null hypothesis of the present study.

2. Materials and Methods

2.1. Study Sample

The research protocol of this retrospective study was approved by the Ethics Review Board of Alberta University (IRB protocol number: Pro00075765) and included a sample of young subjects who completed their orthodontic treatment at the Orthodontic Clinic of the University of Alberta (Edmonton, Canada). Subjects were recruited between September 2019 and August 2021 and randomly assigned to TB-RME or BB-RME. Moreover, the CBCTs used for the present study were obtained from previously published materials [21,22] to avoid unnecessary or additional radiation exposure to the patients. All subjects signed appropriate forms for consent to the treatment.

Inclusion criteria were as follows: (1) age between 11 and 16 years (to avoid extreme differences in the skeletal maturation stage among individuals), registered at the first CBCT acquisition, (2) full permanent dentition (except for the third molar), (3) posterior crossbite, (4) CBCT scans with the field of view (FOV) including all relevant anatomical areas for head orientation and measurements, (5) no artifacts, (6) no temporomandibular joint disorder, (7) no previous orthodontic treatment, (8) no craniofacial anomalies of skeletal and soft-tissue. Figure 1 shows data recruitment process of the present retrospective study.

2.2. Treatment

The TB group received a Hyrax appliance designed with bands on the first permanent molars and first premolars. The design of the expander in the BB group includes two mini-screws (length: 12 mm; diameter: 1.5 mm; Straumann GBR System, Andover, MA, USA) inserted in the basal bone at the level corresponding to the area between the permanent first molars and second premolars and joined by a jackscrew.

In both groups, the activation protocol was 0.25 mm/turn with 2 turns per day (0.5 mm/d) in both groups. Expansion screw activations were stopped when overexpansion was achieved, i.e., when the mesiopalatal cusps of the maxillary first permanent molars were in contact with the buccal cusps of the mandibular first permanent molars. The device was maintained for a further 6 months to maintain the results obtained, and no other orthodontic device/therapy was administered to the patient. Parents received a specific form where they reported each activation performed according to the protocol established. The parents of all included subjects had strictly followed the prescription.

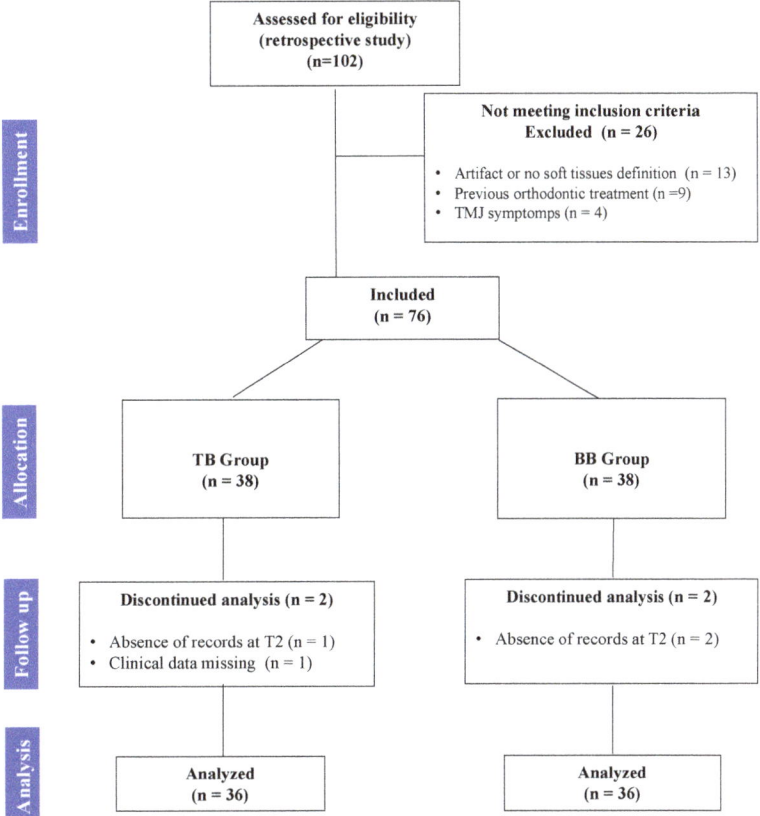

Figure 1. Flowchart showing data recruitment of the present retrospective study.

2.3. Image Acquisition

Cone Beam Computed Tomography (CBCT) was performed before treatment (T0), after 6 months (T1), and one year after retention (T2). Patients were scanned with the same iCAT CBCT unit (Imaging Sciences International, Hartfield, PA, USA). The acquisition protocol was the same for all subjects and included isotropic voxels of 0.3 mm in size, 8.9 s, wide field of view at 120 kV, and 20 mA. The distance between the 2 slices was 0.3 mm.

2.4. Skeletal Measurements

On multiple planar reconstruction images, the skull was reoriented to the Frankfort horizontal (FH) as follows (Figure 2): (1) in the frontal view, the mid-sagittal plane was fixed through the center of the anterior nasal spine (ANS), and the axial plane was constructed through both infraorbital skeletal landmarks; (2) in the right sagittal view, the axial plane was placed through the right porion and right infraorbital landmarks. For standardization, the left sagittal view was not processed to avoid orientation problems due to asymmetrically positioned portions; (3) in the axial view, the mid-sagittal plane was constructed through crista Galli and basion [23].

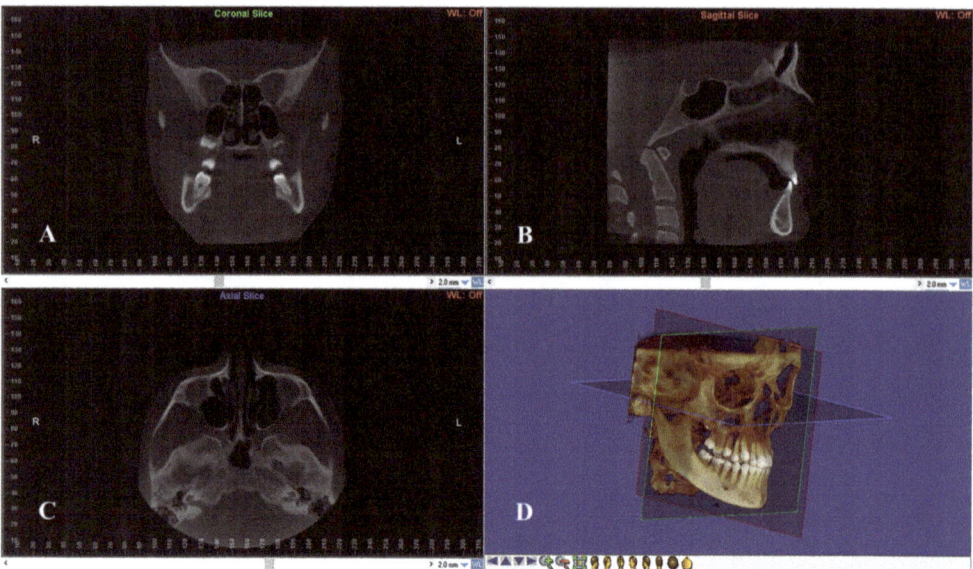

Figure 2. Head re-orientation on coronal (**A**), sagittal (**B**) and axial (**C**) planes of CBCT scans. The 3D image (**D**) shows the head orientation on a 3D space.

Afterward, the transverse dimension of the Apertura Piriformis was measured in the anterior and posterior regions. In the coronal plane passing through the cephalometric point N, the linear measurements of anterior nasal width (ANW) and anterior nasal floor width (ANFW) were performed (Figure 3, Table 1). Similarly, in the coronal plane passing through the upper margin of the mesial aspect of the Sella Turcica, the linear measurements of the posterior nasal width (PNW) and posterior nasal floor width (PNFW) were performed (Figure 4, Table 1). The entire procedure for skeletal measurements was performed by using the Dolphin 3D software (Dolphin Imaging, version 11.0, Chatsworth, CA, USA).

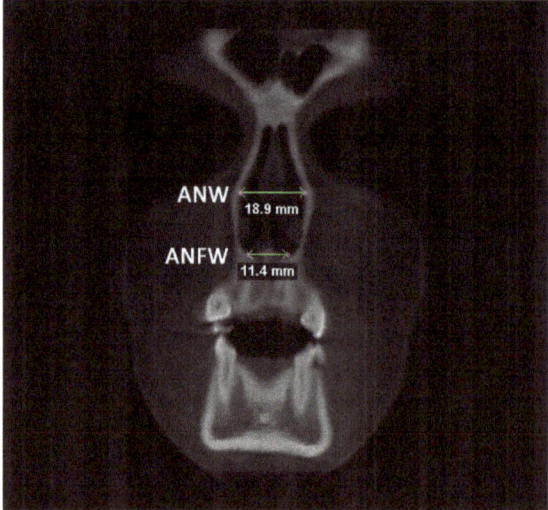

Figure 3. Linear measurements of anterior nasal width (ANW) and anterior nasal floor width (ANFW) in the coronal plane.

Table 1. Description of the linear measurements used in the present study.

	Measurements	Description
Skeletal Measurements	ANW Anterior Nasal Width	Distance between the most lateral points along the inner surface of nasal lateral walls, taken at the coronal plane passing through point N
	ANFW Anterior Nasal Floor Width	Distance between the most lateral points along the inner surface of nasal lateral walls at the nasal floor level, taken at the coronal plane passing through point N
	PNW Posterior Nasal Width	Distance between the most lateral points along the inner surface of nasal lateral walls, taken at the coronal plane passing through point S
	PNFW Posterior Nasal Floor Width	Distance between the most lateral points along the inner surface of nasal lateral walls at the nasal floor level, taken at the coronal plane passing through point S
Soft Tissue Measurements	AW Alar Width	Distance between the most lateral points of the alar curvatures on the right (rLAC) and left (lLAC) sides
	ABW Alar Base Width	Distance between the right point (rAB) and the left point (lAB) of the facial insertion of the alar base
	NL Nasal Lenght	Distance between the soft-tissue N point and PrN points
	NFL Nasal Filter Length	Distance between the PrN and SbN points
	NLA Nasolabial Angle	Angle between nasal filter and the profile of the upper lip

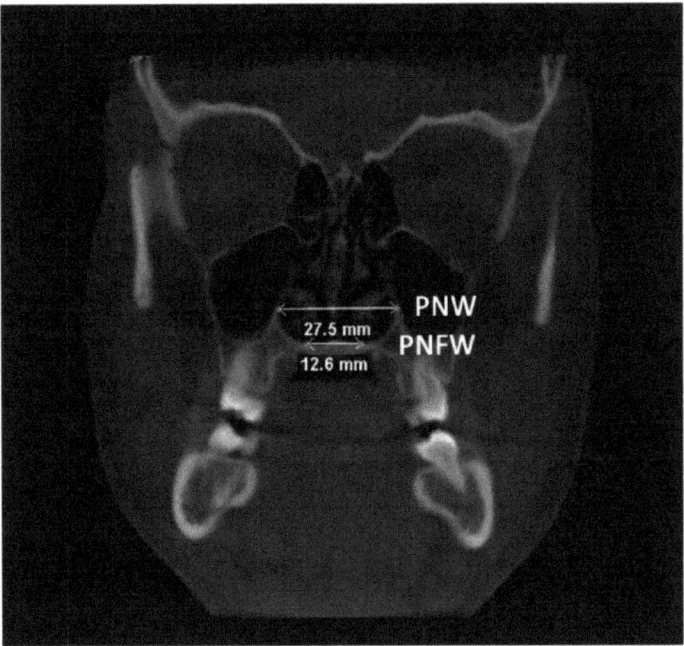

Figure 4. Linear measurements of the posterior nasal width (PNW) and the posterior nasal floor width (PNFW) in the coronal plane.

2.5. Soft Tissue Measurement

The segmentation mask of facial soft-tissue was created, setting the Hounsfield units threshold between −1024 and −200 and then converted into a 3D rendered model. The analysis of the nasal soft-tissue region was performed using the following measurements [17] (Table 1): Alar base width (ABW) (Figure 5), Alar width (AW) (Figure 5), Length of the nose (NL) (Figure 6), Length of the nasal filter (NFL) (Figure 6), Naso-labial angle (NLA) (Figure 7).

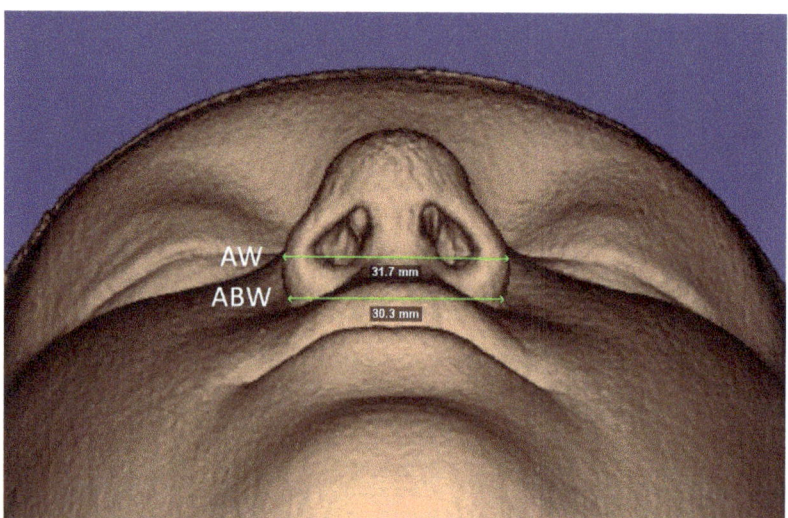

Figure 5. Facial soft-tissue linear measurements of the alar base width (ABW) and the alar width (AW).

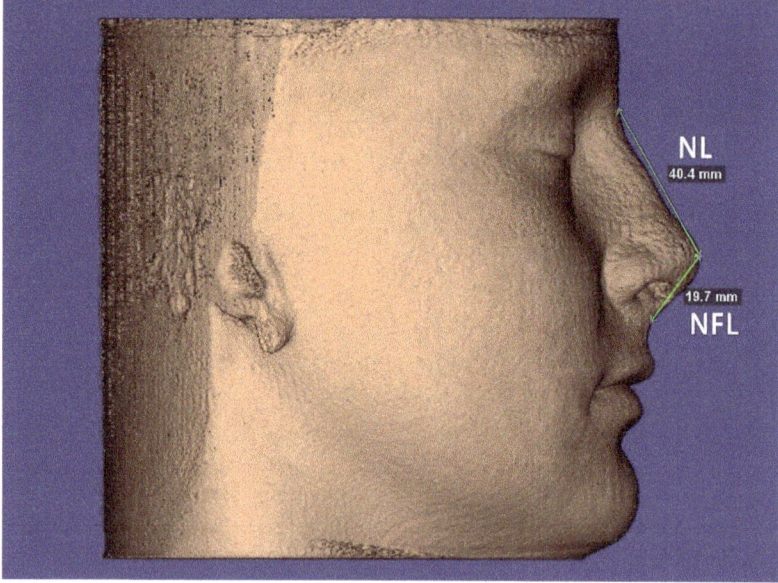

Figure 6. Facial soft-tissue linear measurements of the length of the nose (NL) and length of the nasal filter (NFL).

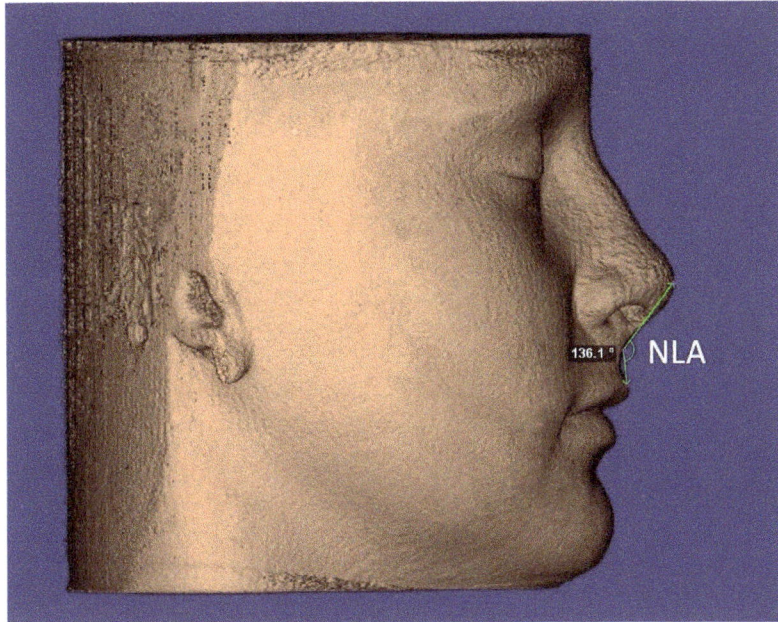

Figure 7. Facial soft-tissue linear measurement of the naso-labial angle (NLA).

The entire procedure for soft tissue measurements was performed by using the Dolphin 3D software (Dolphin Imaging, version 11.0, Chatsworth, CA, USA).

2.6. Statistical Analysis

2.6.1. Sample Size Calculation

In the absence of reference data from the literature, calculation of sample size power was preliminary carried out on 20 subjects (10 in the TB group and 10 in the BB group) using the following settings: primary outcome = measurements of ABW parameter, beta error = 0.20, alpha error = 0.05, comparison = difference in the T0-T1 changes of ABW in the TB group, software = SPSS® version 24 Statistics software (IBM Corporation, 1 New Orchard Road, Armonk, New York, NY, USA). The difference detected in the ABW parameter between T0 and T1 was 0.92 mm (SD = 0.88), and the analysis indicated that 28 patients were required to reach 80% power to detect the same difference. However, according to the inclusion criteria, we were able to include 40 subjects which increased the robustness of the data.

2.6.2. Data Analysis

The normal distribution and equality of variance of the data were preliminarily performed with the Shapiro–Wilk Normality Test and Levene's test. The one-way analysis of variance (ANOVA) and Scheffe's post-hoc comparisons tests were used for inter-timing assessments; instead, the unpaired Student's t-test was used for inter-group comparisons. Linear regression analysis was performed to investigate a cause-effect relationship between skeletal and soft-tissue changes, i.e., expansion of the Apertura piriformis (independent variable) and expansion of the alar width and alar base width (dependent variables). A Chi-square test and Student's *t*-test were used to assess the homogeneous distribution of sex and age variables between the TB and BB groups, respectively.

Ten patients were randomly selected, and the entire procedure was repeated by the same expert investigator (ALG) after 4 weeks. The same patients were also re-measured by a second expert operator (VR). Intra-examiner and inter-examiner reliability for the absolute agreement was assessed for each measurement using the intraclass correlation coefficient (ICC). Data sets were analysed using SPSS® version 24 Statistics software (IBM Corporation, 1 New Orchard Road, Armonk, New York, NY, USA).

3. Results

The demographic characteristics of the study sample are reported in Table 2. No differences were found between TB and BB groups concerning sex distribution. However, differences were detected between the two groups according to age distribution; in this regard, subjects in the TB group were about 1 year younger than those included in the BB group.

Table 2. Demographic characteristics of the study sample.

Sample Characteristics	Total Sample (n = 40)	TB Group (n = 20)	BB Group (n = 20)	Significance
Sex: male/female	17/23	9/11	8/12	$p = 0.21$ *
Age, y: mean (SD)	12.21 (1.46)	11.75 (1.13)	12.68 (1.31)	$p = 0.02$ **

* p value set as ≤ 0.05. and assessed by chi-square test; ** p value set as ≤ 0.05. and assessed by Student's t test.

In both TB and BB groups, there was a statistically significant expansion of the Apertura piriformis (ANW and ANFW) between T0 and T1 ($p < 0.05$), instead no differences were found between T1 and T2 ($p > 0.05$), thus maintaining the post-retention changes (Table 3). The expansion of the Apertura piriformis was significantly greater in the BB group compared to the TB group (TB) ($p < 0.05$) at each time point. The same findings were recorded for the PNW and PNFW measurements (Table 4).

Table 3. Inferential statistics of measurements calculated before treatment (T0), after 6 months (T1) and one year after treatment (T2).

Measurements	N	Groups	T0		T1		T2		Significance
			Mean	SD	Mean	SD	Mean	SD	
ANW	20	TB	28.01 (b,c)	1.69	29.13 (a)	1.81	29.06 (a)	1.77	$p = 0.0003$
	20	BB	28.32 (b,c)	2.07	30.33 (a)	2.11	30.46 (a)	2.14	$p = 0.0002$
ANFW	20	TB	17.09 (b,c)	2.75	18.7 (a)	2.66	18.5 (a)	2.69	$p = 0.0003$
	20	BB	17.75 (b,c)	1.98	20.41 (a)	1.85	20.53 (a)	1.91	$p < 0.0001$
PNW	20	TB	30.26 (b,c)	2.14	31.1 (a)	1.97	31.02 (a)	2.12	$p = 0.0072$
	20	BB	30.6 (b,c)	4.16	32.56 (a)	3.69	32.25 (a)	4.05	$p = 0.0001$
PNFW	20	TB	25.98 (b,c)	3.46	27.09 (a)	3.77	27.22 (a)	3.57	$p < 0.0001$
	20	BB	26.22 (b,c)	4.10	28.71 (a)	4.23	28.93 (a)	4.37	$p < 0.0001$
AW	20	TB	34.6 (b,c)	2.58	35.82 (a)	2.91	35.22 (a)	3.19	$p = 0.0035$
	20	BB	35.52 (b,c)	3.78	37.11 (a)	4.09	36.57 (a)	3.50	$p < 0.0001$
ABW	20	TB	32.53 (b,c)	3.52	33.56 (a)	3.21	33.6 (a)	3.40	$p = 0.0004$
	20	BB	33.24 (b,c)	3,12	34.49 (a)	3.29	34.66 (a)	3.08	$p = 0.0002$
NL	20	TB	44.45	2.93	44.93	3.27	44.40	3.29	$p = 0.0881$
	20	BB	47.12	5.60	47.65	5.44	47.13	5.28	$p = 0.0596$
NFL	20	TB	18.30	1.83	18.55	1.85	18.32	1.73	$p = 0.0743$
	20	BB	20.17	1.45	20.41	1.55	20.16	1.43	$p = 0.1315$
NLA	20	TB	123.49	8.46	124.10	8.36	123.53	7.60	$p = 0.0625$
	20	BB	130.70	10.09	131.44	10.20	130.80	9.49	$p = 0.0564$

TB = Tooth-Borne group; BB = Bone-Borne group; N = sample number; SD = standard deviation; ANW = Anterior nasal width, ANFW = anterior nasal floor width, PNW = posterior nasal width, PNFW = posterior nasal floor width; AW = alar width, ABW = alar base width, NL = nasal lenght, NFL = nasal filter length, NLA = nasolabial angle. Significance set at $p < 0.05$ and based on one-way analysis of variance (ANOVA) and Scheffe's post-hoc comparisons tests; a, b, c = identifiers for post-hoc comparisons tests.

In both TB and BB groups, the alar width (AW) and the alar base width (ABW) slightly increased in both groups between T0 and T1 ($p < 0.05$), while a significant reduction was found at T2, almost reaching pre-treatment values ($p < 0.05$) (Table 3). The increment of the alar width (AW) and the alar base width (ABW) was slightly greater in the BB group compared to the TB group both at 6 months (T0–T1) and 1 year (T0–T2) after maxillary expansion, and such differences were statistically significant ($p < 0.05$) (Table 4).

Table 4. Comparisons of mean changes obtained after 6 months (T0–T1) and one year after treatment (T0–T2) between TB and BB groups.

Measurements	N	Groups	T0–T1			T0–T2		
			Mean	SD	Significance	Mean	SD	Significance
ANW	20	TB	1.12	0.31	$p < 0.0001$	1.05	0.28	$p < 0.0001$
	20	BB	2.01	0.43		2.14	0.37	
ANFW	20	TB	1.61	0.28	$p < 0.0001$	1.41	0.32	$p < 0.0001$
	20	BB	2.66	0.52		2.78	0.53	
PNW	20	TB	0.84	0.21	$p < 0.0001$	0.76	0.25	$p < 0.0001$
	20	BB	1.96	0.27		1.65	0.34	
PNFW	20	TB	1.11	0.19	$p < 0.0001$	1.24	0.24	$p < 0.0001$
	20	BB	2.49	0.51		2.71	0.75	
AW	20	TB	1.22	0.29	$p = 0.0008$	0.62	0.41	$p < 0.0001$
	20	BB	1.59	0.35		1.05	0.31	
ABW	20	TB	1.03	0.17	$p = 0.0014$	1.07	0.15	$p < 0.0001$
	20	BB	1.25	0.23		1.42	0.17	
NL	20	TB	0.48	0.16	$p = 0.314$	−0.05	0.13	$p = 0.4084$
	20	BB	0.53	0.15		0.01	0.17	
NFL	20	TB	0.25	0.21	$p = 0.872$	0.02	0.24	$p = 0.7823$
	20	BB	0.24	0.18		−0.01	0.18	
NLA	20	TB	0.61	0.26	$p = 0.151$	0.04	0.26	$p = 0.45493$
	20	BB	0.74	0.3		0.10	0.36	

TB = Tooth-Borne group; BB = Bone-Borne group; N = sample number; SD = standard deviation. ANW = Anterior nasal width, ANFW = anterior nasal floor width, PNW = posterior nasal width, PNFW = posterior nasal floor width. AW = alar width, ABW = alar base width, NL = nasal length, NFL = nasal filter length, NLA = nasolabial angle. Significance set at $p < 0.05$ and based on Independent Student's t test.

A small increment of nasal length (NL), nasal filter length (NFL), and nasolabial angle (NLA) were found in both groups between T0 and T1; instead, a small reduction in the same measurements was recorded at T2. However, these changes were not statistically significant ($p > 0.05$) (Table 3). Finally, no differences were found between the TB and BB groups in the changes of NL, NFL, and NLA recorded at 6 months (T0–T1) and 1 year (T0–T2) after maxillary expansion ($p > 0.05$) (Table 4).

A high correlation was found between skeletal and soft-tissue expansion in TB group (from 0.903 to 0.941), instead a weaker correlation was found in the BB group (from 0.695 to 0.742) (Table 5).

Table 5. Linear regression tests model using anterior skeletal changes as independent variables (predictor) and soft tissue changes as dependent variables.

Groups	Predictor Variables	Dependent Variables	R	Coefficients	
				Beta	Standard Error
TB	ANW	AW	0.916	0.916	0.020
		ABW	0.903	0.903	0.031
	ANFW	AW	0.927	0.927	0.018
		ABW	0.941	0.941	0.015
BB	ANW	AW	0.716	0.716	0.082
		ABW	0.695	0.695	0.102
	ANFW	AW	0,731	0,731	0.079
		ABW	0.742	0.742	0.068

TB = Tooth-Borne group; BB = Bone-Borne group; ANW = Anterior nasal width; ANFW = anterior nasal floor width; AW = alar width; ABW = alar base width.

Concerning the reliability of the methodology, an excellent correlation was found between intra-operator readings with values ranging from 0.932 to 0.963 for skeletal measurements and from 0.922 to 0.959 for soft-tissue measurements. Inter-operator reliability also showed an excellent correlation between the two readings, with values ranging from 0.901 to 0.916 for skeletal measurements and from 0.915 to 0.928 for soft tissue measurements.

4. Discussion

Several studies have demonstrated that RME, both in the form of tooth-borne and bone-borne anchorage systems, increases the transverse dimension and the volume of the nasal cavity, with a consequent potential improvement of the respiratory function [16]. Although the main goal of RME is to correct the skeletal transverse maxillary deficiency and any consequent functional impairment, it would be interesting to understand if this therapy can determine changes in the soft tissue of the nasal region, being that this aspect is relevant from the patients' aesthetic perspective. To the best of our knowledge, this is the first study in the literature addressing this topic. Previous studies with a similar methodology have been published [17,18]; however, they were focused on changes that occurred after surgically assisted RME, and their findings are far from being comparable to those obtained in the present study, considering the differences between the two treatment approaches. Only two studies have investigated the soft tissue nasal changes after tooth-borne RME using measurements performed on photographic records [24] and in-vivo (clinical inspection using a digital caliper), respectively [25], thus without providing information on the underlying skeletal changes occurring in the tested sample. In this regard, CBCT images allow the analysis of both skeletal and soft tissue changes and perform comparative evaluations, as reported in the present study.

4.1. Post-Retention Transverse Changes

Concerning skeletal measurements, the BB group showed a greater skeletal expansion compared to the TB group, which was consistent with previous findings [8]. The TB group showed a greater expansion of the pyriform aperture width compared to the posterior region confirming the wedge-shaped opening of the suture [4]; instead, BB groups showed a more parallel sutural opening [21]. Furthermore, both groups showed a cranio-caudal pattern of expansion (T0/T1 TB: ANW = 1.12 mm, ANFW = 1.61 mm; T0/T1 BB: ANW = 2.01 mm, ANFW = 2.66 mm), confirming the "V" shape opening of the mid-palatal suture [26]. It should be mentioned that subjects in the BB group were slightly older than those included in the TB group (<1 year); thus, they could present an advanced maturational stage of the mid-palatal suture that would have increased the skeletal resistances compared to TB group [27].

Both TB and BB RME induce a small increment (>1 mm) of the alar base and alar width. Such an increment was slightly greater in the TB group with statistical significance; however, it should be considered irrelevant from the clinical perspective. These data are close to those reported by Johnson et al. [25] and were below the increment of 2 mm of the alar base found by Berger et al. [24] with a TB expander. In the latter study, the authors found that the expansion of the soft tissue alar base was in a 1 to 1 ratio with the skeletal increment. Accordingly, in the TB group of the present study, the expansion of the alar base and of the alar width was similar to that of the Apertura piriformis (T0/T1 ANW= 1.12 mm, ANFW = 1.61mm, AW = 1.22 mm, ABW = 1.03 mm), instead, in the BB group, the expansion of the alar base and of the alar width was remarkable below that of the Apertura piriformis (ANW = 2.01 mm, ANFW = 2.66 mm, AW = 1.39 mm, ABW = 1.25 mm). Considering that the transverse skeletal increment was greater in the BB group while both groups showed a similar amount of expansion of the soft tissue, it can be assumed that the response of the soft tissue of the alar region could follow skeletal expansion up to a certain threshold, beyond that further expansion is prevented. Such limitation can be influenced by intrinsic tissue characteristics, such as tension, tone, and thickness of the soft tissue, which may also contribute to the relapse forces. This assumption would be confirmed by the different values of the linear regression between skeletal and soft-tissue expansion found in this study in the TB group (from 0.903 to 0.941) and BB group (from 0.695 to 0.742).

4.2. Post-Retention Sagittal Changes

Another assumption of this study is the possibility that RME, in the form of TB and/or BB anchorage, can change the sagittal projection of the soft tissue in the nasal region. A small increment of nasio-labial angle, nasal filter, and nasal length was found in both TB and BB groups; however, these findings were not statistically significant as well as they did not differ between the two groups. As far as we know, the only study that looked at the height of soft tissue in the nose was that of Magnonson et al. [18]. In that study, the authors found an insignificant increase ($p > 0.05$) of 0.18 mm, but in contrast to our study that observed changes after RME, they were observing changes following surgical disjunction. Nevertheless, despite being not statistically significant, the increment of nasio-labial angle, nasal filter, and nasal length data were consistent and could be attributed to adaptive postural changes to accommodate the width and thickness of the expander appliance [24].

4.3. Long-Term Changes

One year after appliance removal, all the skeletal and soft-tissue transverse changes obtained after RME were maintained, suggesting that most of the relapse occurred during the retention period, as widely confirmed by literature [10]. Instead, we found a significant reduction in the soft tissue nasolabial angle, nasal length, and nasal filter length, reaching almost pre-treatment values, confirming that the changes recorded during appliance wearing were due to adaptive postural changes of the soft tissue.

Facial aesthetics is a primary concern for patients and clinicians, and consequently, soft-tissue analysis has been integrated into modern orthodontics, being a fundamental aspect of the diagnosis, treatment plan, and decision-making process. Furthermore, in case of documented changes in the facial soft tissue during/after treatment, they should be evaluated and discussed with patients to improve patients' compliance and confidence in the treatment [28]. In this regard, treatment results including nasal proportions, are considered to have an important influence on patients' macro-aesthetic appearance [19].

According to the present findings, RME could induce a small increment of the diameter between alar cartilages, and patients with narrow and constrained nasal structures may benefit from the nasal widening effects of surgically assisted rapid maxillary expansion (SARME). Moreover, patients should not be expected to see relevant changes in the nasal soft tissue when undergoing RME assisted by skeletal anchorage. However, the clinical relevance of these findings remains questionable. It is difficult to judge the patients' perception of the soft tissue changes occurring after RME. There are no established threshold values in the literature for assessing a layperson's perception of variations in nasal width [29]. Different results may be observed in different patients as a result of the same treatment, with deterioration in one case and improvements in another [18]. In this regard, further studies involving patients' self-perception of facial changes after RME are recommended to elucidate this aspect; also, studies with long-term follow-up, even using non-invasive 3D imaging digital technology, are warmly encouraged to evaluate soft-tissue behavior years after RME treatment.

4.4. Limitations

The study sample consisted of CBCT scans taken with Full Filed of View (FOV), which means that the scans included anatomical areas that are beyond the diagnostic and research interest addressed. In this regard, the usage of ionizing radiations beyond the area of interest should be discouraged according to the ALADAIP principle [30]. However, CBCTs used for the present study were obtained from previously published materials [21,22] to avoid unnecessary or additional radiation exposure to the patients.

The comparative data obtained in the present study may be biased by the different craniofacial skeletal patterns and related muscles characteristics [31], as well as patients' ages and skeletal maturation stages. Accordingly, caution must be taken in the interpretation of the present findings, and any generalization should be avoided. The absence of matched groups according to the skeletal growth stages, is another limitation of the present investigation. However, growth should not be considered a significant variable in the changes observed in both TB and BB groups, at least between pre-treatment and post-retention stages.

5. Conclusions

A similar slight increment of the alar width and alar base width was found in growing subjects treated with TB-RME and BB-RME. However, the clinical relevance of these differences, in terms of facial appearance, remains questionable.

Author Contributions: Conceptualization, A.L.G., P.V.; methodology, L.N., S.M., A.M.; software, V.R., V.V.; validation, M.O.L., R.L.; investigation, V.R.; data curation, S.M., A.M.; writing—original draft preparation, A.L.G.; writing—review and editing, A.L.G., G.I. All authors have read and agreed to the published version of the manuscript.

Funding: This research received no external funding.

Institutional Review Board Statement: The study was conducted according to the guidelines of the Declaration of Helsinki and approved by the Institutional Health Research Ethics Board of Alberta University (IRB protocol number: Pro00075765-21/08/17).

Informed Consent Statement: Informed consent was obtained from all subjects involved in the study.

Data Availability Statement: Data are available from the corresponding author upon request.

Conflicts of Interest: The authors declare no conflict of interest.

References

1. Liu, S.; Xu, T.; Zou, W. Effects of rapid maxillary expansion on the midpalatal suture: A systematic review. *Eur. J. Orthod.* **2015**, *37*, 651–655. [CrossRef] [PubMed]
2. Savoldi, F.; Wong, K.K.; Yeung, A.W.K.; Tsoi, J.K.H.; Gu, M.; Bornstein, M.M. Midpalatal suture maturation staging using cone beam computed tomography in patients aged between 9 to 21 years. *Sci. Rep.* **2022**, *12*, 4318. [CrossRef]
3. Bucci, R.; D'Antò, V.; Rongo, R.; Valletta, R.; Martina, R.; Michelotti, A. Dental and skeletal effects of palatal expansion techniques: A systematic review of the current evidence from systematic reviews and meta-analyses. *J. Oral Rehabil.* **2016**, *43*, 543–564. [CrossRef] [PubMed]
4. Celenk-Koca, T.; Erdinc, A.E.; Hazar, S.; Harris, L.; English, J.D.; Akyalcin, S. Evaluation of miniscrew-supported rapid maxillary expansion in adolescents: A prospective randomized clinical trial. *Angle Orthod.* **2018**, *88*, 702–709. [CrossRef]
5. Lo Giudice, A.; Barbato, E.; Cosentino, L.; Ferraro, C.M.; Leonardi, R. Alveolar bone changes after rapid maxillary expansion with tooth-born appliances: A systematic review. *Eur. J. Orthod.* **2018**, *40*, 296–303. [CrossRef]
6. Lo Giudice, A.; Leonardi, R.; Ronsivalle, V.; Allegrini, S.; Lagravère, M.; Marzo, G.; Isola, G. Evaluation of pulp cavity/chamber changes after tooth-borne and bone-borne rapid maxillary expansions: A cbct study using surface-based superimposition and deviation analysis. *Clin. Oral Investig.* **2021**, *25*, 2237–2247. [CrossRef] [PubMed]
7. Garib, D.G.; Henriques, J.F.; Janson, G.; de Freitas, M.R.; Fernandes, A.Y. Periodontal effects of rapid maxillary expansion with tooth-tissue-borne and tooth-borne expanders: A computed tomography evaluation. *Am. J. Orthod. Dentofac. Orthop.* **2006**, *129*, 749–758. [CrossRef]
8. Krusi, M.; Eliades, T.; Papageorgiou, S.N. Are there benefits from using bone-borne maxillary expansion instead of tooth-borne maxillary expansion? A systematic review with meta-analysis. *Prog. Orthod.* **2019**, *20*, 9. [CrossRef]
9. Cozzani, M.; Nucci, L.; Lupini, D.; Dolatshahizand, H.; Fazeli, D.; Barzkar, E.; Naeini, E.; Jamilian, A. The ideal insertion angle after immediate loading in jeil, storm, and thunder miniscrews: A 3d-fem study. *Int. Orthod.* **2020**, *18*, 503–508. [CrossRef]
10. Giudice, A.L.; Spinuzza, P.; Rustico, L.; Messina, G.; Nucera, R. Short-term treatment effects produced by rapid maxillary expansion evaluated with computed tomography: A systematic review with meta-analysis. *Korean J. Orthod.* **2020**, *50*, 314–323. [CrossRef]
11. Savoldi, F.; Massetti, F.; Tsoi, J.K.H.; Matinlinna, J.P.; Yeung, A.W.K.; Tanaka, R.; Paganelli, C.; Bornstein, M.M. Anteroposterior length of the maxillary complex and its relationship with the anterior cranial base. *Angle Orthod.* **2021**, *91*, 88–97. [CrossRef]
12. D'Apuzzo, F.; Minervini, G.; Grassia, V.; Rotolo, R.P.; Perillo, L.; Nucci, L. Mandibular coronoid process hypertrophy: Diagnosis and 20-year follow-up with cbct, mri and emg evaluations. *Appl. Sci.* **2021**, *11*, 4504. [CrossRef]

13. Lo Giudice, A.; Fastuca, R.; Portelli, M.; Militi, A.; Bellocchio, M.; Spinuzza, P.; Briguglio, F.; Caprioglio, A.; Nucera, R. Effects of rapid vs slow maxillary expansion on nasal cavity dimensions in growing subjects: A methodological and reproducibility study. *Eur. J. Paediatr. Dent.* **2017**, *18*, 299–304.
14. Garib, D.G.; Henriques, J.F.; Janson, G.; Freitas, M.R.; Coelho, R.A. Rapid maxillary expansion–tooth tissue-borne versus tooth-borne expanders: A computed tomography evaluation of dentoskeletal effects. *Angle Orthod.* **2005**, *75*, 548–557. [PubMed]
15. Garrett, B.J.; Caruso, J.M.; Rungcharassaeng, K.; Farrage, J.R.; Kim, J.S.; Taylor, G.D. Skeletal effects to the maxilla after rapid maxillary expansion assessed with cone-beam computed tomography. *Am. J. Orthod. Dentofac. Orthop.* **2008**, *134*, 8–9. [CrossRef]
16. Buck, L.M.; Dalci, O.; Darendeliler, M.A.; Papageorgiou, S.N.; Papadopoulou, A.K. Volumetric upper airway changes after rapid maxillary expansion: A systematic review and meta-analysis. *Eur. J. Orthod.* **2017**, *39*, 463–473. [CrossRef]
17. Kayalar, E.; Schauseil, M.; Hellak, A.; Emekli, U.; Fıratlı, S.; Korbmacher-Steiner, H. Nasal soft- and hard-tissue changes following tooth-borne and hybrid surgically assisted rapid maxillary expansion: A randomized clinical cone-beam computed tomography study. *J. Cranio Maxillofac. Surg.* **2019**, *47*, 1190–1197. [CrossRef] [PubMed]
18. Magnusson, A.; Bjerklin, K.; Kim, H.; Nilsson, P.; Marcusson, A. Three-dimensional computed tomographic analysis of changes to the external features of the nose after surgically assisted rapid maxillary expansion and orthodontic treatment: A prospective longitudinal study. *Am. J. Orthod. Dentofac. Orthop.* **2013**, *144*, 404–413. [CrossRef]
19. Sarver, D.M. Interactions of hard tissues, soft tissues, and growth over time, and their impact on orthodontic diagnosis and treatment planning. *Am. J. Orthod. Dentofac. Orthop.* **2015**, *148*, 380–386. [CrossRef]
20. Khosravi, M.; Ugolini, A.; Miresmaeili, A.; Mirzaei, H.; Shahidi-Zandi, V.; Soheilifar, S.; Karami, M.; Mahmoudzadeh, M. Tooth-borne versus bone-borne rapid maxillary expansion for transverse maxillary deficiency: A systematic review. *Int. Orthod.* **2019**, *17*, 425–436. [CrossRef] [PubMed]
21. Kavand, G.; Lagravere, M.; Kula, K.; Stewart, K.; Ghoneima, A. Retrospective cbct analysis of airway volume changes after bone-borne vs tooth-borne rapid maxillary expansion. *Angle Orthod.* **2019**, *89*, 566–574. [CrossRef]
22. Lo Giudice, A.; Ronsivalle, V.; Lagravere, M.; Leonardi, R.; Martina, S.; Isola, G. Transverse dentoalveolar response of mandibular arch after rapid maxillary expansion (rme) with tooth-borne and bone-borne appliances. *Angle Orthod.* **2020**, *90*, 680–687. [CrossRef]
23. Guijarro-Martinez, R.; Swennen, G.R. Three-dimensional cone beam computed tomography definition of the anatomical subregions of the upper airway: A validation study. *Int. J. Oral Maxillofac. Surg.* **2013**, *42*, 1140–1149. [CrossRef] [PubMed]
24. Berger, J.L.; Pangrazio-Kulbersh, V.; Thomas, B.W.; Kaczynski, R. Photographic analysis of facial changes associated with maxillary expansion. *Am. J. Orthod Dentofac. Orthop.* **1999**, *116*, 563–571. [CrossRef]
25. Johnson, B.M.; McNamara, J.A.; Bandeen, R.L.; Baccetti, T. Changes in soft tissue nasal widths associated with rapid maxillary expansion in prepubertal and postpubertal subjects. *Angle Orthod.* **2010**, *80*, 995–1001. [CrossRef] [PubMed]
26. Wertz, R.; Dreskin, M. Midpalatal suture opening: A normative study. *Am. J. Orthod.* **1977**, *71*, 367–381. [CrossRef]
27. Melsen, B. Palatal growth studied on human autopsy material. A histologic microradiographic study. *Am. J. Orthod.* **1975**, *68*, 42–54. [CrossRef]
28. Lee, S.J.; Ahn, S.J.; Kim, T.W. Patient compliance and locus of control in orthodontic treatment: A prospective study. *Am. J. Orthod. Dentofac. Orthop.* **2008**, *133*, 354–358. [CrossRef]
29. Nada, R.M.; van Loon, B.; Schols, J.G.; Maal, T.J.; de Koning, M.J.; Mostafa, Y.A.; Kuijpers-Jagtman, A.M. Volumetric changes of the nose and nasal airway 2 years after tooth-borne and bone-borne surgically assisted rapid maxillary expansion. *Eur. J. Oral Sci.* **2013**, *121*, 450–456. [CrossRef]
30. Oenning, A.C.; Jacobs, R.; Pauwels, R.; Stratis, A.; Hedesiu, M.; Salmon, B. Cone-beam ct in paediatric dentistry: Dimitra project position statement. *Pediatr. Radiol.* **2018**, *48*, 308–316. [CrossRef]
31. Lo Giudice, A.; Rustico, L.; Caprioglio, A.; Migliorati, M.; Nucera, R. Evaluation of condylar cortical bone thickness in patient groups with different vertical facial dimensions using cone-beam computed tomography. *Odontology* **2020**, *108*, 669–675. [CrossRef] [PubMed]

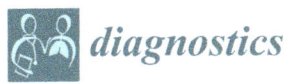

Article

Grade 1 and 2 Chondrosarcomas of the Chest Wall: CT Imaging Features and Review of the Literature

Filippo Del Grande [1,2,*], Shivani Ahlawat [1], Edward McCarthy [3] and Laura M. Fayad [1]

[1] The Russel H. Morgan Department of Radiology and Radiological Science, Johns Hopkins University, Baltimore, MD 21205, USA; sahlawa1@jhmi.edu (S.A.); lfayad1@jhmi.edu (L.M.F.)
[2] Clinica di Radiologia EOC, Via Tesserete, 6900 Lugano, Switzerland
[3] Department of Pathology, Johns Hopkins University, Baltimore, MD 21205, USA; mccarthy@jhmi.edu
* Correspondence: filippo.delgrande@eoc.ch; Tel.: +41-91-811-60-69; Fax: +41-91-811-60-90

Abstract: The purpose of our retrospective article is to review the CT imaging features of chondrosarcomas of the chest wall with pathologic correlation. For 26 subjects with biopsy-proven chondrosarcomas of the chest wall, two musculoskeletal radiologists retrospectively reviewed 26 CT scans in consensus. Descriptive statistics were performed. The mean tumor size was 57 mm. Twenty (20/26, 77%) chondrosarcomas were located in the ribs and six (6/26, 23%) in the sternum. The majority were lytic (19/26, 73%) with <25% calcification (15/26, 58%), and with a soft tissue mass (22/27, 85%). In this study CT features of grade 1 chondrosarcoma overlapped with those of grade 2 tumors. In conclusion, chondrosarcomas of the chest wall are generally lytic with an associated soft tissue mass, showing little calcified matrix and low-to-intermediate grade.

Keywords: chondrosarcoma; chest wall tumor; bone tumor; CT scan

1. Introduction

Chondrosarcomas (CS) of the chest wall are rare lesions, but they represent the most common primary malignant bone tumors of the chest wall [1,2]. Both primary [3–10] and secondary forms of CS [11–13] have previously been reported.

The imaging features of CS of the chest wall have been insufficiently described, with limited reports depicting the imaging features for radiography [6,7,9], cross-sectional imaging [2,4,6–9,12,14], and PET [4,15–17]. There are, however, several reports in the surgical literature regarding the clinical features and prognosis of CS of the chest wall [5,8,13,18–20]. It is important for the imaging interpreter to consider CS in the differential diagnosis of a chest wall mass, especially due to the knowledge that some histologic features of CS can overlap with enchondroma, as has already been described in the extremities [21].

While radiography of a chest wall mass is often the first-line imaging modality for tumor detection, it is often inadequate for characterization. Therefore, cross-sectional imaging techniques are important modalities for the detection and characterization of CS of the chest wall. The purpose of our study was to retrospectively review the CT imaging features of chondrosarcomas (CS) of the chest wall with pathologic correlation.

2. Materials and Methods

2.1. Patients

The study was approved by our institutional review board (IRB). Informed consent was waived. Details of subjects who had a surgical specimen with a diagnosis of chest wall CS at our institution from 1988 to 2016 were retrieved from a pathology database. Inclusion criteria were patients with a histologically proven chest wall CS, cross-sectional imaging with CT exam and no neoadjuvant therapy prior to their imaging studies. Exclusion criteria were patients without histology or CT imaging documentation, and those with imaging that was performed following surgery or other treatments.

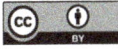

2.2. Image Acquisition

CT protocols were heterogenous, depending on the institution where the exams had been performed. All CT exams included axial CT, and 16/26 (62%) patients had sagittal and coronal reconstructions.

2.3. Image Analysis

Two musculoskeletal radiologists (SA and FDG) with 7 and 17 years of experience in musculoskeletal imaging interpretation, respectively, reviewed the CT imaging features of 26 biopsy-proven chondrosarcomas (CS) of the chest wall in consensus and blinded to clinical information.

The size, location, character (lytic, with chondroid matrix calcification or mixed), calcification percentage (none, 1–25%, 26–50%, 51–75%, >75% lesion calcification), location (central or peripheral, related to the bone), as well as the presence or absence of a soft tissue mass or fracture were recorded. Lesions growing outside the bone with soft tissue Hounsfield units were considered soft tissue masses.

2.4. Pathologic Interpretation

One pathologist (EM) with more than 40 years' experience in bone tumors reviewed all specimens and graded tumors as grade 1, 2, or 3 based on the following scheme: Grade 1 chondrosarcomas showed minimal cellular atypia with occasional binucleated cells; rarely, a few cells had slightly larger nuclei and more cytoplasm. Abundant extracellular matrix was present and there was no evidence of myxoid change or mitotic activity. Grade 2 chondrosarcomas had larger and pale nuclei with visible chromatin. There was mild nuclear polymorphism and the cytoplasm was more abundant. Mitotic figures were extremely rare. Grade 2 lesions were slightly more cellular and, rarely, myxoid change was present. Grade 3 chondrosarcomas had significant cellularity with pleomorphic nuclei. There was often extensive myxoid change with abundant spindle-shaped tumor cells. Mitotic figures were present at the rate of 2 to 10 per high-power field, and, focally, the exterior cellular matrix was sparse. Biopsy material was available, either from surgical excision or percutaneous sampling. In nineteen out of twenty-six (73%) cases, samples from surgical biopsies were available, and in 7/26 (27%) cases, samples from percutaneous core needle biopsies were available. All imaging was available during pathological interpretation.

2.5. Statistical Analysis

Descriptive statistics were tabulated manually in an Excel file for demographics (age with mean and range, and gender), location and size of the lesion, as well as imaging features and histologic grades as detailed above. The Mann–Whitney U test and Fisher's exact test were used to perform comparisons between grade 1 and 2 CS using STATA17 (StataCorp., College Station, TX, USA). Statistical significance was set at 5% ($p < 0.05$).

3. Results

We retrieved reports of 54 subjects with chest wall CS. Twenty-eight subjects (28/54, 52%) were excluded due to the lack of a complete CT. According to our inclusion criteria, we identified 26 (26/54, 48%) patients with CT images and chest wall CS (17/26 males, 9/26 females), with a median age of 61 years (age range: 25–88 years old). A histologic analysis revealed 10 grade 1 CS (10/26, 38%), 16 grade 2 CS (16/26, 62%), and no grade 3 lesions.

No statistically significant differences were detected between grade 1 and 2 CS.

Table 1 summarizes the demographics and general tumor characteristics separated by grade.

The mean tumor size was 57 mm (range: 20–151 mm) (Figure 1).

Table 1. Demographics separated by grade.

Imaging Feature	Variables	Grade 1 11/26 (42%)	Grade 2 15/26 (58%)	p-Value	All CS 26/26 (100%)
Age	Mean and range in years	60 (33–84)	62 (25–88)	0.788	61 (25–88)
Gender	Males	9/11 (82%)	8/15 (53%)	0.217	17/26 (65%)
	Females	2/11 (18%)	7/15 (47%)		9/26 (35%)

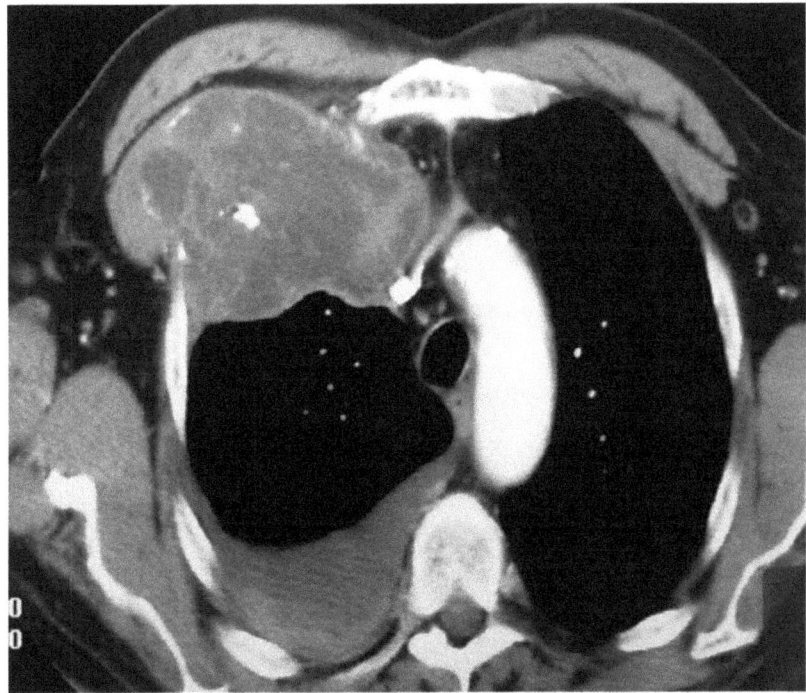

Figure 1. A 72-year-old male patient with grade 2 costochondral junction chondrosarcoma. Contrast-enhanced axial chest CT shows a large (90 mm) soft tissue mass at the right costochondral junction with small calcifications, necrotic areas, mediastinal invasion and right pleural effusion.

Nineteen lesions were located at the costochondral junction (19/26, 73%), six lesions were located in the sternum (6/26, 23%) (Figure 2), and one lesion (1/26, 4%) was located in the posterior rib adjacent to the costovertebral joint (Figure 3).

The typical appearance of CS was lytic (16/26, 62%). More than half of the subjects (15/26, 58%) showed less than 25% calcifications, and only one subject (1/26, 4%) had more than 75% calcifications in the lesion. Commonly, CS were associated with a soft tissue mass (22/26, 85%) (Figure 4), and only two CS (2/26, 8%) had pathological fractures.

Fourteen CS (14/26, 54%) (13 located at the costochondral junction and one on the posterior rib) were considered to be peripherally located, whereas 12 CS (12/26, 46%) were considered to be centrally located (6 located in the sternum and 6 at the costochondral junction). The six CS located in the sternum were all centrally located. Out of 19 CS of the osteochondral junction, 14 (74%) were peripherally located.

The vast majority of the lesions (4/5, 80%) showed less than 25% heterogeneity after contrast medium injection. None of the CS showed evidence of perilesional bone marrow edema, perilesional enhancement, and/or perilesional soft tissue edema. Table 2 shows the CT imaging features separated by the grade of the tumor.

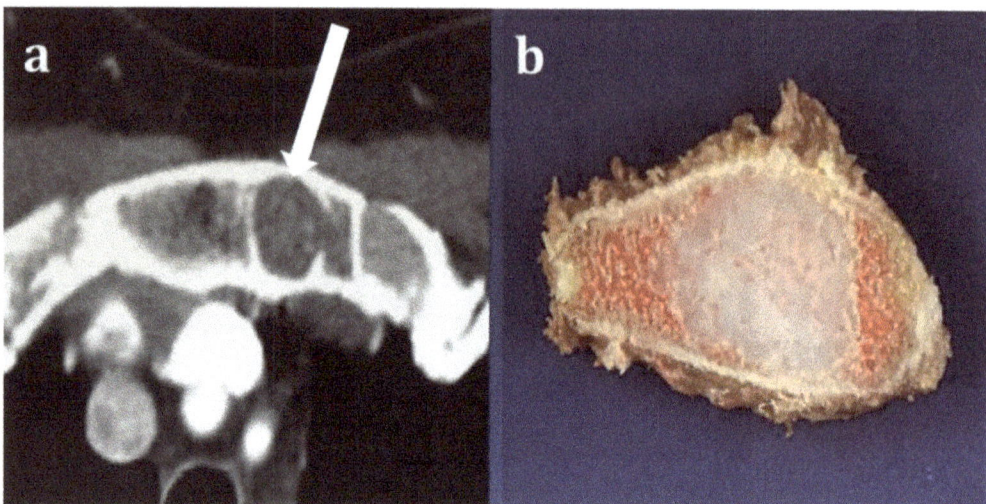

Figure 2. A 49-year-old female patient with grade 2 chondrosarcoma (long white arrow) of the sternum. Contrast-enhancement axial CT with soft tissue window (**a**) shows a lytic lesion with a few punctate calcifications. Gross pathology specimen resection of the sternum (**b**) showing a white-yellow tumor surrounded by bone marrow. Based on imaging, it is not possible to differentiate the lesion from an enchondroma. Enchondromas in the sternum are extremely rare and a solid lesion in the sternum should raise concerns for malignancy until proven otherwise.

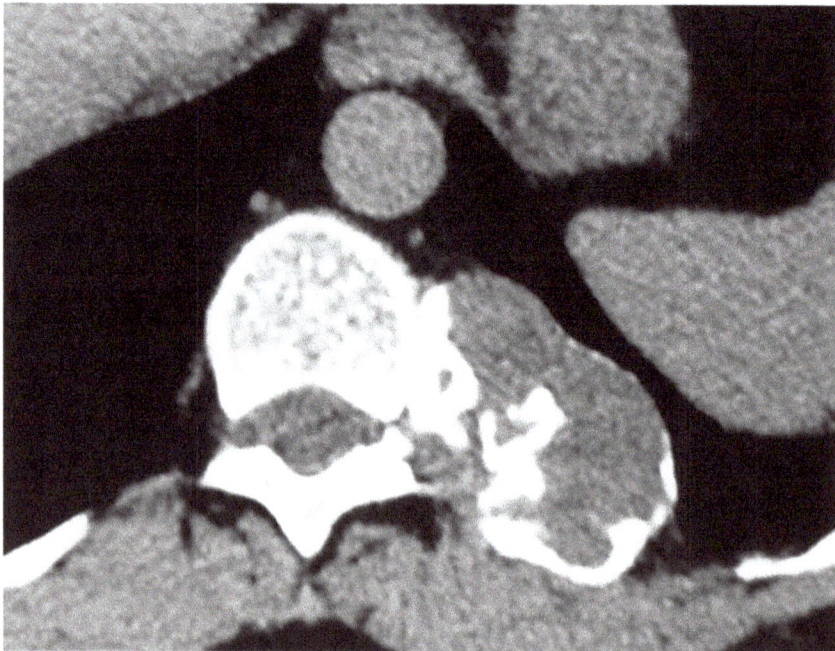

Figure 3. A 62-year-old female patient with grade 2 chondrosarcoma at the posterior rib adjacent to the costovertebral junction. Axial chest CT shows a soft tissue mass at the posterior rib with calcifications.

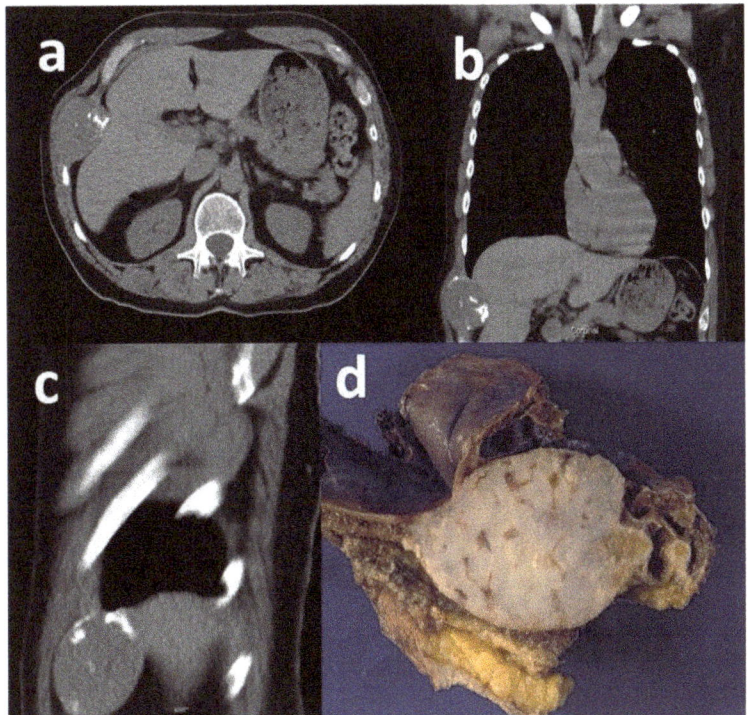

Figure 4. A 74-year-old male patient with grade 1 costochondral junction chondrosarcoma. Axial chest CT (**a**), and coronal (**b**) and sagittal (**c**) multi-planar reconstruction (MPR) CT show a large soft tissue mass at the costochondral junction. Gross pathology specimen (**d**) resection of the rib with chondrosarcoma.

Table 2. CT imaging features of CS, including separation by grade.

Imaging Features	Variables	Grade 1 11/26 (42%)	Grade2 15/26 (58%)	*p*-Value	All CS 26/26 (100%)
Tumor location	Costochondral junction Sternum Posterior rib	9/11 (82%) 2/11 (18%) 0/11 (0%)	10/15 (67%) 4/15 (27%) 1/15 (6%)	0.804	19/26 (73%) 6/26 (23%) 1/26 (4%)
Tumor size	Mean in mm (range) Median in mm (range)	56 (31–151) 40 (31–151)	57 (20–127) 46 (20–127)	0.435	57 (20–151) 45 (20–151)
Character	Lytic only mixed chondroid matrix only	0/11 (0%) 11/11 (100%) 0/11 (0%)	3/15 (20%) 12/15 (80%) 0/15 (0%)	0.238	3/26 (12%) 23/26 (88%) 0/26 (0%)
Chondroid Matrix	0–25% 25–50% 50–75% 75–100%	5/11 (45%) 4/11 (36%) 1/11 (9%) 1/11 (9%)	10/15 (67%) 3/15 (20%) 2/15 (13%) 0/15 (0%)	0.551	15/26 (58%) 7/26 (27%) 3/26 (12%) 1/26 (4%)
Fracture	No Yes	9/11 (82%) 2/11 (18%)	15/15 (100%) 0/15 (0%)	0.169	24/26 (92%) 2/26 (8%)
Tumor location within the bone	Central peripheral	5/11 (45%) 6/11 (55%)	7/15 (47%) 8/15 (53%)	1.000	12/26 (48%) 14/26 (52%)
Soft tissue mass	No Yes	3/11 (27%) 8/11 (73%)	1/15 (7%) 14/15 (93%)	0.279	4/26 (15%) 22/26 (85%)

4. Discussion

In our retrospective series, we found that grade 1 and grade 2 chest wall CS are typically lytic lesions located at the costochondral junction, with an associated soft tissue mass, and with little mineralization. Grade 1 and 2 CS were not statistically different for tumor location in the chest wall, tumor size, tumor location within the bone, presence or absence of chondroid matrix, fractures and/or soft tissue masses.

Compared with prior reports in the literature, our findings are corroborated by Al-Refaie et al., who reported the demographics and treatment of 45 chest wall CS, without a comprehensive assessment of the imaging. The authors found that CS were slightly more common in male than female patients, and were mostly located at the costochondral junction, similarly to our investigation. Histologically, the majority of CS were low-grade lesions, with a minority of intermediate-grade lesions, and no high-grade lesions were reported in the latter study [18].

Cross-sectional imaging features of chest wall CS have only been insufficiently described [2,4,6–9,12,14]. Some cross-sectional imaging features that we observed are similar to the imaging features described in chondrosarcomas elsewhere in the body, and, as such, were expected. In particular, as commonly observed in chondroid lesions, the majority of the lesions showed a low-to-isointense signal on spin-echo T1-weighted sequences and a high signal intensity on fluid-sensitive sequences. Following contrast enhancement, a ring-like pattern was more common than a solid pattern of enhancement.

Several features of CS of the chest wall observed in our study were different from those that have been reported in the aicular skeleton and other sites of the axial skeleton. Unlike CS of the pelvic bones and extremities, in which calcification is common [22,23], in CS of the chest wall, calcification is much less common. In one prior investigation, almost every CS of the aicular skeleton showed more than one third calcified matrix, but the chest wall CS in our series showed surprisingly less calcification, with the majority of the patients having less than 25% of their lesions containing calcification [22]. We can speculate that the difference in calcification pattern between extremity CS and chest wall CS is probably attributed to the overall relatively low percentage of calcification in large chest wall soft tissue masses.

Interestingly, the CT imaging features were similar between low-grade and intermediate-grade lesions. In other words, due to our small series and limited imaging availability, the lesion appearance, percentage of calcification, presence of soft tissue mass, and size of the lesions could not be used to draw any conclusions regarding tumor grade. Furthermore, in some previous reports, the pattern and the degree of contrast medium enhancement did not discriminate between CS and enchondroma [22,24].

In order to avoid unnecessary biopsies or inadequate treatments, it is crucial to identify imaging features in order to discriminate between enchondroma and low-grade CS throughout the body. Similarly to CS, enchondroma are usually located in the rib or at the costochondral junction [2,25], but enchondromas of the sternum are very rare, with only isolated reports [26–29]. In the chest wall, enchondromas generally appear as small (typically less than 3.5 cm), well-defined lytic lesions [30], while we showed that CS of the chest wall are generally associated with more aggressive features, including a soft tissue mass. In addition, demographic and clinical information has been reported to be useful for differentiating between enchondromas and CS elsewhere in the body, including older patient age, male gender, and pain [22]. It is also worth noting that pathologists cannot always differentiate enchondroma from low-grade chondrosarcoma by cytology and histology, further accentuating the importance of imaging features, and the integration of imaging studies and clinical information with a pathologic diagnosis [21]. Therefore, in the management of chondroid lesions, a percutaneous biopsy is not routinely performed in many centers, as it is prone to sampling error and the final histologic diagnosis is strongly reliant on the imaging features.

A correct diagnosis is paramount in starting a correct therapeutic approach, in decreasing the recurrence rate, and in increasing patient survival. Although chest radiography is typically the first-line study of evaluation for osseous lesions, the location of chest wall CS requires cross-sectional imaging for the characterization and definition of tumor extent. CT imaging of the chest is, therefore, the next modality of investigation, as CT offers information for the characterization of the tumor as chondroid. Subsequently, MRI is useful for defining additional aggressive features (such as perilesional edema), as well as the full extent of the tumor within the bone marrow for optimal treatment planning and identification of the margins. It should be noted that CS of the chest wall are relatively resistant to chemotherapy and radiotherapy, and, as such, a radical resection with wide margins is favored [31] (Figures 5 and 6).

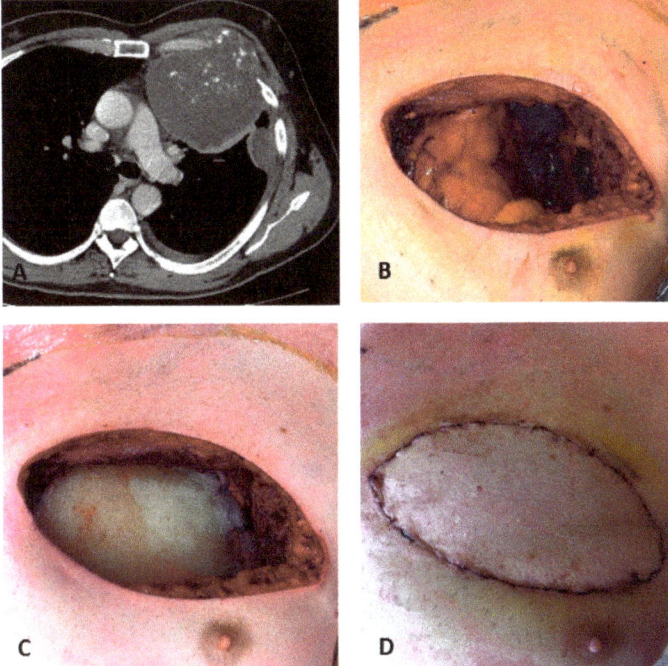

Figure 5. A 67-year-old male patient with a high-grade chondrosarcoma of the costochondral junction. Axial contrast-enhanced CT image (**A**) shows a large chondrosarcoma of the left costochondral junction with less than 25% calcified matrix and a large soft tissue mass. Little left pleural effusion is also present. Intraoperative views show radical resection (**B**), reconstruction by composite rigid prosthesis (**C**), and latissimus dorsi flap reconstruction (**D**). Courtesy of Prof Francesco Petrella, Istituto Europeo di Oncologia (IEO), Milan, Italy.

Following adequate wide-margin resection, patients have been reported to have a 10-year recurrence rate of 7–17%, whereas patients with a local excision only had a reported recurrence rate of 50–57%. Similarly, ten-year survival rates of 96–100% and 65–68% have been reported for patients treated with wide resection and with local excision, respectively [32,33].

Our study has some limitations. Firstly, our sample size is relatively small, but chest wall CS are rare lesions, even in a tertiary referral center. In addition, understanding the proportion of chest wall lesions present with similar features to those we have described as features of chest wall CS would be valuable information, although our study design does not allow exploration of this topic. Secondly, the imaging protocols were heterogeneous, due to the long time span over which the cases were retrieved. Thirdly, clinical presentation, such as the presence of pain, was available for only a small portion of the patients, and was, therefore, not reported.

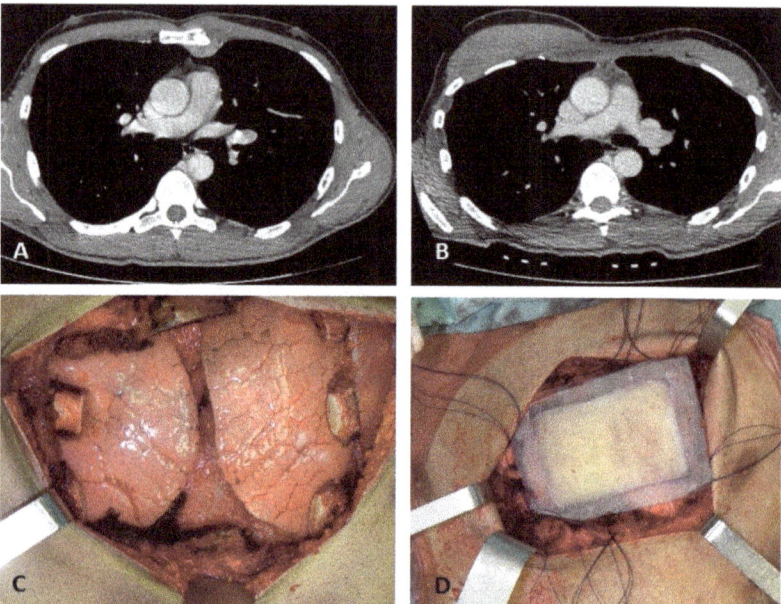

Figure 6. A 35-year-old male patient with a low-grade chondrosarcoma of the sternum. Chondrosarcoma of the sternum with pre- and post-radical resection axial contrast-enhanced CT images (**A**,**B**). Intraoperative views (**C**,**D**) show radical resection and reconstruction by composite rigid prosthesis. Courtesy of Prof Francesco Petrella, Istituto Europeo di Oncologia (IEO), Milan, Italy.

5. Conclusions

In conclusion, chest wall CS are usually lytic lesions with associated soft tissue masses, and have little calcification. The location, lesion size, calcification size and percentage, associated soft tissue mass, and peripheral or central location within the bone are similar for grade 1 and grade 2 CS.

Author Contributions: Conceptualization, L.M.F. and F.D.G.; methodology, L.M.F. and F.D.G.; validation, L.M.F., formal analysis F.D.G., S.A., E.M. and L.M.F. writing—original draft preparation, F.D.G. and L.M.F.; writing—review and editing, F.D.G., S.A., E.M., L.M.F. All authors have read and agreed to the published version of the manuscript.

Funding: This research received no external funding.

Institutional Review Board Statement: The study was conducted according to the guidelines of the Declaration of Helsinki, and approved by the Institutional Review Board of Johns Hopkins Hospital (protocol code IRB-00199443). The protocol was resubmitted on 18 December 2018 and date of approval was 9 January 2019.

Informed Consent Statement: Patient consent was waived because it was not possible to run such a retrospective study with the requirement of a consent form by the patients.

Acknowledgments: We thank Francesco Petrella, Istituto Europeo di Oncologia (IEO), Milan, Italy for providing surgical images and Marilù Garo, for statistical analysis support.

Conflicts of Interest: The authors declare no conflict of interest.

References

1. Liptay, M.J.; Fry, W.A. Malignant bone tumors of the chest wall. *Semin. Thorac. Cardiovasc. Surg.* **1999**, *11*, 278–284. [CrossRef]
2. Tateishi, U.; Gladish, G.W.; Kusumoto, M.; Hasegawa, T.; Yokoyama, R.; Tsuchiya, R.; Moriyama, N. Chest wall tumors: Radiologic findings and pathologic correlation: Part Malignant tumors. *Radiographics* **2003**, *23*, 1491–1508. [CrossRef] [PubMed]
3. Bedard, E.L.; Tang, A.; Johnston, M.R. Massive primary chest wall chondrosarcoma. *Eur. J. Cardiothorac. Surg.* **2004**, *25*, 1124–1125. [CrossRef] [PubMed]
4. He, B.; Huang, Y.; Li, P.; Ye, X.; Lin, F.; Huang, L.; Gao, S.; Shi, H.; Shan, Y. A rare case of primary chondrosarcoma arising from the sternum: A case report. *Oncol. Lett.* **2014**, *8*, 2233–2236. [CrossRef]
5. Kitada, M.; Ozawa, K.; Sato, K.; Hayashi, S.; Sasajima, T. Resection of a chondrosarcoma arising in the right first rib: A case report. *Ann. Thorac. Cardiovasc. Surg.* **2010**, *16*, 119.
6. Lorente, M.P.; De Arriba, C.; Sáenz, J.; Arteche, E.; Abu-Shams, K.; Beloqui, R. An incidental finding in a young woman (2006: 2b). *Eur. Radiol.* **2006**, *16*, 1181–1183. [CrossRef]
7. Rad, M.G.; Mahmodlou, R.; Mohammadi, A.; Mladkova, N.; Noorozinia, F. Spontaneous massive hemothorax secondary to chest wall chondrosarcoma: A case report. *Tuberk Toraks* **2011**, *59*, 168–172. [CrossRef]
8. Sangma, M.M.; Dasiah, S. Chondrosarcoma of a rib. *Int. J. Surg. Case Rep.* **2015**, *10*, 126–128. [CrossRef]
9. Yamamoto, N.; Imai, S.; Motohiro, K.; Shiota, Y.; Sato, N.; Nakayama, H.; Sasaki, N.; Taniyama, K. A case of chondrosarcoma of the low grade malignancy originated in rib. *Kyobu Geka. Jpn. J. Thorac. Surg.* **1995**, *48*, 1141–1143.
10. Zisis, C.; Dountsis, A.; Dahabreh, J. Giant chest wall tumor. *Eur. J. Cardiothorac. Surg.* **2003**, *24*, 825. [CrossRef]
11. Garrison, R.C.; Unni, K.K.; McLeod, R.A.; Pritchard, D.J.; Dahlin, D.C. Chondrosarcoma arising in osteochondroma. *Cancer* **1982**, *49*, 1890–1897. [CrossRef]
12. Nieh, C.C.; Chua, Y.C.; Thirugnanam, A.; Hlwan, M.H. Chest wall secondary chondrosarcoma arising from enchondroma in a young Asian female. *Int. J. Surg. Case Rep.* **2014**, *5*, 968–971. [CrossRef]
13. Rupprecht, H.; Spriewald, B.M.; Hoffmann, A.R. Successful removal of a giant recurrent chondrosarcoma of the thoracic wall in a patient with hereditary multiple exostoses. *Eur. J. Surg. Oncol.* **2001**, *27*, 216–217. [CrossRef]
14. Varma, D.G.; Ayala, A.G.; Carrasco, C.H.; Guo, S.Q.; Kumar, R.; Edeiken, J. Chondrosarcoma: MR imaging with pathologic correlation. *RadioGraphics* **1992**, *12*, 687–704. [CrossRef]
15. Matsuoka, K.; Ueda, M.; Miyamoto, Y. Costal chondrosarcoma requiring differential diagnosis from metastatic tumor. *Asian Cardiovasc. Thorac. Ann.* **2017**, *25*, 154–156. [CrossRef]
16. Park, H.L.; Yoo, I.R.; Lee, Y.; Park, S.Y.; Jung, C.K. Giant Cell Tumor of the Rib: Two Cases of F-18 FDG PET/CT Findings. *Nucl. Med. Mol. Imaging* **2017**, *51*, 182–185. [CrossRef]
17. Saitoh, G.; Yoneshima, Y.; Nakamura, T.; Kitagawa, D.; Kinjo, N.; Ohgaki, K.; Maehara, S.; Teramoto, S.; Adachi, Y.; Ikeda, Y.; et al. Dedifferentiated Chondrosarcoma of the Chest Wall. *Kyobu Geka. Jpn. J. Thorac. Surg.* **2016**, *69*, 764–767.
18. EAl-Refaie, R.; Amer, S.; Ismail, M.; Al-Shabrawy, M.; Al-Gamal, G.; Mokbel, E. Chondrosarcoma of the chest wall: Single-center experience. *Asian Cardiovasc. Thorac. Ann.* **2014**, *22*, 829–834. [CrossRef]
19. Le, H.V.; Wadhwa, R.; Theodore, P.; Mummaneni, P. Excision of Thoracic Chondrosarcoma: Case Report and Review of Literature. *Cureus* **2016**, *8*, e708. [CrossRef]
20. Mori, T.; Suzuki, M. Chest wall tumor, rib tumor. *Kyobu Geka* **2011**, *64*, 725–732.
21. Wang, X.L.; De Beuckeleer, L.H.; De Schepper, A.M.A.; Van Marck, E. Low-grade chondrosarcoma vs enchondroma: Challenges in diagnosis and management. *Eur. Radiol.* **2001**, *11*, 1054–1057. [CrossRef]
22. Murphey, M.D.; Flemming, D.J.; Boyea, S.R.; Bojescul, J.A.; Sweet, D.E.; Temple, H.T. Enchondroma versus chondrosarcoma in the aicular skeleton: Differentiating features. *RadioGraphics* **1998**, *18*, 1213–1237. [CrossRef]
23. Rajiah, P.; Ilaslan, H.; Sundaram, M. Imaging of sarcomas of pelvic bones. *Semin. Ultrasound CT MRI* **2011**, *32*, 433–441. [CrossRef]
24. Aoki, J.; Sone, S.; Fujioka, F.; Terayama, K.; Ishii, K.; Karakida, O.; Imai, S.; Sakai, F.; Imai, Y. MR of enchondroma and chondrosarcoma: Rings and arcs of Gd-DTPA enhancement. *J. Comput. Assist. Tomogr.* **1991**, *15*, 1011–1016. [CrossRef]
25. Nam, S.J.; Kim, S.; Lim, B.J.; Yoon, C.-S.; Kim, T.H.; Suh, J.-S.; Ha, D.H.; Kwon, J.W.; Yoon, Y.C.; Chung, H.W.; et al. Imaging of Primary Chest Wall Tumors with Radiologic-Pathologic Correlation. *RadioGraphics* **2011**, *31*, 749–770. [CrossRef] [PubMed]
26. Brown, A.L.; Barrette, W.C. Enchondroma of the sternum. *Am. J. Surg.* **1958**, *96*, 559–561. [CrossRef]
27. Fink, G.; Bergman, M.; Levy, M.; Avidor, I.; Spitzer, S. Giant chondroma of the sternum mimicking a mediastinal mass. *Thorax* **1990**, *45*, 643–644. [CrossRef]
28. Iartsev, L.P.; Kadyrov, F.A. A case of malignant degeneration of chondroma of the sternum. *Vopr. Onkol.* **1960**, *6*, 80–82.
29. Samberg, C.; Wilson, G.A.; Wilson, G.S. Chondroma of sternum. A case report. *Grace Hosp. Bul.* **1959**, *37*, 93–103.
30. Hughes, E.K.; James, S.L.; Butt, S.; Davies, A.M.; Saifuddin, A. Benign primary tumours of the ribs. *Clin. Radiol.* **2006**, *61*, 314–322. [CrossRef]
31. Marulli, G.; Duranti, L.; Cardillo, G.; Luzzi, L.; Carbone, L.; Gotti, G.; Perissinotto, E.; Rea, F.; Pastorino, U. Primary chest wall chondrosarcomas: Results of surgical resection and analysis of prognostic factors. *Eur. J. Cardiothorac. Surg.* **2014**, *45*, e194–e201. [CrossRef] [PubMed]

32. McAfee, M.K.; Pairolero, P.C.; Bergstralh, E.J.; Piehler, J.M.; Unni, K.K.; McLeod, R.A.; Bernatz, P.E.; Payne, W.S. Chondrosarcoma of the Chest Wall: Factors Affecting Survival. *Ann. Thorac. Surg.* **1985**, *40*, 535–541. [CrossRef]
33. Wang, J.W.; Ger, L.P.; Shih, C.H.; Hsieh, M.C. Chondrosarcoma of bone: A statistical analysis of prognostic factors. *J. Formos. Med. Assoc.* **1991**, *90*, 998–1003. [PubMed]

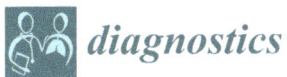

Article

Diagnostic Accuracy of Various Radiological Measurements in the Evaluation and Differentiation of Flatfoot: A Cross-Sectional Study

Fayaz Khan [1,*], Mohamed Faisal Chevidikunnan [1], Mashael Ghazi Alsobhi [1], Israa Anees Ibrahim Ahmed [1], Nada Saleh Al-Lehidan [1], Mohd Rehan [2,3], Hashim Abdullah Alalawi [4] and Ahmed H. Abduljabbar [5]

1 Department of Physical Therapy, Faculty of Medical Rehabilitation Sciences, King Abdulaziz University, Jeddah 22252, Saudi Arabia
2 King Fahd Medical Research Center, King Abdulaziz University, Jeddah 22252, Saudi Arabia
3 Department of Medical Laboratory Sciences, Faculty of Applied Medical Sciences, King Abdulaziz University, Jeddah 22252, Saudi Arabia
4 Department of Radiology, Faculty of Applied Medical Sciences, King Abdulaziz University, Jeddah 22252, Saudi Arabia
5 Department of Radiology, Faculty of Medicine, King Abdulaziz University Hospital, Jeddah 22252, Saudi Arabia
* Correspondence: rkhan2@kau.edu.sa

Abstract: Arch angle is used to indicate flatfoot, but in some cases, it is not easily defined. The presence of flatfoot deformity remains difficult to diagnose due to a lack of reliable radiographic assessment tools. Although various assessment methods for flatfoot have been proposed, there is insufficient evidence to prove the diagnostic accuracy of the various tools. The main purpose of the study was to determine the best radiographic measures for flatfoot concerning the arch angle. Fifty-two feet radiographs from thirty-two healthy young females were obtained. Five angles and one index were measured using weight-bearing lateral radiographs; including arch angle, calcaneal pitch (CP), talar-first metatarsal angle (TFM), lateral talar angle (LTA), talar inclination angle (TIA) and navicular index (NI). Receiver-operating characteristics were generated to evaluate the flatfoot diagnostic accuracy for all radiographic indicators and Matthews correlation coefficient was calculated to determine the cutoff value for each measure. The strongest correlation was between arch angle and CP angle [r = −0.91, $p \leq 0.0001$, 95% confidence interval (CI) (from −0.94 to −0.84)]. Also, significant correlations were found between arch angle and NI [r = 0.62, $p \leq 0.0001$, 95% CI (0.42 to 0.76)], and TFM [r = 0.50, $p \leq 0.0001$, 95% CI (from 0.266 to 0.68)]. Furthermore, CP (cutoff, 12.40) had the highest accuracy level with value of 100% sensitivity and specificity followed by NI, having 82% sensitivity and 89% specificity for the cutoff value of 9.90. In conclusion, CP angle is inversely correlated with arch angle and considered a significant indicator of flatfoot. Also, the NI is easy to define radiographically and could be used to differentiate flat from normal arched foot among young adults.

Keywords: flatfoot; X-rays; pes planus; diagnosis; evaluation

1. Introduction

Flatfoot is a common foot pathology characterized by a collapse of the medial longitudinal arch (MLA) of the foot. As a result, the entire sole of the foot makes total contact with the ground [1]. Additionally, it is characterized by the abduction of the forefoot and eversion of the calcaneus [2]. The MLA has a concave shape that acts as a shock absorber during walking, jumping, and running on different surfaces [3]. The prevalence of flatfoot was reported to be approximately 3–10% among the adult population [4]. Among adults, flatfoot can be asymptomatic or symptomatic, resulting in various clinical consequences [5]. Flatfoot may lead to many deformities or disabilities if it remains undiagnosed [6], and

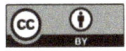

Citation: Khan, F.; Chevidikunnan, M.F.; Alsobhi, M.G.; Ahmed, I.A.I.; Al-Lehidan, N.S.; Rehan, M.; Alalawi, H.A.; Abduljabbar, A.H. Diagnostic Accuracy of Various Radiological Measurements in the Evaluation and Differentiation of Flatfoot: A Cross-Sectional Study. *Diagnostics* **2022**, *12*, 2288. https://doi.org/10.3390/diagnostics12102288

Academic Editor: Majid Chalian

Received: 1 September 2022
Accepted: 16 September 2022
Published: 22 September 2022

Publisher's Note: MDPI stays neutral with regard to jurisdictional claims in published maps and institutional affiliations.

Copyright: © 2022 by the authors. Licensee MDPI, Basel, Switzerland. This article is an open access article distributed under the terms and conditions of the Creative Commons Attribution (CC BY) license (https://creativecommons.org/licenses/by/4.0/).

further consequences may include pain in the lower extremities [7], back pain [8], stress fractures [9], and hallux valgus deformities [10].

The foot is an important component of the body that maintains adequate balance when people move in their gaits. Individuals with foot deformities are more susceptible to falls and loss of balance, which affect their quality of life (QoL) [11–13]. In clinical practice, foot structural deformities have a high prevalence of 50% to 80% among adults [14]. Several studies reported the negative impacts of different foot deformities on the QoL. A recent study conducted by López-López et al. (2021) [15] investigated the relationship between QoL and foot health among individuals with and without foot pathologies. The researchers stated that foot disorders negatively affect people's daily life activities. Additionally, another study highlighted the importance of considering the relationship between QoL and foot structure deformities [16]. In that context, the present study was conducted to discover the best radiographic measure for detecting flatfoot, which may assist in improving the quality of care among young adults.

Clinically, there are several approaches to identifying flatfoot deformity, including clinical diagnosis [17], footprint, and radiologic assessment [18]. In radiographic assessment, the weight-bearing MLA has been utilized as a diagnostic assessment tool to determine the presence of flatfoot [19]. While it is considered the standard diagnostic method, numerous studies have found discrepancies in MLA radiographic measurements among subjects [20–23]. Many radiological measurements can be determined from the weight-bearing X-ray [24]. A set of radiological measurements can be defined from a posterior or lateral radiographic view of the weight-bearing foot to identify flatfoot deformity. The arch angle and calcaneal pitch angle (CP) have been used radiographically to evaluate the MLA [25]. In a study conducted in Taiwan, military recruits were determined to have flatfoot if the arch angle was $\geq 165°$. However, researchers revealed that the assessment of arch angle was restricted because the image quality was affected by the superimposition of the metatarsal bones [6]. It was recommended that the CP angle should be measured to distinguish flatfoot from a normal arch when it is challenging to define the arch angle.

Today, several radiographic assessment techniques are proposed for use in the MLA assessment, such as: talar-first metatarsal angle (TFM), lateral talar angle (LTA), talar inclination angle (TIA), and navicular index (NI) [22,23,26,27], however none of these measures are universally agreed on. In this study, we aimed to find the best radiographic measurement for diagnosing flatfoot among healthy females. According to the available studies, there is limited literature regarding the measurement of flatfoot angles among healthy, young females. This study was conducted to provide information about cutoff values for the five radiographic measures (CP, TFM, LTA, TIA, and NI), to facilitate the improved interpretation and evaluation of flatfoot radiographs. Additionally, we aimed to identify the relationship between these sets of radiographic measures by keeping the arch angle as the reference value. This study hypothesized that radiographic measures represent simple and easy tools to use to diagnose flatfoot with a high level of sensitivity and specificity. Furthermore, the researchers of this study hypothesized that relationships exist between the five radiographic measures (CP, TFM, LTA, TIA, and NI) and the arch angle.

2. Materials and Methods
2.1. Subjects and Setting

Researchers of this study used the Foot Posture Index (FPI $\geq$ +6) to screen for the flatfoot. Subjects who scored +6 or above on the FPI for one or both feet were included in the study. Subjects who had any history of surgery or restricted foot and/or ankle range of motion were excluded from the study. After fulfilling the criteria, only thirty-two healthy young females aged between 18 to 25 years were recruited for the study. The minimum sample size was calculated by using G-power 3.1 software (G-power v3.1. https://gpower.software.informer.com/3.1/ (accessed on 28 March 2022)) to achieve a power of 0.80. In G-power, a correlation test was selected for a priori power calculation with a medium effect size of 0.7 and significance level of 0.05. Thirty-nine feet were estimated to be the minimum sample needed to reach a power of 0.8 and in the current study fifty two feet were included for the analysis. This cross-sectional study was conducted in the Department of Physical Therapy, King Abdulaziz University. The report of this study has been written according to the Standards for Reporting Diagnostic accuracy studies (STARD) [28] and the Strengthening the Reporting of Observational Studies in Epidemiology (STROBE) guidelines (Table S1) [29].

2.2. Procedure

Ethical approval was obtained from the Center of Excellence in Genomic Medical Research (number: 05-CEGMR-Bioeth-2019), approved by the National Committee of Bioethics (KACST: HA-02-J-003). Also, a written informed consent was obtained from each subject before they were included in the study. Demographic characteristics of the subjects including age, gender, BMI, and FPI-6 were documented for each of the subjects. Then, subjects were asked to take off their shoes and socks for barefoot examination to determine subjects' eligibility for the study. FPI-6 is considered a good reliable clinical flatfoot measurement tool with inter-rater reliability between 0.62 to 0.91 and intra-rater reliability of 0.81 to 0.91 [30], and it is used to determine the presence of flatfoot in either right or left foot. The first author F.K, who is a senior author with 15 years of experience, screened the subjects. Also, an experienced radiologist who was blinded to the study took the foot X-rays. The first and second author M.C, who has 20 years of experience in the musculoskeletal field, measured the angles using RadiAnt DICOM software (RadiAnt DICOM v4.2. https://www.radiantviewer.com/ (accessed on 12 April 2022)).

Figure 1 shows a flowchart of the subject selection process. All subjects were instructed to walk a few steps, then stand in a relaxed–static standing position with head in a neutral position and both arms by their sides. The six components of the FPI-6 are: (a) palpation of the talonavicular head, (b) observation and comparison of the superior and inferior lateral malleolus curves, (c) observation of the inversion and eversion of the calcaneus in the frontal plane, (d) protrusions in the region of the talonavicular joint, (e) height and congruence of the medial longitudinal arch, and (f) abduction/adduction of the forefoot on the rearfoot. Each component of the six observations was measured and graded as 0 for a neutral foot position, at least -2 for a clear indication of foot supination, and at most $+2$ for a clear indication of foot pronation. The total FPI score for all components was between -12 and $+12$. Foot posture was classified as normal if the total score was between 0 and $+5$, supinated if the score was between -1 and -12, or pronated if it was scored from $+6$ to $+12$. Only subjects who scored $+6$ and above were included in the study [31,32].

After determining the eligibility of the subjects, foot X-rays were taken by an experienced radiologist who was blinded to the study. A lateral weight-bearing radiograph was taken for each foot separately while the subject was standing straight (in an upright neutral position) on a table and the other foot was raised. The X-ray system used for the study was a DR Definum 6000 machine (General Electric Company, Boston, USA) with a 17×14-inch cassette. The placement of the cassette was between the medial borders of the hindfoot, maintained vertically in the groove. From a fixed distance of 100 cm, the X-ray tube was directed vertically toward the cassette. The exposure was set at 52 kV and 4.5 mA for the lateral projection. The central X-ray beam was aimed toward the navicular bone.

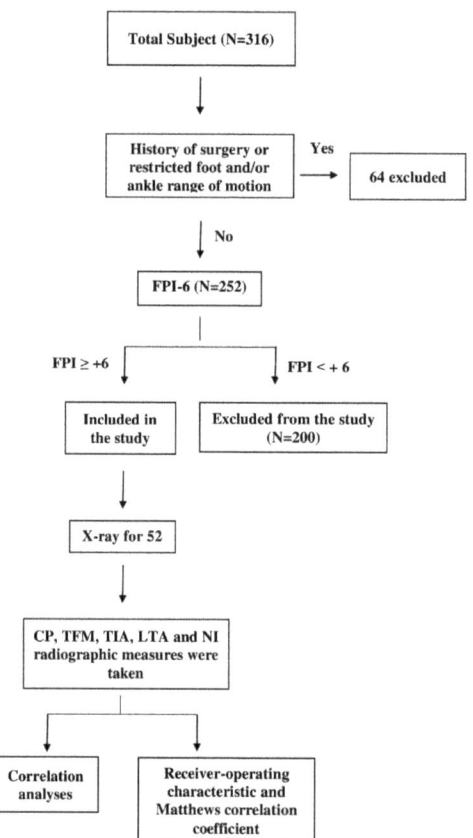

Figure 1. Flowchart of the study selection procedure and design.

In our study, five angles and one index were measured to determine flatfoot on the radiographs, including the arch angle, CP, TFM, LTA, TIA, and NI. The arch angle was used as the reference standard for all other radiographic measures in this study. The arch angle was measured at the intersection of two lines: the calcaneal line (a line drawn along the inferior surface of the calcaneus) and the fifth metatarsal line (a line drawn along the inferior edge of the fifth metatarsal bone) [33]. Subjects were determined to have flatfoot if the arch angle was ≥165° [34]. The CP angle was drawn by a horizontal line (a line drawn horizontally from calcaneus to the inferior surface of the 5th metatarsal head inferior surface) and the calcaneal line [33]. The TFM angle was made by the intersection of the two longitudinal axes of the first metatarsal and talus. The talus longitudinal axis was the line connecting the centers of the talar head and neck parts in its narrowest width [35,36]. The lateral talar angle was the angle created between the talus line, which runs through the center point of the body and neck of the talus, and the calcaneal line. The talar inclination angle was made between the horizontal line and the talar line [22]. To determine the NI, the longitudinal arch length was divided by the navicular height measured from the floor [26] (Figure 2a,b).

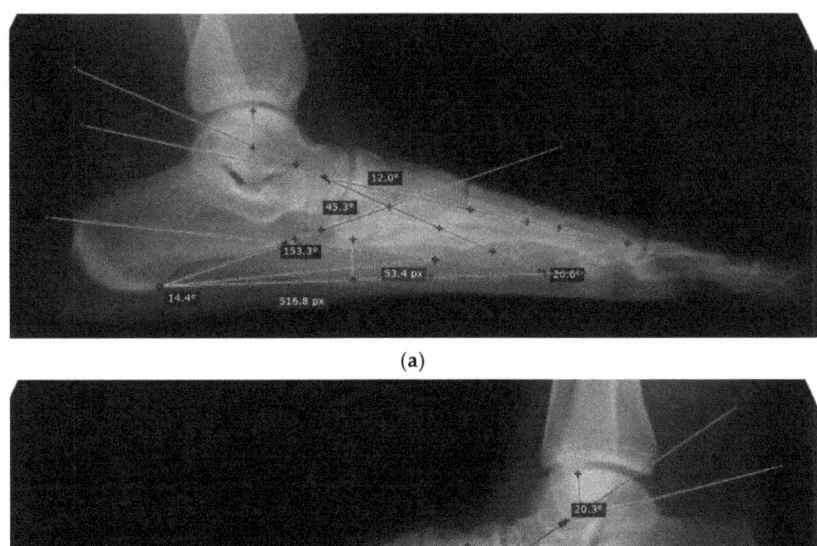

Figure 2. (a): Lateral radiographic assessment of a normal weight-bearing foot demonstrating the arch angle = 153.3°, CP angle = 26.6°, TFM = 12°, TIA = 14.4°, LTA = 45.3°, and NI = 9.68. (b): Lateral radiographic assessment of a flatfoot weight-bearing foot demonstrating the arch angle = 168.7°, CP angle = 7.8°, TFM = 20.3°, TIA = 33.5°, LTA = 43.4°, and NI =19.5.

2.3. Statistical Analysis

The data were analyzed using the Statistical Package for Social Sciences version 21.0 (Statistical Package for Social Sciences v21.0. https://www.ibm.com/support/pages/downloading-ibm-spss-statistics-21 (accessed on 24 May 2022) and GraphPad Prism (GraphPad Prism v7.0. https://www.graphpad.com/guides/prism/7/user-guide/ (accessed on 18 June 2022)). Descriptive statistics were used to describe the demographic characteristics of the sample. Mean, median and standard deviation were calculated for age, BMI, FPI and all radiographic measurements. Correlation analyses were used to identify the associations between arch angle and the five radiographic measurements. Correlation coefficients (r) were classified as follows: little or no association (r = 0–0.24), fair (r = 0.25–0.49), moderate–good (r = 0.50–0.74), and good–excellent association (r = 0.75–1) [37]. Before conducting the correlation analysis, data were checked for normality to perform the suitable test by conducting the Shapiro–Wilk test. The receiver-operating characteristic (ROC) test was conducted for the CP, TFM, LTA, TIA and NI measures, compared to the arch angle for predicting flatfoot. Matthews correlation coefficient (MCC) was used to define the cutoff value for all flatfoot radiographic measurements. A p-value of 0.05 or less was considered statistically significant for all analyses.

2.4. Receiver-Operating Characteristic (ROC) Curve

The ROC test is a popular and widely used method to evaluate the performance of a binary classifier model. The ROC curve is generated by plotting the true positive rate (TPR) versus the false positive rate (FPR) with various cutoff settings for the binary classifier.

The area under the curve (AUC) or ROC space provides a measure of the effectiveness of the binary classifier. An ideal classifier will cover 100% area (AUC = 1.0) and a random classifier will cover 50% area (AUC = 0.5) with all the points along the diagonal.

2.5. Matthews Correlation Coefficient (MCC)

The MCC or phi coefficient is a measure of the quality of a binary classifier, calculated as follows:

$$\text{MCC} = \frac{TP \times TN - FP \times FN}{\sqrt{(TP+FP)(TP+FN)(TN+FP)(TN+FN)}}$$

The value of MCC ranges between −1 and +1. The value of MCC + 1 represents an ideal classifier, 0 a random classifier, and −1 a total disagreement between prediction and observation. The maximum value of MCC was used to determine the cutoff value for each classifier.

3. Results

The radiographic data of fifty-two feet images were included in the analysis. The mean age of the subjects was 20.69 ± 1.15 years (range = 18–25 years) and their mean BMI was 23.02 ± 3.79 kg/m^2 (range = 16.20–33.30). The mean values of the five radiographic angles and the NI are illustrated in Table 1.

Table 1. Demographic characteristics and baseline scores (n = 52).

Variables	Mean ± SD	Median (Range)	95% CI
Age (years)	20.69 ± 1.15	21 (18–25)	20.37–21.01
BMI (kg/m^2)	23.02 ± 3.79	23.01 (16.20–33.30)	21.96–24.08
FPI-6	7.22 ± 2.76	9 (6–11)	6.45–7.99
Arch angle	159.1 ± 6.74	157.8 (141–171.6)	157.2–161
CP	15.14 ± 4.66	15.70 (5.2–24.9)	13.85–16.44
TFMA	11.06 ± 5.37	10.50 (1.5–26.00)	9.56–12.55
LTA	43.50 ± 6.04	44.45 (25.60–54.60)	25.29–27.82
TIA	26.56 ± 4.54	26.65 (14.10–36.40)	25.29–27.82
NI	9.54 ± 5.82	8.03 (4.42–39.44)	7.92–11.16

SD: standard deviation; 95% CI: confidence interval.

All radiographic measurements were significantly correlated with the arch angle ($p \leq 0.05$). All the angles and NI had a positive correlation with the arch angle, except for the CP angle, which had a negative relationship. We found the strongest correlation was between the arch angle and the CP angle (r = −0.91, $p \leq 0.0001$, 95% CI (from 0.94 to −0.84)). Additionally, a significant relationship was found between the arch angle and the NI (r = 0.62, $p \leq 0.0001$, 95% CI (from 0.42 to 0.76)), and the TFM (r = 0.50, $p \leq 0.0001$, 95% CI (from 0.27 to 0.68)). However, we found a weak relationship was found between the arch angle and the LTA (r = −0.49, p = 0.0002, 95% CI (from −0.67 to −0.24)), and the TIA (r = 0.32, p = 0.021, 95% CI (from 0.05 to 0.55)) (Figure 3).

The ROC test showed that the CP angle and NI were perfect classifiers for flatfoot, with AUCs of 1 and 0.9, respectively (Figure 4 and Table 2). We found a CP angle cutoff of 12.40 yielded high accuracy, with a sensitivity and specificity of 1 for the flatfoot diagnosis, while NI with a cutoff value of 9.90 yielded 0.82 sensitivity and 0.89 specificity. Meanwhile, the LTA (0.76 sensitivity and 0.83 specificity) had a cutoff value of 41.8 and MCC of 0.58, while the TFM angle (0.65 sensitivity and 0.86 specificity) had a cutoff value of 13.4 and MCC of 0.51. Similarly, the TIA angle (0.88 sensitivity and 0.37 specificity) had a cutoff value of 24.60 and MCC of 0.26 (Table 2).

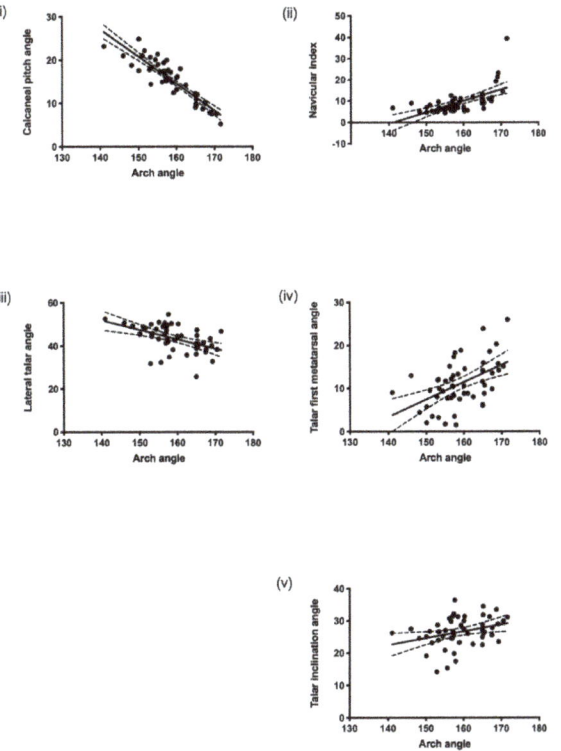

Figure 3. Correlation of arch angle with (**i**) calcaneal pitch angle, (**ii**) navicular index, (**iii**) lateral talar angle, (**iv**) talar-first metatarsal angle, and (**v**) talar inclination angle.

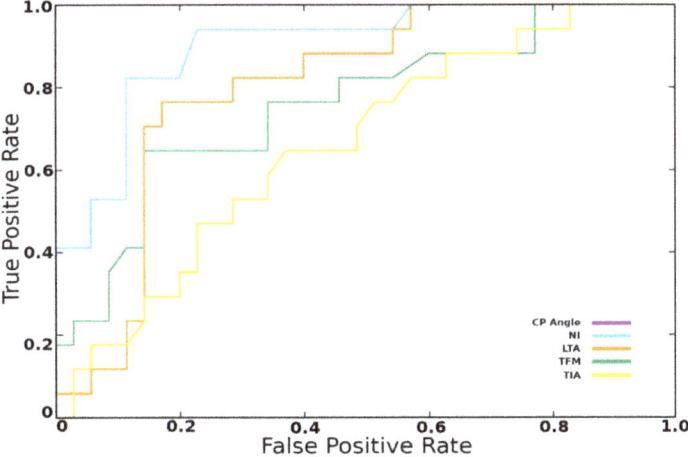

Figure 4. Receiver-operating characteristic (ROC) curves demonstrating the sensitivity (true positive rate) and specificity (1—false positive rate) of the arch angle, calcaneal pitch angle (CP), talar-first metatarsal angle (TFM), talar inclination angle (TIA), and lateral talar angle (LTA) when used for predicting flatfoot.

Table 2. ROC measures including AUC or ROC space and MCC cutoff values for the four radiographic parameters. The MCC cutoff column shows the cutoff values, with the MCC values in parentheses.

Parameter	AUC	MCC Cutoff	FPR (1-Specificity)	TPR (Sensitivity)	PPV	NPV
CP	1.00	12.40 (1.00)	0	1	1	1
NI	0.90	9.90 (0.70)	0.11	0.82	0.78	0.91
LTA	0.8	41.8 (0.58)	0.17	0.76	0.68	0.88
TFM	0.76	13.4 (0.51)	0.14	0.65	0.69	0.83
TIA	0.66	24.60 (0.26)	0.63	0.88	0.40	0.87

4. Discussion

The aim of this study was to determine the best radiographic measures for diagnosing flatfoot concerning arch angle measurements. Although numerous flatfoot diagnostic procedures have been proposed in the literature, there remains no standard diagnostic measure to determine the presence of flatfoot. According to the available studies, the accuracy levels of these flatfoot diagnostic measures have not yet been determined [25]. In our study, we discovered that the CP angle was the best flatfoot indicator among all radiographic measures, which was indicated by its perfect sensitivity and specificity, as well as its PPV and NPV values. In addition, the CP angle had a strong negative correlation with the arch angle, and it had an AUC value equal to 1. Our findings were consistent with the results of Huan-Chu Lo et al., who found that the CP angle was a significant indicator of flatfoot. Our findings further suggested that the CP angle might be the best radiographic measure to predict flatfoot after the arch angle. In our study, the CP angle cutoff of <12.40° was determined to identify flatfoot, with a sensitivity and specificity of 1, which was in line with the results of Huan-Chu Lo et al., who determined the cutoff value for the CP angle to be <12.30°. The CP angle represents a useful indicator to distinguish a normal foot from flatfoot because it can be defined easily on the foot radiograph by the intersection of the calcaneal and horizontal lines [6].

An important finding of this study was the significant association between the NI and arch angle. The NI had a cutoff value of 9.90, with 0.82 sensitivity and 0.89 specificity. To the best of our knowledge, no previous studies assessed the NI as a diagnostic measure for adult flatfoot. However, a study was conducted by Roth et al. on children to identify the association of NI with other flatfoot diagnostic measurement angles, and they stated that a NI cutoff value of 6.74 distinguished flatfeet from normal feet among children, with 0.86 sensitivity and 0.75 specificity, which was similar to our findings [26]. Amongst the different flatfoot measuring angles described in the literature, the NI represents an easy and quick method to determine flatfoot because the determination procedure does not require high-quality X-ray images; instead, the NI can simply be obtained by dividing the height of the longitudinal arch by the navicular bone height. Therefore, the NI might offer a valuable radiographic measuring tool to determine flatfoot among young adults.

On the lateral radiographic view, the TFM angle was determined by measuring the talar inclination and heel pronation, and it was moderately associated with the arch angle. In this study, the TFM cutoff value was found to be 13.4°, with 0.65 sensitivity and 0.86 specificity, which was a slightly higher cutoff value than that found previously in the literature (9.58, with a high specificity of 0.90) [6]. The cutoff value discrepancy might be attributable to the different flatfoot screening criteria used, i.e., FPI $\geq$ 6 in our study vs. arch angle $\geq$165° in the study of Huan-Chu Lo et al. [6].

In contrast to all other radiographical measures, the LTA and TIA were weakly correlated with the arch angle reference. Additionally, the AUC values for both angles were below 0.9, signaling they were inefficient indicators of flatfoot, in keeping with the previous findings [20,23,27]. The LTA was not easily determined because of the irregular shape of the calcaneus and talus. This was highlighted in a recent study by Hamel et al., who noted the difficulty of defining this angle on foot radiographs [27].

It is not easy to identify adult flatfoot and there are no definitive diagnostic tools for that purpose. The results of this study defined several radiographic measures that can be used in clinical settings. A key strength of this study was discovering that the NI offers an easy and precise radiographic measure for flatfoot thanks to the simplicity of its measurement, i.e., dividing the length of the foot arch by the navicular height. Yet, as with any research, there were some limitations to the findings of this study. Our sample was limited to healthy, young females, which may limit the applicability of the findings to other populations. Future studies may compare males and females to assess and confirm the results of this study. Additionally, further research could include a wide range of ages among both genders, which is recommended to confirm the results presented in this report. Furthermore, our study was limited to the radiographic assessment methods; to go beyond this, future studies may compare the radiographic measures with other flatfoot diagnostic methods such as footprint analysis. Additionally, this study failed to investigate whether there was a significant difference in radiographic or demographic features of adult flatfoot, which could be investigated in the future.

In conclusion, the study findings suggest that the CP angle and the NI can be used as indicators to determine the presence of flatfoot. Moreover, the study findings demonstrate strong correlations between the arch angle, CP angle, TFM angle, and NI. The CP angle and NI may represent the best radiographic measuring tools to evaluate the presence of flatfoot among young adults. The results of this study produce a baseline for the radiographic measures that can be used to indicate flatfoot. The CP angle and NI are simple and accurate identifiers of flatfoot that can be easily applied in clinical settings. It is essential to highlight the importance of determining flatfoot because of its association with fall risk and balance problems among adults.

Supplementary Materials: The following supporting information can be downloaded at: https://www.mdpi.com/article/10.3390/diagnostics12102288/s1, Table S1: STROBE Statement—Checklist of items that should be included in reports of cross-sectional studies.

Author Contributions: Conceptualization, F.K., M.F.C., M.G.A. and N.S.A.-L.; data collection, F.K., N.S.A.-L., H.A.A., A.H.A. and I.A.I.A.; methodology, F.K., M.F.C., M.G.A., I.A.I.A., N.S.A.-L., M.R., H.A.A. and A.H.A.; writing—original draft preparation, F.K., M.F.C., M.G.A., I.A.I.A., N.S.A.-L., M.R., H.A.A. and A.H.A.; writing—review and editing, F.K., M.F.C. and M.G.A.; supervision, F.K., M.F.C., M.R. and A.H.A.; project administration, F.K., M.F.C., M.R., H.A.A. and A.H.A.; funding acquisition, F.K. and M.F.C. All authors have read and agreed to the published version of the manuscript.

Funding: This project was funded by the Deanship of Scientific Research (DSR) at King Abdulaziz University, Jeddah (under grant number G-621-142-38). The authors acknowledge with thanks the DSR for the technical and financial support it provided. The funders had no role in the design of the study; in the collection, analyses, or interpretation of data; in the writing of the manuscript, or in the decision to publish the results.

Institutional Review Board Statement: The study was conducted according to the guidelines of the Declaration of Helsinki, and it was approved by the Center of Excellence in Genomic Medical Research (number 05-CEGMR-Bioeth-2019) and the National Committee of Bioethics (KACST: HA-02-J-003).

Informed Consent Statement: Informed consent was obtained from all subjects involved in the study.

Data Availability Statement: The data presented in this study are available on request from the corresponding author. The data are not publicly available due to privacy restrictions.

Conflicts of Interest: The authors declare no conflict of interest.

References

1. Lin, Y.-C.; Ni Mhuircheartaigh, J.; Lamb, J.; Kung, J.W.; Yablon, C.M.; Wu, J.S. Imaging of Adult Flatfoot: Correlation of Radiographic Measurements With MRI. *Am. J. Roentgenol.* **2015**, *204*, 354–359. [CrossRef] [PubMed]
2. Flores, D.V.; Gómez, C.M.; Hernando, M.F.; Davis, M.A.; Pathria, M.N. Adult Acquired Flatfoot Deformity: Anatomy, Biomechanics, Staging, and Imaging Findings. *RadioGraphics* **2019**, *39*, 1437–1460. [CrossRef] [PubMed]

3. Yang, C.-H.; Chou, K.-T.; Chung, M.-B.; Chuang, K.S.; Huang, T.-C. Automatic Detection of Calcaneal-Fifth Metatarsal Angle Using Radiograph: A Computer-Aided Diagnosis of Flat Foot for Military New Recruits in Taiwan. *PLoS ONE* **2015**, *10*, e0131387. [CrossRef]
4. Martinelli, N.; Bianchi, A.; Prandoni, L.; Maiorano, E.; Sansone, V. Quality of Life in Young Adults after Flatfoot Surgery: A Case-Control Study. *J. Clin. Med.* **2021**, *10*, 451. [CrossRef] [PubMed]
5. Lee, M.S.; Vanore, J.V.; Thomas, J.L.; Catanzariti, A.R.; Kogler, G.; Kravitz, S.R.; Miller, S.J.; Gassen, S.C. Diagnosis and treatment of adult flatfoot. *J. Foot Ankle Surg.* **2005**, *44*, 78–113. [CrossRef]
6. Lo, H.-C.; Chu, W.-C.; Wu, W.-K.; Hsieh, H.; Chou, C.-P.; Sun, S.-E.; Chou, P.-Y.; Liao, C.-H.; Guan, X.-Y.; Li, S.-C. Comparison of radiological measures for diagnosing flatfoot. *Acta Radiol.* **2012**, *53*, 192–196. [CrossRef]
7. Uden, H.; Scharfbillig, R.; Causby, R. The typically developing paediatric foot: How flat should it be? A systematic review. *J. Foot Ankle Res.* **2017**, *10*, 37. [CrossRef]
8. Buldt, A.K.; Murley, G.S.; Butterworth, P.; Levinger, P.; Menz, H.B.; Landorf, K.B. The relationship between foot posture and lower limb kinematics during walking: A systematic review. *Gait Posture* **2013**, *38*, 363–372. [CrossRef]
9. Cheng, Y.; Yang, H.; Ni, L.; Song, D.; Zhang, H. Stress fracture of the distal fibula in flatfoot patients: Case report. *Int. J. Clin. Exp. Med.* **2015**, *8*, 6303–6307.
10. Nguyen, U.-S.; Hillstrom, H.; Li, W.; Dufour, A.; Kiel, D.; Procter-Gray, E.; Gagnon, M.; Hannan, M. Factors associated with hallux valgus in a population-based study of older women and men: The MOBILIZE Boston Study. *Osteoarthr. Cartil.* **2010**, *18*, 41–46. [CrossRef]
11. López-López, D.; Expósito-Casabella, Y.; Iglesias, M.E.L.; Vallejo, R.B.D.B.; Saleta-Canosa, J.L.; Alonso-Tajes, F. Impact of shoe size in a sample of elderly individuals. *Rev. Assoc. Med. Bras.* **2016**, *62*, 789–794. [CrossRef] [PubMed]
12. Irving, D.B.; Cook, J.L.; Young, M.A.; Menz, H. Impact of Chronic Plantar Heel Pain on Health-Related Quality of Life. *J. Am. Podiatr. Med. Assoc.* **2008**, *98*, 283–289. [CrossRef]
13. Menz, H.B.; Morris, M.; Lord, S.R. Foot and Ankle Characteristics Associated with Impaired Balance and Functional Ability in Older People. *J. Gerontol. A Biol. Sci. Med. Sci.* **2005**, *60*, 1546–1552. [CrossRef] [PubMed]
14. Santos, A.D.; Prado-Rico, J.M.; Cirino NT de, O.; Perracini, M.R. Are foot deformity and plantar sensitivity impairment associated with physical function of community-dwelling older adults? *Braz. J. Phys. Ther.* **2021**, *25*, 846–853. [CrossRef] [PubMed]
15. López-López, D.; Pérez-Ríos, M.; Ruano-Ravina, A.; Losa-Iglesias, M.E.; Becerro-De-Bengoa-Vallejo, R.; Romero-Morales, C.; Calvo-Lobo, C.; Navarro-Flores, E. Impact of quality of life related to foot problems: A case–control study. *Sci. Rep.* **2021**, *1451*, 14515. [CrossRef] [PubMed]
16. López-López, D.; Vilar-Fernández, J.M.; Barros-García, G.; Losa-Iglesias, M.E.; Palomo-López, P.; Becerro-De-Bengoa-Vallejo, R.; Calvo-Lobo, C. Foot Arch Height and Quality of Life in Adults: A Strobe Observational Study. *Int. J. Environ. Res. Public Health* **2018**, *15*, 1555. [CrossRef]
17. Menz, H.B.; Fotoohabadi, M.R.; Wee, E.; Spink, M. Visual categorisation of the Arch Index: A simplified measure of foot posture in older people. *J. Foot Ankle Res.* **2012**, *5*, 10. [CrossRef]
18. Murley, G.S.; Menz, H.B.; Landorf, K.B. A protocol for classifying normal- and flat-arched foot posture for research studies using clinical and radiographic measurements. *J. Foot Ankle Res.* **2009**, *2*, 22. [CrossRef]
19. Aenumulapalli, A.; Kulkarni, M.M.; Gandotra, A.R. Prevalence of Flexible Flat Foot in Adults: A Cross-sectional Study. *JCDR* **2017**, *11*, AC17. [CrossRef]
20. Chen, C.-H.; Huang, M.-H.; Chen, T.-W.; Weng, M.-C.; Lee, C.-L.; Wang, G.-J. The Correlation Between Selected Measurements from Footprint and Radiograph of Flatfoot. *Arch. Phys. Med. Rehabil.* **2006**, *87*, 235–240. [CrossRef]
21. Kanatli, U.; Yetkin, H.; Cila, E. Footprint and Radiographic Analysis of the Feet. *J. Pediatr. Orthop.* **2001**, *21*, 225–228. [CrossRef] [PubMed]
22. Pehlivan, O.; Cilli, F.; Mahirogullari, M.; Karabudak, O.; Koksal, O. Radiographic correlation of symptomatic and asymptomatic flexible flatfoot in young male adults. *Int. Orthop.* **2009**, *33*, 447–450. [CrossRef] [PubMed]
23. Younger, A.S.; Sawatzky, B.; Dryden, P. Radiographic Assessment of Adult Flatfoot. *Foot Ankle Int.* **2005**, *26*, 820–825. [CrossRef]
24. Agoada, D.; Kramer, P.A. Radiographic measurements of the talus and calcaneus in the adult pes planus foot type. *Am. J. Phys. Anthr.* **2020**, *171*, 613–627. [CrossRef] [PubMed]
25. Kao, E.-F.; Lu, C.-Y.; Wang, C.-Y.; Yeh, W.-C.; Hsia, P.-K. Fully automated determination of arch angle on weight-bearing foot radiograph. *Comput. Methods Programs Biomed.* **2018**, *154*, 79–88. [CrossRef]
26. Roth, S.; Roth, A.; Jotanovic, Z.; Madarevic, T. Navicular index for differentiation of flatfoot from normal foot. *Int. Orthop.* **2013**, *37*, 1107–1112. [CrossRef]
27. Hamel, J.; Hörterer, H.; Harrasser, N. Is it possible to define reference values for radiographic parameters evaluating juvenile flatfoot deformity? A case-control study. *BMC Musculoskelet. Disord.* **2020**, *21*, 838. [CrossRef]
28. Bossuyt, P.M.; Reitsma, J.B.; Bruns, D.E.; Gatsonis, C.A.; Glasziou, P.P.; Irwig, L.; Lijmer, J.G.; Moher, D.; Rennie, D.; de Vet, H.C.W.; et al. STARD 2015: An updated list of essential items for reporting diagnostic accuracy studies. *BMJ* **2015**, *351*, h5527. [CrossRef]
29. Von Elm, E.; Altman, D.G.; Egger, M.; Pocock, S.J.; Gøtzsche, P.C.; Vandenbroucke, J.P.; STROBE Initiative. The Strengthening the Reporting of Observational Studies in Epidemiology (STROBE) statement: Guidelines for reporting observational studies. *J. Clin. Epidemiol.* **2008**, *61*, 344–349. [CrossRef]

30. Redmond, A.C.; Crosbie, J.; Ouvrier, R.A. Development and validation of a novel rating system for scoring standing foot posture: The Foot Posture Index. *Clin. Biomech.* **2006**, *21*, 89–98. [CrossRef]
31. Khan, F.; Chevidikunnan, M.; Mazi, A.; Aljawi, S.; Mizan, F.; BinMulayh, E.; Sahu, K.S.; Al-Lehidan, N. Factors affecting foot posture in young adults: A cross sectional study. *J. Musculoskelet Neuronal. Interact.* **2020**, *20*, 216–222. [PubMed]
32. Lee, J.S.; Kim, K.B.; Jeong, J.O.; Kwon, N.Y.; Jeong, S.M. Correlation of Foot Posture Index With Plantar Pressure and Radiographic Measurements in Pediatric Flatfoot. *Ann. Rehabil. Med.* **2015**, *39*, 10–17. [CrossRef] [PubMed]
33. DiGiovanni, J.; Smith, S. Normal biomechanics of the adult rearfoot: A radiographic analysis. *J. Am. Podiatr. Med. Assoc.* **1976**, *66*, 812–824. [CrossRef] [PubMed]
34. Kaschak, T.J.; Laine, W. Radiology of the diabetic foot. *Clin. Podiatr. Med. Surg.* **1988**, *5*, 849–857.
35. Shakoor, D.; Netto, C.D.C.; Thawait, G.K.; Ellis, S.J.; Richter, M.; Schon, L.C.; Demehri, S. Weight-bearing radiographs and cone-beam computed tomography examinations in adult acquired flatfoot deformity. *Foot Ankle Surg.* **2020**, *27*, 201–206. [CrossRef]
36. Sensiba, P.R.; Coffey, M.J.; Williams, N.E.; Mariscalco, M.; Laughlin, R.T. Inter- and Intraobserver Reliability in the Radiographic Evaluation of Adult Flatfoot Deformity. *Foot Ankle Int.* **2010**, *31*, 141–145. [CrossRef]
37. Inui, K.; Ikoma, K.; Imai, K.; Ohashi, S.; Maki, M.; Kido, M.; Hara, Y.; Oka, Y.; Fujiwara, H.; Kubo, T. Examination of the Correlation Between Foot Morphology Measurements Using Pedography and Radiographic Measurements. *J. Foot Ankle Surg.* **2017**, *56*, 298–303. [CrossRef]

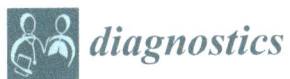

Article

Myeloma Spine and Bone Damage Score (MSBDS) on Whole-Body Computed Tomography (WBCT): Multiple Reader Agreement in a Multicenter Reliability Study

Alberto Stefano Tagliafico [1,2,*], Clarissa Valle [3,4], Pietro Andrea Bonaffini [3,4], Ali Attieh [2], Matteo Bauckneht [1,2], Liliana Belgioia [1,2], Bianca Bignotti [2], Nicole Brunetti [1,2], Alessandro Bonsignore [1,2], Enrico Capaccio [2], Sara De Giorgis [1,2], Alessandro Garlaschi [2], Silvia Morbelli [1,2], Federica Rossi [5], Lorenzo Torri [6], Simone Caprioli [2,7], Simona Tosto [2], Michele Cea [2,7] and Alida Dominietto [2]

1. Department of Health Sciences, University of Genoa, 16132 Genoa, Italy
2. Ospedale Policlinico San Martino, 16132 Genoa, Italy
3. School of Medicine, University Milano Bicocca, 20126 Milan, Italy
4. Department of Diagnostic Radiology, Papa Giovanni XXIII Hospital, 24127 Bergamo, Italy
5. Department of Radiology, Ospedale Santa Corona, 17027 Pietra Ligure, Italy
6. Department of Vascular Surgery, AOU Pisana, 56124 Pisa, Italy
7. Department of Internal Medicine, University of Genoa, 16132 Genoa, Italy
* Correspondence: alberto.tagliafico@unige.it

Abstract: **Objective:** To assess the reliability of the myeloma spine and bone damage score (MSBDS) across multiple readers with different levels of expertise and from different institutions. **Methods:** A reliability exercise, including 104 data sets of static images and complete CT examinations of patients affected by multiple myeloma (MM), was performed. A complementary imaging atlas provided detailed examples of the MSBDS scores, including low-risk and high-risk lesions. A total of 15 readers testing the MSBDS were evaluated. ICC estimates and their 95% confidence intervals were calculated based on mean rating (k = 15), absolute agreement, a two-way random-effects model and Cronbach's alpha. **Results:** Overall, the ICC correlation coefficient was 0.87 (95% confidence interval: 0.79–0.92), and the Cronbach's alpha was 0.93 (95% confidence interval: 0.94–0.97). Global inter- and intra-observer agreement among the 15 readers with scores below or equal to 6 points and scores above 6 points were 0.81 (95% C.I.: 0.72–0.86) and 0.94 (95% C.I.:0.91–0.98), respectively. **Conclusion:** We present a consensus-based semiquantitative scoring systems for CT in MM with a complementary CT imaging atlas including detailed examples of relevant scoring techniques. We found substantial agreement among readers with different levels of experience, thereby supporting the role of the MSBDS for possible large-scale applications. **Significance and Innovations** • Based on previous work and definitions of the MSBDS, we present real-life reliability data for quantitative bone damage assessment in multiple myeloma (MM) patients on CT. • In this study, reliability for the MSBDS, which was tested on 15 readers with different levels of expertise and from different institutions, was shown to be moderate to excellent. • The complementary CT imaging atlas is expected to enhance unified interpretations of the MSBDS between different professionals dealing with MM patients in their routine clinical practice.

Keywords: multiple myeloma; computed tomography; quantitative imaging; bone

Citation: Tagliafico, A.S.; Valle, C.; Bonaffini, P.A.; Attieh, A.; Bauckneht, M.; Belgioia, L.; Bignotti, B.; Brunetti, N.; Bonsignore, A.; Capaccio, E.; et al. Myeloma Spine and Bone Damage Score (MSBDS) on Whole-Body Computed Tomography (WBCT): Multiple Reader Agreement in a Multicenter Reliability Study. *Diagnostics* 2022, 12, 1894. https://doi.org/10.3390/diagnostics12081894

Academic Editor: Majid Chalian

Received: 16 May 2022
Accepted: 2 August 2022
Published: 4 August 2022

Publisher's Note: MDPI stays neutral with regard to jurisdictional claims in published maps and institutional affiliations.

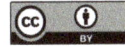

Copyright: © 2022 by the authors. Licensee MDPI, Basel, Switzerland. This article is an open access article distributed under the terms and conditions of the Creative Commons Attribution (CC BY) license (https://creativecommons.org/licenses/by/4.0/).

1. Introduction

In multiple myeloma (MM), there is an abnormal and excessive production of monoclonal immunoglobulin M derived from plasma cells. The pathological alteration of bone marrow, shown in both histopathology and medical imaging, is due to the increased presence of plasma cells, which is the main feature of MM [1–6]. In addition, in MM, there is an imbalance in the activation of osteoclasts and osteoblasts often, but not only, derived from a single tumoral clone. Medical imaging, such as computed tomography (CT), is normally used to detect bone disease in MM, which is responsible for a reduction in quality of life mainly due to pain and pathological fractures. Bone disease is also related to increased mortality. In addition, new therapies for MM are going to be developed and tested in clinical trials, where imaging techniques can be considered as a surrogate endpoint, especially in patients with early disease [2,3,6–10]. Alongside these developments in medical therapies, imaging tools have been showing progressive improvements over the last decades, with increased complexity. Indeed, imaging is clearly crucial in the diagnosis, management, and follow-up of patients with MM, as has been reported in the most recent guidelines [1,5,6,9,11]. Due to these developments, numerous randomized controlled trials on disease-modifying drugs and other treatment strategies for MM are expected to be implemented or are already under preparation. The use of CT for MM is widespread in most oncological centers, is readily available and is amenable to second-look evaluations in order to increase reliability [12]. Therefore, CT-based scoring systems could be suitable instruments for use in clinical trials if reliability is assured. Unfortunately, there is little or even no consensus yet on CT scoring systems, even with regards to the most elementary MM lesions [1,8,12]. In 2020, a preliminary CT-based scoring system, called the *"myeloma spine and bone damage score"* (MSBDS), was developed and included semi-quantitative assessments of elementary lesions using descriptive criteria with the aim of harmonizing total body CT interpretation in MM [13]. Despite the good results obtained by the authors, it should be noted that this scoring system was tested by a limited number of readers [3] on a small series of patients. Therefore, the aim of the current study was to test the reliability and the inter- and intra-observer agreement of the MSBDS with multiple readers with different levels of expertise and from different institutions in order to simulate the real-life application of this system.

2. Methods

2.1. Patients

Approval from the institutional review board was obtained (054REG2019). The patients involved in this study provided written informed consent for this retrospective research before CT examinations were performed. Due to the nature of this study, data analysis for this study was not used to influence patient care. CT examinations were acquired with different CT scanners: (1) two 128-slice scanners (Siemens SOMATOM Definition Flash), using the following parameters adjusted according to patients' characteristics: collimation 64×0.6 mm; spatial resolution: 0.30 mm; scanning time: 36 s; length of scanning: 650 mm; rotating time: 0.33 s; tube current: 100/140 kV, 50/60 mAs; effective dose: 2.6 mSv, (2) one 64-slice scanner (GE Optima 660) and (3) one 16-slice scanner (GE Lightspeed). Of the 150 consecutive patients (mean age, 59 years; range, 35–79 years; 72 females; 78 males) admitted to the hospital (BLIND for REVIEW) in the last three years, because of suspicions of MM that were later confirmed by bone biopsy, anonymized images and complete CT examinations were collected from 104 patients with relevant bone abnormalities (diffuse pattern or focal lesions). This pool of 104 patients with complete CT examinations was selected by two authors (who were not involved in the reading sessions) to represent all degrees of pathology related to the osseous involvement of MM, including localizations with extraosseous extension. The proportion of CT images acquired using different scanners was balanced across all of the images that were evaluated in this study: 30% of the images were obtained using the 128-slice CT, 30% with the 64-slice CT and 40% with the 16-slice CT. A lytic lesion, in both axial and extra-axial skeletons, had to be >5 mm in diameter to be considered significant, as per the most recent guidelines [2,4–7,11–13]. Patient risk stratification was performed using the Revised International Staging System (ISS), combining serum beta2-microglobulin and serum albumin, lactate dehydrogenase for three-stage classification and cytogenetics to determine a binary normal–high risk stadiation [5–7].

2.2. CT Imaging Atlas

A preliminary CT atlas was developed for use in the web-based evaluation (see further) and was edited according to evaluations made by three radiologists with expertise in musculoskeletal imaging (F.R, B.B and C.V. with 5, 6 and 7 years of experience, respectively). Images were collected from the inpatients who underwent a whole-body CT at the university and hospital Hematologic Unit. After collection, the CT images were anonymized for the web-based evaluation.

2.3. Web-Based Evaluation

A web-based reliability study was performed using the CT atlas containing a pool of 104 CT exams that were selected by a radiologist with 15 years of experience in musculoskeletal radiology (A.T.) who was not involved in the MSBDS assessment. The CT images and exams were selected to have a balanced degree of pathology involving the bones and the adjacent tissue. For the inter-reader reliability assessment, the MSBDS was assigned to every item available to readers. Subsequently, for intra-reader reliability, 44 images were randomly chosen and redistributed two months after the first round in order to guarantee sufficient wash-out. In this way, each reader evaluated a reduced sample of CT images that were randomly selected from the previous patient's cohort. MSBDS is a semiquantitative additive scale where the total score is the sum of the single items related to the abnormalities detected. MSBDS values range from 0 (minimum) to values >10, where 10 or more is represented by high-risk patients requiring immediate surgical or radiation oncologist evaluation [13]. The MSBDS scoring systems are briefly recalled in Table 1. In this study, 15 readers were selected from different institutions and with different expertise, not only regarding their expertise in bone evaluation using CT images, but also regarding their medical specializations. Among these readers, there were eleven radiologists (three of whom subspecialized in musculoskeletal radiology), one vascular surgeon, one radiation oncologist, one expert in legal medicine and one hematologist. An expert with 15 years of experience in musculoskeletal radiology (with a strong track record and a diploma from the European Society of Musculoskeletal Radiology) led a training session for every reader before they commenced the web-based reliability exercise, a number of whom were present for the training (10/15 readers) and a number completed the training remotely (5/15 readers).

Table 1. MSBDS (Myeloma Spine and Bone Damage Score). Interpretation: High-risk: >10, requiring immediate surgical or radiation oncologist consultation. Medium risk: ≥5–10, possible instability and a medium risk of pathological fracture. Low-risk: <5. * Bone abnormalities not sufficient to give high-risk scores, if isolated. ** 1 point for every segment according to MY-RADS [13].

Location	Points
Junctional Spine (C0-C2, C7-T2, T11-L1, L5-S1)	3
Mobile Spine (C3-C6, L2-L4) * only 1 point for semi-rigid (T3-T10)	2
Collapse/involvement >50%	3
Collapse <50% *	2
Posterolateral (facet, pedicle) involvement monolateral	2
Posterolateral (facet, pedicle) bilateral monolateral	3
Spinal Canal involvement	5
Trochanteric region focal lesions <10 mm	2
Femoral neck or entire trochanteric region	5
More than 2/3 of bone diameter	3
Focal lesion >5 mm at any site *	1
Diffuse Pattern	1 **

2.4. Statistical Analysis

As a measure of MSBDS reliability for both the degree of correlation and agreement between measurements, the intraclass correlation coefficient (ICC) was calculated as an index [14]. The aim of this paper was to generalize the results from our reliability exercise to any raters or readers who possess the same characteristics of expertise as the selected raters in this reliability study. Therefore, we used a two-way random-effects model according to Shoukri [15] MM et al. [15]. As a commonly suggested rule of thumb, we obtained far more than 30 heterogeneous samples (104 samples in this study) and involved more than 3 raters (15 raters) to conduct this reliability study. ICC values that were less than 0.5 were considered indicative of poor reliability. ICC values between 0.5 and 0.75 indicated moderate reliability, whereas ICC values between 0.75 and 0.9 indicated good reliability. Finally, ICC values greater than 0.90 indicated excellent reliability [16]. In this study, ICC estimates and their 95% confidence intervals were calculated based on a mean rating (k = 15), absolute agreement and a two-way random-effects model. Cronbach's alpha was used to assess the internal consistency of the method; values of alpha that were above or equal to 0.90 were considered useful for clinical purposes. Statistical analyses were performed using software for Windows (MedCalc—version 12.3.0) [17].

3. Results

The main characteristics of the 104 MM patients enrolled in the study, including clinical data, are shown in Table 2.

Table 2. Clinical data of the 104 MM patients included in the study. High-risk defines MM patients carrying HR features, including del17p, t(4;14) or t(14,16), according to the FISH analysis. International Staging System includes stage I-III based on beta2-microglobulin and albumin levels.

	Number	Percentage
Patients	104	100
Age (mean years)	58	
Age Standard Deviation	8.1	
Males	62	59.6
Females	42	40.4
Cytogenetics		
Normal	72	69.2
High-risk	32	30.8
Relapsed		
	71/104	68
Days before relapse (mean)	1173	
Days of follow-up (mean)	1466	
International Staging System		
Stage I	48	46
Stage II	28	27
Stage III	28	27

3.1. CT Imaging Atlas

A CT imaging atlas of lesions that were detectable using the MSBDS was prepared, including a comprehensive version that was available for the reliability assessment, and was prepared using a complete spectrum of lesions broad enough to give coverage of all possible lesions, ranging from small lytic (<5 mm), diffuse patterns to large lesions with destructive and extra-medullary patterns (Figure 1).

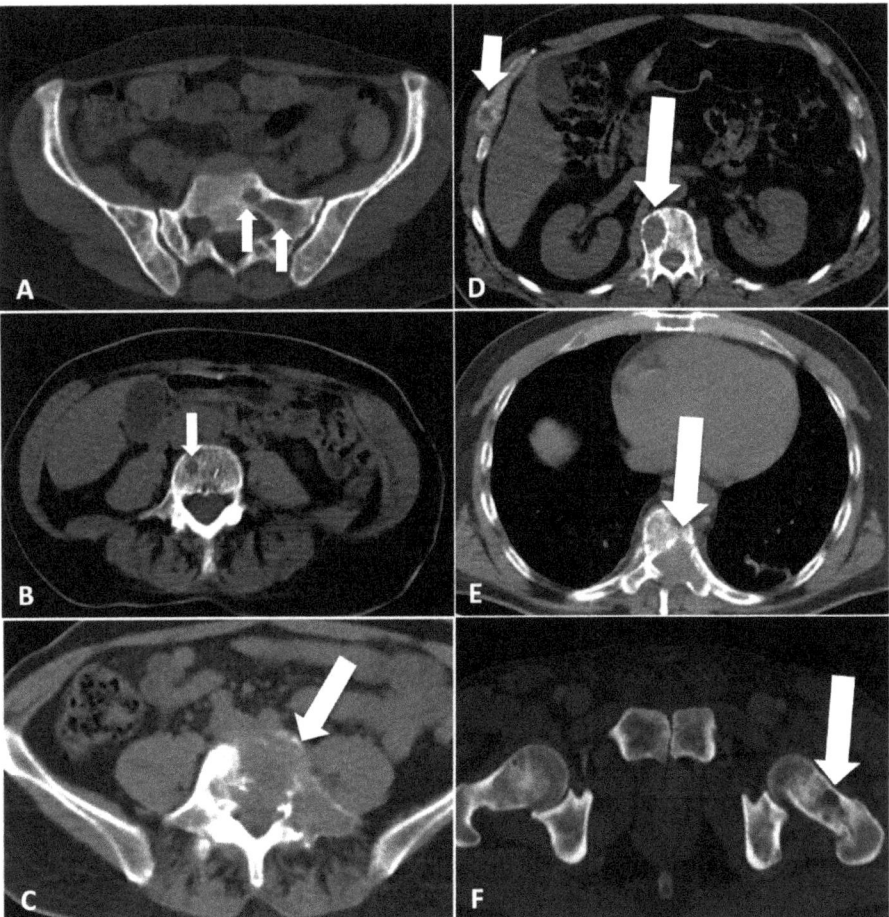

Figure 1. Scoring bone damage and instability: spectrum of findings. (**A**) Focal lytic lesions >5 mm in diameter located at the left sacrum (white arrows). In this case the MSBDS was 2 (1 + 1). (**B**) Single focal lytic lesion >5 mm in the vertebral body (white arrow) with no vertebral collapse (sagittal not shown). The adjacent smaller focal lytic lesion (green line) is <5 mm (no points in the MSBDS). In this case, the MSBDS was 1. (**C**) Large lytic lesion at the junctional spine (L5-S1) with cortical erosion, collapse/involvement >50%, posterolateral (facet, pedicle) involvement and more than 2/3 of bone diameter. In this case, the MSBDS was 11 (3 + 3 + 2 + 3): the lesion was considered "high-risk" and immediate surgical or radiation oncologist consultation was warranted. In this case, there was also possible spinal canal involvement. (**D**) Lytic lesion >5 mm (white arrow) at the junctional spine (thoracic spine) with collapse/involvement <50% and a small (small white arrow) focal lesion at the anterior arch of the right rib cage with extraosseous extension. In this case, the MSBDS was 6 (3 + 2 + 1): the lesion was considered "medium-risk" (5–10 with medium risk of pathologic fracture). (**E**) Large lytic lesion at the junctional spine (thoracic spine) with collapse/involvement >50%, posterolateral (facet, pedicle) involvement and more than 2/3 of bone diameter. In this case, the MSBDS was 11 (3 + 3 + 2 + 3): the lesion was considered "high-risk" and immediate surgical or radiation oncologist consultation was warranted. In this case, there is spinal canal involvement. (**F**) Lytic lesion at the left femoral neck (white arrow). This lesion alone warrants 5 points in the MSBDS: the lesion was considered "medium-risk", although immediate fracture seems unlikely.

3.2. Web-Based Reliability Assessment

Overall, the 15 readers completed the web-based reliability assessment of the scoring systems. The staging and the spectrum of bone lesions were sufficiently broad in order to give acceptable coverage of the severity of the disease as reported in the staging system. The distribution of the degree of pathological findings according to the MSBDS is reported in Figure 2. The coefficient of variation of the lesions analyzed was 0.8, the mean score was 5.5 and the interquartile range (25–75) was 6. The entire spectrum of possible bone disease, according to the MSBDS, was present, but there was a low prevalence of the highest score, thus reflecting the peculiar robustness of the method and the possible clinical impact, particularly in the lower stages. The mean time to perform the analysis was 2 min per patient.

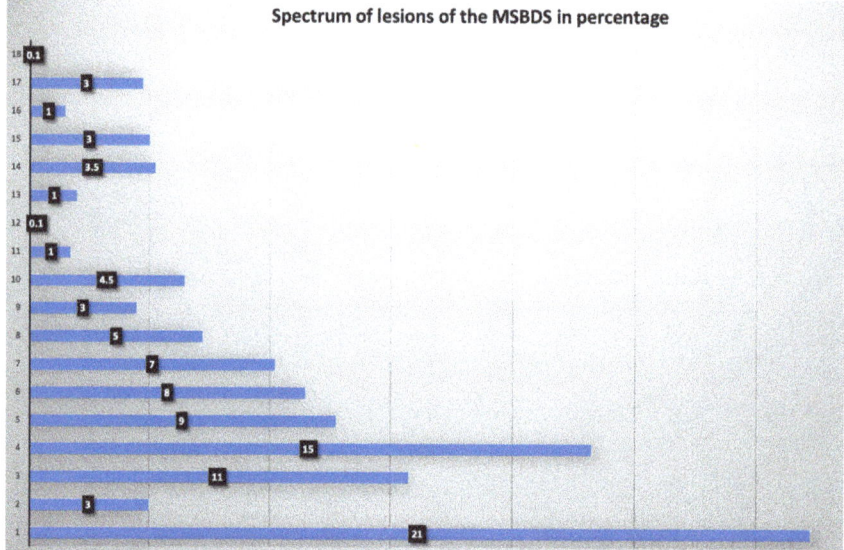

Figure 2. Frequency of bone lesions in the web-based reliability assessment. In this graph, the distribution of the degree of pathological findings, according to the MSBDS, is presented. The range of the MSBDSs was between 1 and 18. Most lesions (21%) were small lesions with an MSBDS of 1.

3.3. Overall Agreement for MSBDS

Overall, the ICC correlation coefficient was 0.87 (95% confidence interval: 0.79–0.92), reflecting the degree of consistency among measurements. The ICC for the single measure was 0.69 (0.61–0.77). Overall, Cronbach's alpha was 0.93 (95% confidence interval: 0.94–0.97). The inter-reader agreement was 0.68 (0.56–0.79) with a standard error of 0.05. Global inter- and intra-observer agreement among the 15 readers considering the MSBDS with scores below or equal to 6 points and scores above 6 points are reported in Table 3. Some examples of images where maximal discrepancies were found are reported in Figure 3. The ICC was not influenced by different CT scanners.

Table 3. Global inter- and intra-observer agreement among the 15 readers considering the MSBDS with scores below or equal to 6 points and scores above 6 points. K values are reported as weighed with linear weights.

Inter-observer	ICC	95% Confidence Interval
MSBDS ≤ 6 points	0.81	0.72–0.86
Intra-observer	**ICC**	**95% Confidence Interval**
MSBDS ≥ 6 points	0.94	0.91–0.98

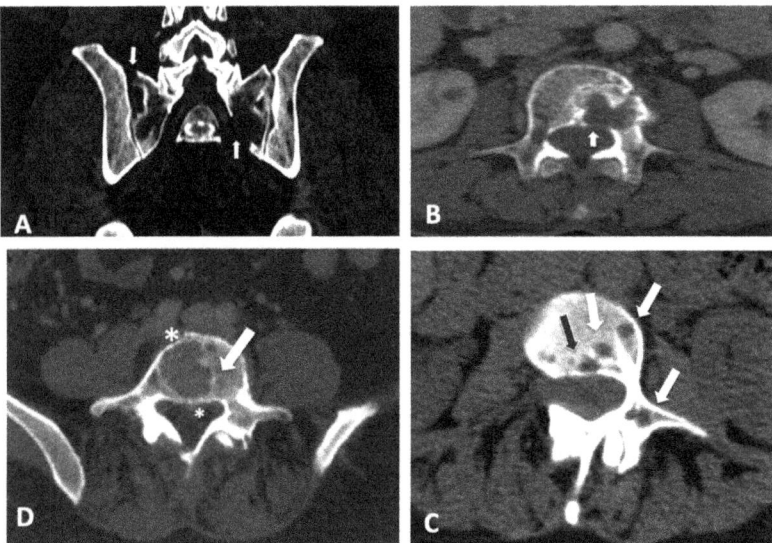

Figure 3. Scoring bone damage and instability: spectrum of findings with maximum disagreement among readers. Discrepancies with an MSBDS > 6. (**A**) Focal lytic lesions >5 mm in diameter located at the left sacrum (white arrow) with another small lesion in the sacrum near the sacroiliac joint. In this case, the MSBDS was 7 with a standard deviation of 4.9. (**B**) Single large focal lytic lesion >5 mm in the vertebral body (white arrow) with no vertebral collapse (sagittal not shown) but possible spinal canal infiltration. In this case, the MSBDS was 11 with a standard deviation of 5.3 due to difficulties in spinal canal assessment mainly by non-specialists. In these cases, a sub-specialized second reading should be recommended. Discrepancies with an MSBDS < 6. (**C**) Multiple lytic lesions >5 mm (white arrows and the black arrow) at the junctional spine (T11-L1 level) with involvement of the vertebral body and pedicle. In this case, the MSBDS was 4 with a standard deviation of 2.6. (**D**) Single large focal lytic lesion >5 mm in the vertebral body (white arrow) with no vertebral collapse. In this case, the MSBDS was 5.7 with a standard deviation of 3.3 due to difficulties in spinal canal assessment, bone diameter and extraosseous involvement (asterisks).

4. Discussion

In this study, we developed and assessed a consensus-based scoring system for MM bone lesions detectable with CT using a previously validated methodology [18,19].

Based on previous CT evaluations of MM-related lesions, we scored the clinically relevant lytic lesions, which are >5 mm in diameter, with the aim of creating a simple, reliable, reproducible and semiquantitative method consistent in radiological reporting [13]. This scoring system is a novel scoring system of bone lesions tailored specifically for use in MM with the purpose of being used with standard whole-body CT in daily clinical practice and to complement common evaluations. Indeed, bone damage is a typical target area in patients who are affected by MM, and numerous trials investigating potential structure-modifying or bone-protective treatments and other management strategies for MM are anticipated. Our scoring system may be an instrument for the domains determined by the Revised International Staging System. Bone lesions, such as lytic lesions detected by radiography, CT or PET/CT, are the myeloma-defining events belonging to the standard CRAB criteria (calcium elevation, renal failure, anemia, lytic bone lesions) [6,20]. In MM patients, imaging the bone is crucial because the detection of an osteolytic lesion provides a reason to treat. In patients with confirmed MM, medical imaging can be used to localize the source of pain and to prevent any eventual complications that are usually related to bone destruction [21]. The focal lesions detected on medical imaging are a strong prognostic marker and mark the need for treatment, even in the absence of cortical bone destruction [22–24]. Despite the diagnostic value of CT for the detection of bone marrow lesions, it is limited and MRI is superior. However, the possibility to use a reliable score to evaluate computed tomography images with acceptable agreement among different readers, such as the MSBDS, could be clinically helpful. In addition, the complementary CT imaging atlas is expected to enhance unified interpretations of the grading scales between radiologists and clinicians across countries and departments. Indeed, MM-associated bone disease impacts quality of life, with increases in both morbidity and mortality [3,25–29]. CT, as well MRI, is important when diagnosing MM, especially in the detection of bone lesions when they are small and when they are amenable to intervention, even to prevent pathological fractures or neurological complications due to the compression of the medulla or nerves [3,5,7,10,25–32]. CT-proven MM lesions were tested in a web-based exercise with substantial to excellent agreement. The CT images selected for the web-based exercises were of high quality, were pre-selected and did not include image selection and acquisition. The current semiquantitative score may be more helpful in clarifying the role of CT in MM bone and bone marrow imaging compared to the standard reporting of CT imaging, which is improved by sub-specialized second-opinion reading [12]. Indeed, in MM CT evaluation, discrepancies when interpreting a clinically important abnormality, such as the presence of a lytic lesion >5 mm, could be present in up to 21% of patients and has the potential to impact treatment planning [12]. The database was comprised mostly of stage I and II lesions, and most of them (22%) were small lesions (MSBDS 1), as is expected in normal clinical practice. Some variation in intra-class reliability is probably due to initial difficulty in applying new definitions of the 'real life' application of anatomical terms which are not so defined when dealing with 5 mm lesions. For example, it is difficult to clearly define the borders or limits of a posterolateral facet or pedicle involvement, the limit of spinal canal involvement or the "entire" trochanteric region, especially when the readers are not radiologists involved in medical imaging assessment and reporting on a daily basis. To reduce further variability when reading CT images, we believe that appropriate training could be useful, but, when possible, double reading of CT images could be the best choice, even for lesion identification. In this study, the MSBDS scoring system had a high concordance among many readers. The number of readers involved in this study and their different levels of expertise is very high, which is a strength of the current analysis. In addition, the scoring system was fast and suitable for routine clinical practice, and can be applied in clinical practice when reading or reporting CT in patients with MM. As opposed to the first application of the MSBDS, which was performed on a relatively high number of patients with advanced stages of disease for demonstrative and academic applications [13], in this work, the majority of lesions (22%) were small lesions with an MSBDS of 1, and we aimed to enhance the clinical utility of the scoring systems. Indeed, at least in theory, it is very important to correctly stratify patients at early stage of disease. We have to remember that MSBDS is strongly correlated with the Myeloma Response Assessment and Diagnosis System (MY-RADS) [13], confirming the relevance of the MSBDS scoring system [33–36]. The MSBDS is suitable for CT images, is typically more available than MRI and has the potential to be highly applicable for large scale clinical trials with imaging parameters as endpoints. The prospective clinical validation of MSBDS criteria regarding its clinical impact on patients is underway.

In conclusion, we presented a consensus-based semiquantitative scoring system for CT in MM together with a complementary CT imaging atlas, in which detailed examples of relevant scoring techniques are provided. We found substantial agreement among readers with different levels of experience, supporting the role of MSBDS for large scale applications. MSBDS is specifically tailored for use with patients who are affected by MM and differs from other scoring systems that have been developed in orthopedic literature for bone metastasis [37].

Author Contributions: Conceptualization, A.S.T., A.D., B.B. and M.C.; methodology, A.S.T., B.B., F.R. and M.C.; validation, all authors; formal analysis, B.B., F.R. and A.S.T.; investigation, all authors; resources, A.D., M.C. and A.S.T.; data curation, A.S.T., B.B. and F.R.; writing—original draft preparation, A.S.T.; writing—review and editing, all authors; supervision, A.S.T., M.C. and A.D.; project administration, A.S.T., M.C. and A.D.; funding acquisition, A.S.T. All authors have read and agreed to the published version of the manuscript.

Funding: This work was partially supported by grants from the Italian Ministry of Health (Ricerca Corrente; grant to A.S.T. and 5 × 1000 grant to A.S.T.) and FRA (Fondi Ricerca di Ateneo; grant to A.S.T.).

Institutional Review Board Statement: The study was conducted according to the guidelines of the Declaration of Helsinki and was approved by the Institutional Review Board (or Ethics Committee) of Comitato Etico Regionale Regione Liguria (protocol codes 0077 and 22 January 2020).

Informed Consent Statement: Informed consent was obtained from all subjects involved in the study.

Data Availability Statement: The datasets generated during and/or analyzed during the current study are available from the corresponding author on reasonable request.

Conflicts of Interest: The authors declare no conflict of interest.

Abbreviations

MM	multiple myeloma
CT	computed tomography
ISS	Revised International Staging System
ICC	intraclass correlation coefficient
MSBDS	Myeloma Spine and Bone Damage Score
MRI	magnetic resonance imaging
MY-RADS	Myeloma Response Assessment and Diagnosis System

References

1. Nassar, S.; Taher, A.; Spear, R.; Wang, F.; Madewell, J.E.; Mujtaba, B. Multiple Myeloma: Role of Imaging in Diagnosis, Staging, and Treatment Response Assessment. *Semin. Ultrasound CT MR* **2021**, *42*, 184–193. [CrossRef]
2. Mosebach, J.; Thierjung, H.; Schlemmer, H.P.; Delorme, S. Multiple Myeloma Guidelines and Their Recent Updates: Implications for Imaging. *Rofo* **2019**, *191*, 998–1009. [CrossRef] [PubMed]
3. Salwender, H.; Bertsch, U.; Weisel, K.; Duerig, J.; Kunz, C.; Benner, A.; Blau, I.W.; Raab, M.S.; Hillengass, J.; Hose, D.; et al. Rationale and design of the German-Speaking myeloma multicenter group (GMMG) trial HD6: A randomized phase III trial on the effect of elotuzumab in VRD induction/consolidation and lenalidomide maintenance in patients with newly diagnosed myeloma. *BMC Cancer* **2019**, *19*, 504. [CrossRef] [PubMed]
4. Tagliafico, A.S.; Cea, M.; Rossi, F.; Valdora, F.; Bignotti, B.; Succio, G.; Gualco, S.; Conte, A.; Dominietto, A. Differentiating diffuse from focal pattern on Computed Tomography in multiple myeloma: Added value of a Radiomics approach. *Eur. J. Radiol.* **2019**, *121*, 108739. [CrossRef] [PubMed]
5. Joseph, N.S.; Gentili, S.; Kaufman, J.L.; Lonial, S.; Nooka, A.K. High-Risk Multiple Myeloma: Definition and Management. *Clin. Lymphoma Myeloma Leuk.* **2017**, *17*, S80–S87. [CrossRef]
6. Palumbo, A.; Avet-Loiseau, H.; Oliva, S.; Lokhorst, H.M.; Goldschmidt, H.; Rosinol, L.; Richardson, P.; Caltagirone, S.; Lahuerta, J.J.; Facon, T.; et al. Revised International Staging System for Multiple Myeloma: A Report From International Myeloma Working Group. *J. Clin. Oncol.* **2015**, *33*, 2863–2869. [CrossRef]

7. Liu, J.; Zeng, P.; Guo, W.; Wang, C.; Geng, Y.; Lang, N.; Yuan, H. Prediction of High-Risk Cytogenetic Status in Multiple Myeloma Based on Magnetic Resonance Imaging: Utility of Radiomics and Comparison of Machine Learning Methods. *J. Magn. Reson. Imaging* **2021**, *54*, 1303–1311. [CrossRef]
8. Mosci, C.; Pericole, F.V.; Oliveira, G.B.; Delamain, M.T.; Takahashi, M.E.S.; Carvalheira, J.B.C.; Etchebehere, E.C.S.C.; Santos, A.O.; Miranda, E.C.M.; Lima, M.C.L.; et al. 99mTc-sestamibi SPECT/CT and 18F-FDG-PET/CT have similar performance but different imaging patterns in newly diagnosed multiple myeloma. *Nucl. Med. Commun.* **2020**, *41*, 1081–1088. [CrossRef]
9. Tagliafico, A.S. Imaging in multiple myeloma: Computed tomography or magnetic resonance imaging? *World J. Radiol.* **2021**, *13*, 223–226. [CrossRef]
10. Yoshihara, S.; Yoshihara, K.; Shimizu, Y.; Imado, T.; Takatsuka, H.; Kawamoto, H.; Misawa, M.; Ifuku, H.; Ohe, Y.; Okada, M.; et al. Feasibility of six cycles of lenalidomide-based triplet induction before stem cell collection for newly diagnosed transplant-eligible multiple myeloma. *Hematology* **2021**, *26*, 388–392. [CrossRef]
11. Tagliafico, A.S.; Dominietto, A.; Belgioia, L.; Campi, C.; Schenone, D.; Piana, M. Quantitative Imaging and Radiomics in Multiple Myeloma: A Potential Opportunity? *Medicina* **2021**, *57*, 94. [CrossRef] [PubMed]
12. Tagliafico, A.S.; Belgioia, L.; Bonsignore, A.; Rossi, F.; Succio, G.; Bignotti, B.; Dominietto, A. Subspecialty Second-Opinion in Multiple Myeloma CT: Emphasis on Clinically Significant Lytic Lesions. *Medicina* **2020**, *56*, 195. [CrossRef] [PubMed]
13. Tagliafico, A.S.; Belgioia, L.; Bonsignore, A.; Signori, A.; Formica, M.; Rossi, F.; Piana, M.; Schenone, D.; Dominietto, A. Development and definition of a simplified scoring system in patients with multiple myeloma undergoing stem cells transplantation on standard computed tomography: Myeloma spine and bone damage score (MSBDS). *Cancer Imaging* **2020**, *20*, 31. [CrossRef] [PubMed]
14. Koo, T.K.; Li, M.Y. A Guideline of Selecting and Reporting Intraclass Correlation Coefficients for Reliability Research. *J. Chiropr. Med.* **2016**, *15*, 155–163. [CrossRef] [PubMed]
15. Shoukri, M.M.; Colak, D.; Kaya, N.; Donner, A. Comparison of two dependent within subject coefficients of variation to evaluate the reproducibility of measurement devices. *BMC Med. Res. Methodol.* **2008**, *8*, 24. [CrossRef] [PubMed]
16. Shrout, P.E.; Fleiss, J.L. Intraclass correlations: Uses in assessing rater reliability. *Psychol. Bull.* **1979**, *86*, 420–428. [CrossRef]
17. Landis, J.R.; Koch, G.G. The measurement of observer agreement for categorical data. *Biometrics* **1977**, *33*, 159–174. [CrossRef]
18. Christiansen, S.N.; Østergaard, M.; Slot, O.; Fana, V.; Terslev, L. Retrospective longitudinal assessment of the ultrasound gout lesions using the OMERACT semi-Quantitative scoring system. *Rheumatology* **2022**. [CrossRef]
19. Di Matteo, A.; Cipolletta, E.; Destro Castaniti, G.M.; Smerilli, G.; Airoldi, C.; Aydin, S.Z.; Becciolini, A.; Bonfiglioli, K.; Bruns, A.; Carrara, G.; et al. Reliability assessment of the definition of ultrasound enthesitis in SpA: Results of a large, multicentre, international web-Based study. *Rheumatology* **2022**. [CrossRef]
20. Rajkumar, S.V. Updated Diagnostic Criteria and Staging System for Multiple Myeloma. *Am. Soc. Clin. Oncol. Educ. Book* **2016**, *35*, e418–e423. [CrossRef]
21. Derlin, T.; Bannas, P. Imaging of multiple myeloma: Current concepts. *World J. Orthop.* **2014**, *5*, 272–282. [CrossRef] [PubMed]
22. Hillengass, J.; Moehler, T.; Hundemer, M. Monoclonal gammopathy and smoldering multiple myeloma: Diagnosis, staging, prognosis, management. *Recent Results Cancer Res.* **2011**, *183*, 113–131. [PubMed]
23. Lecouvet, F.E.; Vekemans, M.C.; Van Den Berghe, T.; Verstraete, K.; Kirchgesner, T.; Acid, S.; Malghem, J.; Wuts, J.; Hillengass, J.; Vandecaveye, V.; et al. Imaging of treatment response and minimal residual disease in multiple myeloma: State of the art WB-MRI and PET/CT. *Skelet. Radiol.* **2022**, *51*, 59–80. [CrossRef] [PubMed]
24. Merz, A.M.A.; Merz, M.; Hillengass, J.; Holstein, S.A.; McCarthy, P. The evolving role of maintenance therapy following autologous stem cell transplantation in multiple myeloma. *Expert Rev. Anticancer Ther.* **2019**, *19*, 889–898. [CrossRef]
25. Chen, F.; Leng, Y.; Ni, J.; Niu, T.; Zhang, L.; Li, J.; Zheng, Y. Symptom clusters and quality of life in ambulatory patients with multiple myeloma. *Support. Care Cancer* **2022**, *30*, 4961–4970. [CrossRef]
26. Efficace, F.; Cottone, F.; Sparano, F.; Caocci, G.; Vignetti, M.; Chakraborty, R. Patient-Reported Outcomes in Randomized Controlled Trials of Patients with Multiple Myeloma: A Systematic Literature Review of Studies Published Between 2014 and 2021. *Clin. Lymphoma Myeloma Leuk.* **2022**, *22*, 442–459. [CrossRef]
27. LeBlanc, M.R.; Bryant, A.L.; LeBlanc, T.W.; Yang, Q.; Sellars, E.; Chase, C.C.; Smith, S.K. A cross-Sectional observational study of health-Related quality of life in adults with multiple myeloma. *Support. Care Cancer* **2022**, *30*, 5239–5248. [CrossRef]
28. Nicol, J.L.; Woodrow, C.; Cunningham, B.J.; Mollee, P.; Weber, N.; Smith, M.D.; Nicol, A.J.; Gordon, L.G.; Hill, M.M.; Skinner, T.L. An Individualized Exercise Intervention for People with Multiple Myeloma-Study Protocol of a Randomized Waitlist-Controlled Trial. *Curr. Oncol.* **2022**, *29*, 901–923. [CrossRef]
29. Piechotta, V.; Skoetz, N.; Engelhardt, M.; Einsele, H.; Goldschmidt, H.; Scheid, C. Clinical Practice Guideline: Patients With Multiple Myeloma or Monoclonal Gammopathy of Undetermined Significance-Diagnosis, Treatment, and Follow Up. *Dtsch. Arztebl. Int.* **2022**, *119*, 253–260.
30. Feroz, I.; Makhdoomi, R.H.; Khursheed, N.; Shaheen, F.; Shah, P. Utility of Computed Tomography-Guided Biopsy in Evaluation of Metastatic Spinal Lesions. *Asian J. Neurosurg.* **2018**, *13*, 577–584.
31. Toocheck, C.; Pinkhas, D. Treatment of relapsed multiple myeloma complicated by cardiac extramedullary plasmacytoma with D-PACE chemotherapy. *BMJ Case Rep.* **2018**, *2018*, bcr2017223611. [CrossRef] [PubMed]
32. Yang, W.; Zheng, J.; Li, R.; Ren, H.; Hou, B.; Zhao, Z.; Wang, D.; Wang, G.; Liu, J.; Yan, J.; et al. Multiple myeloma with pathologically proven skull plasmacytoma after a mild head injury: Case report. *Medicine* **2018**, *97*, e12327. [CrossRef]

33. Dong, H.; Huang, W.; Ji, X.; Huang, L.; Zou, D.; Hao, M.; Deng, S.; Shen, Z.; Lu, X.; Wang, J.; et al. Prediction of Early Treatment Response in Multiple Myeloma Using MY-RADS Total Burden Score, ADC, and Fat Fraction From Whole-Body MRI: Impact of Anemia on Predictive Performance. *AJR Am. J. Roentgenol.* **2022**, *218*, 310–319. [CrossRef] [PubMed]
34. Messiou, C.; Hillengass, J.; Delorme, S.; Lecouvet, F.E.; Moulopoulos, L.A.; Collins, D.J.; Blackledge, M.D.; Abildgaard, N.; Østergaard, B.; Schlemmer, H.-P.; et al. Guidelines for Acquisition, Interpretation, and Reporting of Whole-Body MRI in Myeloma: Myeloma Response Assessment and Diagnosis System (MY-RADS). *Radiology* **2019**, *291*, 5–13. [CrossRef] [PubMed]
35. Mulligan, M.E. Myeloma Response Assessment and Diagnosis System (MY-RADS): Strategies for practice implementation. *Skelet. Radiol.* **2022**, *51*, 11–15. [CrossRef]
36. Rossi, F.; Torri, L.; Dominietto, A.; Tagliafico, A.S. Spectrum of magnetic resonance imaging findings in transplanted multiple myeloma patients with hip/pelvic pain (according to MY-RADS): A single center experience. *Eur. J. Radiol.* **2020**, *130*, 109154. [CrossRef]
37. Fisher, C.G.; DiPaola, C.P.; Ryken, T.C.; Bilsky, M.H.; Shaffrey, C.I.; Berven, S.H.; Harrop, J.S.; Fehlings, M.G.; Boriani, S.; Chou, D.; et al. A novel classification system for spinal instability in neoplastic disease: An evidence-Based approach and expert consensus from the Spine Oncology Study Group. *Spine* **2010**, *35*, E1221–E1229. [CrossRef]

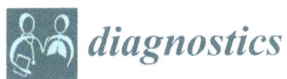

Article

Osteonecrosis of the Femoral Head: A Multidisciplinary Approach in Diagnostic Accuracy

Adrián Cardín-Pereda [1,*], Daniel García-Sánchez [1], Nuria Terán-Villagrá [2], Ana Alfonso-Fernández [3], Michel Fakkas [3], Carlos Garcés-Zarzalejo [3] and Flor María Pérez-Campo [1,*]

[1] Departamento de Bioquímica y Biología Molecular, Facultad de Medicina, Universidad de Cantabria-IDIVAL, 39012 Santander, Spain; daniel.garcias@alumnos.unican.es

[2] Servicio de Anatomía Patológica, Hospital UM Valdecilla, Universidad de Cantabria, 39008 Santander, Spain; nuriateran@unican.es

[3] Servicio de Traumatología y Ortopedia, Hospital Universitario Marqués de Valdecilla-IDIVAL, Universidad de Cantabria, 39008 Santander, Spain; anaalfonso@scsalud.es (A.A.-F.); michelfakkas@scsalud.es (M.F.); carlosgarces@scsalud.es (C.G.-Z.)

* Correspondence: adrianalbertocardinpereda@osakidetza.eus (A.C.-P.); f.perezcampo@unican.es (F.M.P.-C.); Tel.: +34-942200958 (F.M.P.-C.)

Abstract: Osteonecrosis of the Femoral Head (ONFH) is a disabling disease affecting up to 30,000 people yearly in the United States alone. Diagnosis and staging of this pathology are both technically and logistically challenging, usually relying on imaging studies. Even anatomopathological studies, considered the gold standard for identifying ONFH, are not exempt from problems. In addition, the diagnosis is often made by different healthcare specialists, including orthopedic surgeons and radiologists, using different imaging modes, macroscopic features, and stages. Therefore, it is not infrequent to find disagreements between different specialists. The aim of this paper is to clarify the association and accuracy of ONFH diagnosis between healthcare professionals. To this end, femoral head specimens from patients with a diagnosis of ONFH were collected from patients undergoing hip replacement surgery. These samples were later histologically analyzed to establish an ONFH diagnosis. We found that clinico-radiological diagnosis of ONFH evidences a high degree of histological confirmation, thus showing an acceptable diagnostic accuracy. However, when the diagnoses of radiologists and orthopedic surgeons are compared with each other, there is only a moderate agreement. Our results underscore the need to develop an effective diagnosis based on a multidisciplinary approach to enhance currently limited accuracy and reliability.

Keywords: avascular necrosis of the hip; diagnosis; radiological tests; reproducibility; reliability; accuracy; histopathology

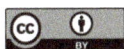

1. Introduction

Osteonecrosis of the Femoral Head (ONFH) is a disabling condition that usually results in the collapse of the femoral head and secondary osteoarthritis (OA) in young adults and middle-aged individuals, with a mean age of presentation of 38 years [1]. To date, there is no epidemiological report on ONFH worldwide, however, some countries have already performed studies on the incidence of this disease. In the United States the number of new cases each year is estimated to be greater than 30,000 [2], with these numbers steadily increasing yearly. Importantly, ONFH seems to be the direct cause of between 5 and 18% of all the hip arthroplasties performed annually in the United States [3]. Apart from the important healthcare costs associated with the surgical treatment of the ONFH, the fact that this disease causes severe pain and disability mainly in adults at a productive age also translates into an important socioeconomic burden [4]. Clinical presentation of ONFH is generally asymptomatic in early stages, although occasionally patients could indicate hip or groin pain. At initial stages, negative plain radiographs are common, therefore,

ONFH must be suspected if patients present any of the reported risk factors [5]. Thus, a precise diagnosis and staging of ONFH to treat our patients optimally becomes critical. Presumably, the optimal therapeutic approach might include a multimodal treatment regime, or a patient tailored plan from hip surgery to rehabilitation [6–8].

In the early stages the disease can be treated with conservative approaches, such as drugs, biological therapies, or extracorporeal shock wave therapy, to delay or stop its progression. Unfortunately in many cases this condition will lead to loss of integrity of the subchondral bone, requiring surgical treatments, typically a total hip arthroplasty within two years after the development of hip pain [9]. To avoid this outcome, an early and accurate diagnosis that would allow us to treat this pathology in its early stages is key [10]. However, the early diagnosis of ONFH is highly challenging, as the onset of symptoms and imaging characteristics are insidious and subtle [11], frequently posing a diagnostic problem to orthopedic surgeons. The difficulty associated with ONFH diagnosis often results in the presentation of advanced cases of this disease, when femoral-head-conserving surgical treatment is no longer indicated [12].

Longitudinal studies of patients with various forms of osteonecrosis and osteochondritis show that the history of mild cases of ONFH (abnormal alterations in soft tissues observable only by MRI) is to naturally heal, with only the most severe cases requiring a hip arthroplasty and being susceptible to histological studies [13]. Ideally, therefore, ONFH diagnosis should be made by non-invasive means, such as imaging techniques. However, to be able to perform an accurate diagnosis using these non-invasive tests, an adequate correlation with the gold standard, the anatomopathological exam [13], should be clearly stablished. ONFH diagnosis currently relies largely on imaging techniques. The imaging study is usually initiated by a common radiographical analysis. However, as previously mentioned, plain radiographs are usually negative in early disease, since only a minor osteopenia might be present at this stage. If the findings are inconclusive, more imaging techniques, such as magnetic resonance imaging (MRI), computerized tomography (CT), or bone scan are normally requested. MRI is considered the method of choice for ONFH diagnosis, with the highest sensitivity and specificity [1]. In recent decades, various scientific societies have developed different classification systems for grading the evolution of the process [14]. However, despite these efforts, the controversy regarding the optimal way for classifying osteonecrosis of the femoral head remains. Apart from data such as the etiology, age, occupation, or hip functionality, clearly clarifying the staging of the osteonecrosis is also key in the diagnosis as well as in developing treatment strategies.

The fact that the diagnosis of the ONFH can be performed by different specialists, using different diagnostic tools adds to the challenge of the diagnosis itself. The aim of this paper is to clarify the association and accuracy of ONFH diagnosis between all the professionals involved in its diagnosis including orthopedic surgeons, radiologists, and pathologists.

2. Materials and Methods

2.1. Study Design

This was a prospective case-control study conducted at the Marqués de Valdecilla University Hospital, in which femoral heads of image-diagnosed ONFH and OA patients undergoing arthroplasty were collected from the operating room for 3 years, to later perform a confirmatory histological analysis. The study sample was determined following the guidelines of other studies in this line made in the field of osteonecrosis [15–21].

2.2. Patients

Patients who met the following criteria were included: (1) between 40 and 90 years old, (2) clinico-radiological diagnosis of ONFH or hip OA, (3) indication of hip replacement surgery [2,22]. Exclusion criteria included: (1) systemic glucocorticoids and/or bisphosphonates treatment history, (2) past or present heavy alcohol consumption, (3) hip trauma or radiation history, (4) storage disorders, pancreatitis, hemoglobinopathies, or dysbarisms history; as we intended to study idiopathic cases of AVNH, with no obvious etiologic factor [10,23] (secondary osteonecrosis).

All patients gave informed written consent. Study protocol was approved by the institutional review board (Comité de Ética en Investigación Clínica de Cantabria, February 2018). Identification Code 2018.014.

2.3. Diagnosis

Our study population was triply diagnosed by experienced and certified orthopedic surgeons, radiologists, and pathologists. Orthopedic surgeons diagnosed patients according to signs and symptoms, imaging studies, and macroscopic evaluation of femoral head specimens from the operating room. Plain radiographs and/or MR images were reported by general and musculoskeletal radiologists. Radiographic scoring by the Ficat and Arlet system was used.

From all femoral head specimens macroscopically affected, cylindrical samples underwent anatomopathological analysis. From the histological point of view, a positive diagnosis of ONFH was considered as the presence of significant and diffuse trabecular necrosis (>50% of empty osteocytic lacunae) and necrotic hematopoietic bone marrow in the absence of other specific lesions [18]. For a better histological characterization, other degenerative signs, such as fatty infiltration and medullary fibrosis or heterotopic ossification presence, were graded in qualitative manner ("1-absence", "2-presence", "3-moderate", and "4-intense") [16].

2.4. Histological Analysis

Samples of bone were isolated from the macroscopically affected areas of femoral head specimens (Figure 1A), sectioned in the coronal plane. Bone cylinders were extracted from the sample with the help of a trephine. These samples were preserved and subsequently used for the anatomopathological analyses. For preservation, the cylindrical biopsies were immediately placed in 10% neutral buffered formalin at room temperature for 24 h and subsequently decalcified in 10% ethylenediaminetetraacetic acid at room temperature following standard procedures [24,25]. Decalcified specimens were embedded in paraffin and paraffin sections (4 mm thick) were cut using conventional methods. Sections were stained with Mayer hematoxylin and eosin and Masson trichrome [15,16]. The total number of empty osteocyte lacunae was quantified by two unaware examiners in four non-overlapping regions of interest. At least 300 osteocyte lacunae were quantified in each specimen.

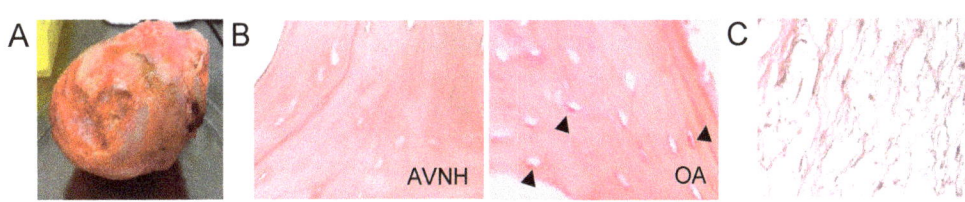

Figure 1. (**A**) Gross specimen of advanced femoral head osteonecrosis with associated osteoarthritis, showing complete loss of articular surface and collapse of the central region of the head. (**B**) Hematoxylin and eosin-stained sections showing trabeculae; (**A**) partially necrotic trabecula: bone showing empty lacunae in ONFH samples. (20×). (**B**) Osteoarthritis (control group) trabecula showing lacunae containing viable osteocytes, necrotic osteocytes, and empty lacunae (20×). (**C**) Hematoxylin and eosin-stained section showing dense medullary fibrosis in ONFH bone samples (20×).

2.5. Statistical Analysis

Statistical comparison was performed using chi-square and Fisher's exact test analysis for categorical data, Student's t-test for mean comparison (for normally distributed variables), Spearman's coefficient for rank correlation, the Mann–Whitney U test to compare two related samples (for non-normally distributed variables), and Cohen's kappa coefficient for inter-rater and intra-rater reliability. A P value probability threshold of less than 0.05 was considered statistically significant. All statistical analyses were performed using SPSS software (SPSS Inc, Chicago, IL, USA).

3. Results

Between 2017 and 2020, a total of sixty femoral head specimens were collected from patients undergoing hip replacement surgery at the Marqués de Valdecilla University Hospital. Of those sixty samples, twenty-six corresponded to patients that have had a previous diagnosis of ONFH and thirty-four of them, used as controls in this study, corresponded to patients that have been diagnosed with OA. Clinico-radiological diagnosis was confirmed by anatomopathological analysis which was considered the definitive reference diagnosis. Of all the collected samples, only twelve ONFH and twelve OA specimens met further selection criteria, that is, to have a radiologist-reported imaging study, and a correctly preserved bone sample with enough quality to perform an appropriate histological analysis. Samples lacking a certified radiologist report or showing poor histological quality were excluded.

Histological examination of the femoral head specimens collected confirmed radiological diagnosis in twenty of the twenty-four hips analyzed (84%) (Table 1). Regarding the samples with a diagnosis of ONFH that comply with our selection criteria, only one of the twelve radiologically diagnosed cases of ONFH (8%) was not confirmed by anatomopathological analysis. Interestingly, we found that three of the twelve samples with a radiological diagnosis of OA, representing a 25% of the OA analyzed samples, met the histological diagnosis criteria for ONFH. Furthermore, only 25% of the patients misdiagnosed had been subjected to an MRI scan, highlighting the early reported superior diagnostic capability of this technique. This result, however, could not be considered statistically significant.

Table 1. From the initial sixty femoral heads collected, only twenty-four met our selection criteria, twelve with a previous diagnosis of ONFH and twelve controls with an OA diagnosis. The table illustrates the diagnosis of every sample according to different specialists: orthopedic surgeons, radiologists, and pathologists.

Specimen	Surgeon Pre-Surgery	Surgeon Post-Surgery	Radiologist	Pathologist	Disagreement
1 (CASE)	AVNH	AVNH	AVNH	AVNH	NO
2 (CASE)	AVNH	AVNH	AVNH	AVNH	NO
3 (CASE)	AVNH	AVNH	OA	AVNH	Radiologist vs. others
4 (CASE)	AVNH	AVNH	AVNH	AVNH	NO
5 (CASE)	AVNH	AVNH	AVNH	AVNH	NO
6 (CASE)	AVNH	AVNH	AVNH	AVNH	NO
7 (CASE)	AVNH	AVNH	AVNH	AVNH	NO
8 (CASE)	OA	OA	OA	AVNH	Pathologist vs. others
9 (CASE)	OA	OA	AVNH	AVNH	Surgeon vs. others
10 (CASE)	AVNH	AVNH	AVNH	AVNH	NO
11 (CASE)	AVNH	AVNH	AVNH	AVNH	NO
12 (CASE)	OA	OA	OA	AVNH	Pathologist vs. others
13 (CONTROL)	OA	AVNH	OA	OA	Surgeon vs. others
14 (CONTROL)	OA	OA	OA	OA	NO
15 (CONTROL)	OA	OA	OA	OA	NO
16 (CONTROL)	OA	OA	OA	OA	NO
17 (CONTROL)	OA	OA	OA	OA	NO
18 (CONTROL)	OA	OA	OA	AVNH	Pathologist vs. others
19 (CONTROL)	OA	OA	OA	OA	NO
20 (CONTROL)	OA	OA	OA	OA	NO
21 (CONTROL)	OA	OA	OA	OA	NO
22 (CONTROL)	OA	OA	OA	AVNH	Pathologist vs. others
23 (CONTROL)	OA	OA	OA	OA	NO
24 (CONTROL)	OA	OA	OA	OA	NO

A statistically significant difference in the number of empty osteocytic lacunae (t = 5.13; $p < 0.05$) was found between the ONFH (mean ± SE = 68.16 ± 10.57) and the control group (mean ± SE = 40.91 ± 15.03) (Figure 1B and Table 2). There was also a statistically significant difference (U = 35; $p < 0.05$) between medullary fibrosis (Figure 1C) presence between the ONFH (mean ± SE = 2.75 ± 1.21) and the control (mean ± SE = 1.66 ± 0.98) group (Table 2). The histological analysis of other degenerative signs, such as fatty infiltration and heterotopic ossification, indicated no statistically significant differences between the two groups analyzed.

Table 2. Histological analysis data from femoral head specimens.

	ONFH (Mean ± SE)	Control (Mean ± SE)	p Value Intergroup Differences
Age (years)	65.88 ± 12.6	63.84 ± 10.9	0.262991
Empty osteocytic lacunae (%)	68.16 ± 10.57	40.91 ± 15.03	0.000019
Fatty infiltration (1–4) *	3.5 ± 0.9	2.83 ± 0.83	0.08914
Medullary fibrosis (1–4) *	2.75 ± 1.21	1.66 ± 0.98	0.03486
Heterotopic ossification (%) †	25 ± 0.45	25 ± 0.45	1
Age (years)	65.88 ± 12.6	63.84 ± 10.9	-

*: "1-absence", "2-presence", "3-moderate", and "4-intense". †: significative presence yes/no.

Importantly, the association between the number of empty osteocytic lacunae with the Ficat and Arlet staging could not be considered statistically significant (Table 3). When the diagnoses of radiologists and orthopedic surgeons were compared with each other, twenty-one of the twenty-four diagnoses agreed (k = 0.58; percentage agreement of 85.71%), expressing moderate agreement. Interobserver diagnosis reliability did not differ significantly between the different Ficat and Arlet stages.

Table 3. Data comparing Ficat and Arlet imaging stage and the average number of empty osteocytic lacunae in our ONFH specimens.

Ficat and Arlet Stage	Number of Samples Analyzed	Empty Osteocytic Lacunae (%)
I	2	63
II	1	80
III	3	73
IV	6	65

For orthopedic surgeons, the rate of agreement between the pre-surgery and the post-surgery diagnosis was 91.67% (kappa value for intra-observer reproducibility of 0.75), expressing substantial agreement.

When the diagnoses of radiologists and orthopedic surgeons were compared with each other, twenty-one of the twenty-four diagnoses agreed (k = 0.58; percentage agreement of 85.71%), expressing moderate agreement. Interobserver diagnosis reliability did not differ significantly between the different Ficat and Arlet stages.

4. Discussion

Early diagnosis of ONFH is key to achieving satisfactory therapeutic results that allow prompt selection of an effective joint-preserving treatment. However, accurate diagnosis of ONFH is challenging, especially at the early stages. Normal plain radiographs and physical exams can be falsely reassuring and delay appropriate referral [11,26]. In this context, several studies have found suboptimal diagnostic accuracy, reproducibility, and reliability [13,14,25,27–29]. The aim of this paper is to specifically clarify the association and accuracy of ONFH diagnosis between orthopedic surgeons, radiologists, and pathologists, considering imaging modes, microscopic and macroscopic bone features, and disease staging.

Non-specific initial imaging findings and confusing prevalence data are probably the most important causes of ONFH diagnosis disregard. In addition, imaging pitfalls and lack of anatomopathological analysis consensus led to misdiagnosis. Regarding histological diagnosis, there are no established quantitative criteria (number of blocks, trabeculae, or lacunae to quantify) and surgeons' requisition forms usually lack important information. Therefore, there is a need for a consensus definition of the histological features of ONFH and improvement of samples collection [13].

Empty osteocytic lacunae evaluation is a legitimate method for ONFH diagnosis, not always related directly to age and without a clear relationship with disease stage. In our study, there was a statistically significant difference in the number of empty osteocytic lacunae found between the ONFH and the control group, thus contributing to validate our samples and their histological diagnosis. However, in the present work, the association between age and empty osteocytic lacunae, widely described in the literature [15,30], could not be considered statistically significant. These findings might be explained by the fact that the distribution of empty lacunae in relation to age is quite heterogeneous, compared to the complete loss of osteocytes observed in ONFH [30]. On the other hand, no statistically significant difference was found between the number of empty osteocytic lacunae and Ficat and Arlet stage for ONFH [20]. Although several studies have shown the link between imaging features and osteonecrosis severity [17,20,31], a direct relationship between the proportion of empty osteocytic lacunae and radiological staging has not yet been reported.

The presence of dense medullary fibrosis is significantly greater in necrotic femoral heads when compared to osteoarthritic ones. These results agree with previous findings that describe this degenerative sign in advanced stages of the disease [16,17,20]. In addition, necrosis of the fatty marrow was consistently present in most of the ONFH samples. This result is part of the histological features spectrum of osteonecrosis, with fatty and haemopoietic marrow becoming ghosted [16,30]. Other non-specific degenerative signs examined, such as fatty infiltration and heterotopic ossification, showed no statistically significant difference between both groups (Supplementary Table S1).

Importantly, three of the twelve osteoarthritis controls (25%) met the histological diagnosis criteria for ONFH. This finding agrees with previous works, in which 21–31% of cases of ONFH were seen pathologically but not radiographically [27,32]. A study investigating the presence of secondary osteonecrosis in osteoarthritis of the hip confirmed it microscopically in 38.2% of the femoral heads, identifying two different histological patterns: 'shallow' osteonecrosis (probably pressure necrosis as a result of eburnation) and 'deep wedge-shaped' osteonecrosis (a less frequent, independent phenomena related to primary osteonecrosis) [33].

The ONFH diagnosis varies among medical specialties, and it is not uncommon to find literature failing to mention which methods were used for the diagnosis. Previous works have evidenced a distribution of ONFH diagnosis by specialty of 13% for pathologists (pathology report), 15% for orthopedic surgeons (clinical record), and 19% for radiologists (radiology report) [13]. In our specimen selection, we found a proportion in ONFH diagnosis of 26% for pathologists, 46% for surgeons, and 26% for radiologists.

ONFH diagnosis relies mostly on the assessments performed by the orthopedic surgeon, involving physical examination, medical history, and plain radiographs, or on the radiologist report [27]. However, histological, or even gross pathologic evaluation of hip arthroplasty specimens, is not consistently practiced in medical centers, since the implementation of those analyses is not considered cost-effective [4]. Thus, clinical diagnosis of ONFH remains most of the time unconfirmed. In the hips, a concordance rate of 81.2% in clinical diagnosis verified histologically has been reported [4]. According to the literature, in ONFH this concordance rate varies from 68% to 93% [4,27,31,32]. In the present study, histologic examination of the femoral head specimens confirmed clinico-radiological diagnosis of ONFH in 84% of the cases, hence showing correlation with previous reports. On the other hand, we found that 25% of samples with a radiological diagnosis of OA met histologic diagnosis criteria for ONFH. Previous works have evidenced this kind of false positive in 16% of cases. Misdiagnosis of ONFH can occur if clinician is unaware of potential pitfalls, such as persistent hematopoietic red marrow, the fovea centralis or synovial herniation pits, or existence of pathologic processes that can mimic osteonecrosis, such as subchondral cysts, transient osteoporosis, insufficiency subchondral fractures, osteochondral lesions, and metastasis [10]. Additionally, in agreement with previous reports, we verified that MRI improves diagnostic performance and reduces misdiagnosis of ONFH, with the highest sensitivity and specificity compared to plain radiographs, computed tomography, or scintigraphy. MRI is also highly effective in depicting the early stage and staging lesions accurately [9].

In the present study, when diagnoses of radiologists and orthopedic surgeons were compared with each other, there was only a moderate agreement. Twenty-one of the twenty-four diagnoses agreed (interobserver kappa reliability coefficient of 0.58; percentage agreement of 85.71%), expressing moderate agreement. Literature regarding ONFH interobserver reliability has focused mainly on imaging staging correlation, with average kappa values ranging from 0.39 to 0.56, thus evidencing a poor interobserver reliability, especially among the intermediate stages [25,29,34,35]. In the present work, interobserver diagnosis reproducibility did not show a statistically significant difference when considering the different Ficat and Arlet stages.

Reported evaluations of intra-observer diagnosis variation in ONFH, based mainly in disease imaging staging, have evidenced fair reproducibility, with mean kappa values ranging from 0.43 to 0.88 [25,29,34,35]. Regarding histology, we are not aware of any studies that have looked at intra- or inter-observer variability in the pathological diagnosis of avascular necrosis of the femoral head. This diagnosis was based on macroscopic features of the resected femoral head, an information usually overlooked in literature. Preservation of femoral head sphericity, the presence of degenerative changes or identification of necrotic areas are some of the useful data that a gross evaluation in the operating room can provide, thus contributing to a better diagnosis [30]. In summary, diagnosis of ONFH requires a multidisciplinary approach to enhance currently limited accuracy and reliability. Prompt diagnosis of ONFH may lead to morbidity and costs avoidance, and due to an increased risk of developing the disease contralaterally, an accurate postoperative pathologic diagnosis may be essential [18].

Study limitations: Albeit the aim of the present work was to underline the key role of multidisciplinary diagnoses of patients with ONFH suspicion, some limitations should be considered before drawing conclusions. The complexity of the process of samples collection, preservation, and preparation allowed us to analyze only twenty-four suitable specimens, and thus, the limitations of a small sample size and that of it being a monocentric study should be considered.

5. Conclusions

To enhance current diagnostic precision of ONFH we propose a closer collaboration between clinicians and a greater participation of pathologists. Macroscopic evaluation of the femoral head in the operating room and a more extended use of MRI are also suggested.

Regarding anatomopathological analyses of ONFH, our findings support the quantification of diffuse empty osteocytic lacunae as a valid diagnostic criterion of trabecular necrosis. According to our results, this parameter is not directly related to age or imaging stage significantly. Further investigation of intra- or inter-observer variability in the pathological diagnosis of ONFH is needed.

Supplementary Materials: The following supporting information can be downloaded at: https://www.mdpi.com/article/10.3390/diagnostics12071731/s1, Table S1: Anatomopathological exam from selected bone samples.

Author Contributions: Conceptualization, A.C.-P. and F.M.P.-C.; Methodology, A.C.-P., N.T.-V., A.A.-F. and F.M.P.-C.; Validation, A.C.-P., D.G.-S., N.T.-V., A.A.-F. and F.M.P.-C.; Formal analysis, A.C.-P., N.T.-V. and F.M.P.-C.; Investigation, A.C.-P., D.G.-S., N.T.-V., A.A.-F. and F.M.P.-C.; Resources, A.A.-F.,

M.F. and C.G.-Z.; Writing—original draft preparation, A.C.-P. and F.M.P.-C.; Writing—review and editing, A.C.-P. and F.M.P.-C.; Visualization, F.M.P.-C.; Supervision F.M.P.-C.; Project administration, F.M.P.-C.; Funding acquisition, F.M.P.-C. All authors have read and agreed to the published version of the manuscript.

Funding: This research was funded by a grant from the Instituto de Investigación Marqués de Valdecilla-IDIVAL (PREVAL19/02).

Institutional Review Board Statement: Institutional review board (Comité de Ética en Investigación Clínica de Cantabria). Approved on February 2018. Identification Code 2018.014.

Informed Consent Statement: Informed consent was obtained from all subjects involved in the study.

Conflicts of Interest: The authors declare no conflict of interest.

References

1. Mont, M.A.; Salem, H.S.; Piuzzi, N.S.; Goodman, S.B.; Jones, L.C. Nontraumatic Osteonecrosis of the Femoral Head: Where Do We Stand Today?: A 5-Year Update. *J. Bone Joint Surg. Am.* **2020**, *102*, 1084–1099. [CrossRef]
2. Lavernia, C.J.; Villa, J.M. Total hip arthroplasty in the treatment of osteonecrosis of the femoral head: Then and now. *Curr. Rev. Musculoskelet. Med.* **2015**, *8*, 260–264. [CrossRef]
3. Vail, T.P.; Covington, D.B. *The incidence of osteonecrosis. Osteonecrosis: Etiology, Diagnosis, Treatment*; Urbaniak, J.R., Jones, J.R., Eds.; American Academy of Orthopedic Surgeons: Rosemont, IL, USA, 1997; pp. 43–49.
4. DiCarlo, E.F.; Klein, M.J. Comparison of clinical and histologic diagnoses in 16,587 total joint arthroplasties: Implications for orthopedic and pathologic practices. *Am. J. Clin. Pathol.* **2014**, *141*, 111–118. [CrossRef]
5. Moya-Angeler, J.; Gianakos, A.L.; Villa, J.C.; Ni, A.; Lane, J.M. Current concepts on osteonecrosis of the femoral head. *World J. Orthop.* **2015**, *6*, 590–601. [CrossRef]
6. Luan, S.; Wang, S.; Lin, C.; Fan, S.; Liu, C.; Ma, C.; Wu, S. Comparisons of Ultrasound-Guided Platelet-Rich Plasma Intra-Articular Injection and Extracorporeal Shock Wave Therapy in Treating ARCO I-III Symptomatic Non-Traumatic Femoral Head Necrosis: A Randomized Controlled Clinical Trial. *J. Pain Res.* **2022**, *15*, 341–354. [CrossRef]
7. Sconza, C.; Coletta, F.; Magarelli, N.; D'Agostino, M.C.; Egan, C.G.; Di Matteo, B.; Respizzi, S.; Mazziotti, G. Multimodal conservative treatment of migrating bone marrow edema associated with early osteonecrosis of the hip. *SAGE Open Med. Case Rep.* **2022**, *10*, 2050313X211067617. [CrossRef]
8. de Sire, A.; Invernizzi, M.; Baricich, A.; Lippi, L.; Ammendolia, A.; Grassi, F.A.; Leigheb, M. Optimization of transdisciplinary management of elderly with femur proximal extremity fracture: A patient-tailored plan from orthopaedics to rehabilitation. *World J. Orthop.* **2021**, *12*, 456–466. [CrossRef]
9. Karantanas, A.H. Accuracy and limitations of diagnostic methods for avascular necrosis of the hip. *Expert. Opin. Med. Diagn.* **2013**, *7*, 179–187. [CrossRef]
10. Jackson, S.M.; Major, N.M. Pathologic conditions mimicking osteonecrosis. *Orthop. Clin. N. Am.* **2004**, *35*, 315–320. [CrossRef]
11. Larson, E.; Jones, L.C.; Goodman, S.B.; Koo, K.H.; Cui, Q. Early-stage osteonecrosis of the femoral head: Where are we and where are we going in year 2018? *Int. Orthop.* **2018**, *42*, 1723–1728. [CrossRef]
12. Papakostidis, C.; Tosounidis, T.H.; Jones, E.; Giannoudis, P.V. The role of "cell therapy" in osteonecrosis of the femoral head. A systematic review of the literature and meta-analysis of 7 studies. *Acta Orthop.* **2016**, *87*, 72–78. [CrossRef]
13. Parajuli, S.; Fowler, J.R.; Balasubramanian, E.; Reinus, W.R.; Gaughan, J.P.; Rosenthal, D.I.; Khurana, J.S. Problems with the pathological diagnosis of osteonecrosis. *Skelet. Radiol.* **2016**, *45*, 13–17. [CrossRef]
14. Sultan, A.A.; Mohamed, N.; Samuel, L.T.; Chughtai, M.; Sodhi, N.; Krebs, V.E.; Stearns, K.L.; Molloy, R.M.; Mont, M.A. Classification systems of hip osteonecrosis: An updated review. *Int. Orthop.* **2019**, *43*, 1089–1095. [CrossRef]
15. Humphreys, S.; Spencer, J.D.; Tighe, J.R.; Cumming, R.R. The femoral head in osteonecrosis. A quantitative study of osteocyte population. *J. Bone Joint. Surg. Br.* **1989**, *71*, 205–208. [CrossRef]
16. Kim, Y.H.; Kim, J.S. Histologic analysis of acetabular and proximal femoral bone in patients with osteonecrosis of the femoral head. *J. Bone Joint. Surg. Am.* **2004**, *86*, 2471–2474. [CrossRef]
17. Lang, P.; Jergesen, H.E.; Moseley, M.E.; Block, J.E.; Chafetz, N.I.; Genant, H.K. Avascular necrosis of the femoral head: High-field-strength MR imaging with histologic correlation. *Radiology* **1988**, *169*, 517–524. [CrossRef]
18. Mukisi-Mukaza, M.; Gomez-Brouchet, A.; Donkerwolcke, M.; Hinsenkamp, M.; Burny, F. Histopathology of aseptic necrosis of the femoral head in sickle cell disease. *Int. Orthop.* **2011**, *35*, 1145–1150. [CrossRef]
19. Plenk, H., Jr.; Gstettner, M.; Grossschmidt, K.; Breitenseher, M.; Urban, M.; Hofmann, S. Magnetic resonance imaging and histology of repair in femoral head osteonecrosis. *Clin. Orthop. Relat. Res.* **2001**, *386*, 42–53. [CrossRef]
20. Simmons, D.J.; Daum, W.J.; Totty, W.; Murphy, W.A. Correlation of MRI images with histology in avascular necrosis in the hip. A preliminary study. *J. Arthroplast.* **1989**, *4*, 7–14. [CrossRef]
21. Yeh, L.R.; Chen, C.K.; Huang, Y.L.; Pan, H.B.; Yang, C.F. Diagnostic performance of MR imaging in the assessment of subchondral fractures in avascular necrosis of the femoral head. *Skelet. Radiol.* **2009**, *38*, 559–564. [CrossRef]

22. Pang, Y.; Zheng, X.; Pei, F.; Chen, Y.; Guo, K.; Zhao, F. A Retrospective Study to Compare the Efficacy and Postoperative Outcome of Total Hip Arthroplasty with Internal Screw Fixation in Patients with Avascular Necrosis of the Femoral Head. *Med. Sci. Monit.* **2019**, *25*, 3655–3661. [CrossRef]
23. Bradway, J.K.; Morrey, B.F. The natural history of the silent hip in bilateral atraumatic osteonecrosis. *J. Arthroplast.* **1993**, *8*, 383–387. [CrossRef]
24. Bone, M.R. *Laboratory Histopathology*; Woods AE and Ellis RC: New York, NY, USA, 1994; Volume 7, pp. 2–10.
25. Hesketh, K.; Sankar, W.; Joseph, B.; Narayanan, U.; Mulpuri, K. Inter-observer and intra-observer reliability in the radiographic diagnosis of avascular necrosis of the femoral head following reconstructive hip surgery in children with cerebral palsy. *J. Child. Orthop.* **2016**, *10*, 143–147. [CrossRef]
26. Li, W.L.; Tan, B.; Jia, Z.X.; Dong, B.; Huang, Z.Q.; Zhu, R.Z.; Zhao, W.; Gao, H.H.; Wang, R.T.; Chen, W.H. Exploring the Risk Factors for the Misdiagnosis of Osteonecrosis of Femoral Head: A Case-Control Study. *Orthop. Surg.* **2020**, *12*, 1792–1798. [CrossRef]
27. Dermawan, J.K.; Goldblum, A.; Reith, J.D.; Kilpatrick, S.E. Accurate and Reliable Diagnosis of Avascular Necrosis of the Femoral Head From Total Hip Arthroplasty Specimens Requires Pathologic Examination. *Am. J. Clin. Pathol.* **2021**, *155*, 565–574. [CrossRef]
28. Narayanan, A.; Khanchandani, P.; Borkar, R.M.; Ambati, C.R.; Roy, A.; Han, X.; Bhoskar, R.N.; Ragampeta, S.; Gannon, F.; Mysorekar, V.; et al. Avascular Necrosis of Femoral Head: A Metabolomic, Biophysical, Biochemical, Electron Microscopic and Histopathological Characterization. *Sci. Rep.* **2017**, *7*, 10721. [CrossRef]
29. Plakseychuk, A.Y.; Shah, M.; Varitimidis, S.E.; Rubash, H.E.; Sotereanos, D. Classification of osteonecrosis of the femoral head. Reliability, reproducibility, and prognostic value. *Clin. Orthop. Relat. Res.* **2001**, *386*, 34–41. [CrossRef]
30. Fondi, C.; Franchi, A. Definition of bone necrosis by the pathologist. *Clin. Cases Miner. Bone Metab.* **2007**, *4*, 21–26.
31. Crim, J.; Layfield, L.J.; Stensby, J.D.; Schmidt, R.L. Comparison of Radiographic and Pathologic Diagnosis of Osteonecrosis of the Femoral Head. *AJR Am. J. Roentgenol.* **2021**, *216*, 1014–1021. [CrossRef]
32. Layfield, L.J.; Crim, J.R.; Oserowsky, A.; Schmidt, R.L. Pathology Assessment of Femoral Head Resection Specimens: An Important Quality Assurance Procedure. *Arch. Pathol. Lab. Med.* **2020**, *144*, 580–585. [CrossRef]
33. Yamamoto, T.; Yamaguchi, T.; Lee, K.B.; Bullough, P.G. A clinicopathologic study of osteonecrosis in the osteoarthritic hip. *Osteoarthr. Cartil.* **2000**, *8*, 303–308. [CrossRef]
34. Schmitt-Sody, M.; Kirchhoff, C.; Mayer, W.; Goebel, M.; Jansson, V. Avascular necrosis of the femoral head: Inter- and intraobserver variations of Ficat and ARCO classifications. *Int. Orthop.* **2008**, *32*, 283–287. [CrossRef]
35. Smith, S.W.; Meyer, R.A.; Connor, P.M.; Smith, S.E.; Hanley, E.N., Jr. Interobserver reliability and intraobserver reproducibility of the modified Ficat classification system of osteonecrosis of the femoral head. *J. Bone Joint. Surg. Am.* **1996**, *78*, 1702–1706. [CrossRef]

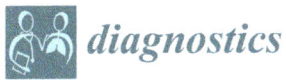

Article

Prevalence of Monosodium Urate (MSU) Deposits in Cadavers Detected by Dual-Energy Computed Tomography (DECT)

Andrea S. Klauser [1], Sylvia Strobl [1], Christoph Schwabl [1,*], Werner Klotz [2], Gudrun Feuchtner [1], Bernhard Moriggl [3], Julia Held [2], Mihra Taljanovic [4], Jennifer S. Weaver [5], Monique Reijnierse [6], Elke R. Gizewski [1] and Hannes Stofferin [3]

1 Department of Radiology, Medical University Innsbruck, 6020 Innsbruck, Austria; andrea.klauser@i-med.ac.at (A.S.K.); gudrun.feuchtner@i-med.ac.at (G.F.); elke.gizewski@i-med.ac.at (E.R.G.)
2 Department of Internal Medicine II, Medical University Innsbruck, 6020 Innsbruck, Austria; werner.klotz@tirol-kliniken.at (W.K.); julia.held@tirol-kliniken.at (J.H.)
3 Department of Anatomy, Histology and Embryology, Institute of Clinical and Functional Anatomy, Medical University Innsbruck, 6020 Innsbruck, Austria; bernhard.moriggl@i-med.ac.at (B.M.); hannes.stofferin@i-med.ac.at (H.S.)
4 Department of Medical Imaging, Banner University Medical Center, College of Medicine, The University of Arizona, Tucson, AZ 85724, USA; mihrat@radiology.arizona.edu
5 Department of Radiology, University of New Mexico, Albuquerque, NM 87131, USA; jsweaver@salud.unm.edu
6 Division of Musculoskeletal Radiology, Department of Radiology, Leiden University Medical Center, 2333 ZC Leiden, The Netherlands; m.reijnierse@lumc.nl
* Correspondence: christoph.schwabl@i-med.ac.at

Abstract: Background: Dual-energy computed tomography (DECT) allows direct visualization of monosodium urate (MSU) deposits in joints and soft tissues. Purpose: To describe the distribution of MSU deposits in cadavers using DECT in the head, body trunk, and feet. Materials and Methods: A total of 49 cadavers (41 embalmed and 8 fresh cadavers; 20 male, 29 female; mean age, 79.5 years; SD ± 11.3; range 52–95) of unknown clinical history underwent DECT to assess MSU deposits in the head, body trunk, and feet. Lens, thoracic aorta, and foot tendon dissections of fresh cadavers were used to verify MSU deposits by polarizing light microscopy. Results: 33/41 embalmed cadavers (80.5%) showed MSU deposits within the thoracic aorta. 11/41 cadavers (26.8%) showed MSU deposits within the metatarsophalangeal (MTP) joints and 46.3% of cadavers demonstrated MSU deposits within foot tendons, larger than and equal to 5 mm. No MSU deposits were detected in the cranium/intracerebral vessels, or the coronary arteries. Microscopy used as a gold standard could verify the presence of MSU deposits within the lens, thoracic aorta, or foot tendons in eight fresh cadavers. Conclusions: Microscopy confirmed the presence of MSU deposits in fresh cadavers within the lens, thoracic aorta, and foot tendons, whereas no MSU deposits could be detected in cranium/intracerebral vessels or coronary arteries. DECT may offer great potential as a screening tool to detect MSU deposits and measure the total uric acid burden in the body. The clinical impact of this cadaver study in terms of assessment of MSU burden should be further proven.

Keywords: gout; monosodium urate deposits; cardiovascular; musculoskeletal; dual-energy computed tomography; ocular lense; tendons; kidney

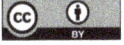

1. Introduction

Gout is a crystal-induced inflammatory arthritis with increasing incidence and prevalence in recent decades [1]. It represents a major healthcare burden, given its association with metabolic syndrome, coronary heart disease, and diabetes mellitus [1].

Dual-energy computed tomography (DECT) is a well-established method for the detection of MSU deposits in peripheral joints and tendons and has been implemented in the American College of Radiology/European League Against Rheumatism (ACR/EULAR) 2018 gout classification criteria [2–5].

Chhana et al. [6] described DECT as an advanced imaging method for the assessment of crystal proven tophaceous gout in 12 different joints but only in one cadaveric specimen. A recent study by Klauser et al. [7] demonstrated the usefulness of DECT for the detection of cardiovascular MSU deposits in patients with gout and a control group of patients without a previous history of gout or inflammatory rheumatic disease, as verified by microscopy in fresh cadavers. Especially in the last few years, studies concerning extraarticular gout manifestations have become more and more frequent [8,9]. Nevertheless, there is still a broad discussion regarding subclinical or vascular deposits [10–12]. A general consensus regarding the optimal DECT protocol has not yet been established. it remains questionable how many of the MSU deposits found in the DECT are actual urate or merely artifacts [13–16].

To our knowledge, direct imaging of MSU deposits of the head, body trunk, and feet in embalmed cadavers by DECT has not been reported to date.

The detection of artefacts in DECT is a frequent point of discussion and several typical artefacts have been well described in the literature, e.g., finger nails [17,18]. Due to the lack of verification by microscopy, we do not yet know, if the MSU deposits are always true or artefacts. To exclude artefacts and verify the MSU deposits found with DECT, crystal characterization with polarizing light microscopy was performed in the lens, aorta, and feet tendons in fresh cadavers.

2. Materials and Methods

2.1. Cadavers

A total of 49 cadavers, 41 embalmed (16 male, 25 female, mean age, 82 years; SD ± 16.4; range 52–91) and 8 fresh (4 male, 4 female, mean, 75 years; SD ± 13.2; range 72–95) were enrolled from 1 January 2017, and through 1 November 2018.

Informed consent was provided according to the last wills of the donors, who had donated their bodies to human research studies. Institutional review board approval was obtained. All embalmed and fresh cadavers were referred to DECT after death and were in legal custody of the Anatomy institution.

No medical history was available including gouty arthritis or hyperuricemia. DECT examinations of the head, body trunk, and feet were performed.

2.2. DECT Scan Parameters

The evaluation was performed with a 128-row dual-source CT scanner (Somatom Definition Flash; Siemens Healthineers, Forchheim, Germany) at two energy levels (80 and 140 kV) using two separate sets of X-ray tubes and detectors positioned 90 to 95 degrees apart without the use of contrast media. The standardized protocol settings included 80 kV/100–140 mAs for tube A and 140 kV/200–250 mAs for tube B, with a ratio of 1.36, range of 4, minimum HU of 150, and maximum HU of 500. Scan parameters were $2 \times 64 \times 0.625$ mm acquisition, rotation time of 1 s, DLP 219 mGycm, CTDI vol 11.01 L, total mAs 3415, slice thickness of 0.75 mm, and increment of 0.5 mm. Axial, coronal, and sagittal reformations were reconstructed from the DE datasets at a resolution of 0.4 mm with soft tissue kernel (D30) and bone kernel (B60). D30 kernel was used for DE processing and MSU detection.

The acquired datasets were reconstructed in the desired planes and processed with dual-energy software utilizing a standardized two-material decomposition algorithm designed for specific clinical applications [19]. The two-material decomposition algorithm is based on the principle that materials with a high atomic number such as calcium would demonstrate a higher increase in attenuation at higher photon energies than does a material composed of low atomic number materials such as MSU crystals. Once separated and characterized, the materials were color-coded and overlaid on multi-planar reformatted cross-sectional images [19]. We choose green pixels for MSU deposit demonstration when using the software of the Syngovia workstation (Siemens Healthineers).

Pre-processed and processed images were transferred to the picture archiving system (PACS). Corresponding pre-processed grey-scale images are reviewed for the presence of deposits (8).

2.3. CT and DECT Scoring

Two radiologists with experience in gout imaging by DECT of 5 and 7 years evaluated the DECT images in consensus.

Anatomic locations of calcified plaques and MSU deposits were determined as follows:

+ Head/Neck:
1. Cranium/intracerebral vessels, ear cartilage and orbits (lens)
2. Supraaortal vessels (Subclavian and Carotid arteries)

+ Body trunk
1. Ascending aorta, descending aorta, aortic arch, aortic root, abdominal aorta
2. Right coronary artery (RCA), left main artery (LM), circumflex artery (CX) and left anterior descending artery (LAD)
3. Tricuspid valve and mitral valve
4. Iliac vessels
5. Rib cartilages
6. Kidney

Cardiovascular calcified plaques with a CT attenuation >130 Houndsfield Units (HU) [20] and MSU deposits in the thoracic aorta, coronary arteries, valves, abdominal aorta, and iliac vessels were graded according to Gondrie et al. [21] as follows:

Score 0 = absent, score 1 = 5 or fewer foci, score 2 = between 6–8 foci and extending over 3 section, score 3 = more than 9 foci extending over 3 sections.

+ Feet:
1. Joints: Metatarsophalangeal (MTP) joints, interphalangeal joints (IP), tibiotalar joint.
2. Tendons: Extensor hallucis longus tendon (EHL), tibialis anterior tendon (TAT), tibialis posterior tendon (TPT), flexor hallucis longus tendon (FHL), peroneal tendons (PT), and Achilles tendon (AT).

MSU deposits in MTP joints and foot tendons were graded as follows:

Score 0 = absent, Score 1 = MSU deposits < 5 mm, Score 2 = MSU deposits between 5–10 mm, Score 3 = MSU deposits $\geq$ 10 mm.

According to ACR/EULAR guidelines nail bed deposits, submillimeter deposits, skin deposits, and deposits by beam hardening and vascular artefacts were not classified as positive findings in our study [3].

2.4. Polarizing Microscopic Evaluation

In 8 fresh cadavers with DECT positive MSU deposits within the lens, thoracic aorta, or foot tendons, gross anatomical sectioning according to defined landmark was performed, cut unfixed to pieces of 5 mm × 5 mm, embedded using Tissue-Tek®® O.C.T.™ compound medium and sectioned at 5 µm using a Leica CM1950 S cryostat. After mounting on microscope slides and covering using Glycerine/Phosphate-Buffered Saline (PBS) solution, cryostat section examination was performed with compensated polarized light microscopy at 400× magnification. First order red compensation was performed to recognize MSU crystals by their needle-like appearance and strong negative birefringence.

2.5. Statistical Analysis

Statistical analysis was performed using R Project for Statistical Computing 3.5.1 [R Core Team (2013). R: A language and environment for statistical computing. R Foundation for Statistical Computing, Vienna, Austria. http://www.R-project.org]. The presence of MSU deposits and calcified plaques for the different anatomical locations was tabulated together with the individual scores. To analyze the relationship between MSU deposits and the occurrence of calcified plaques contingency tables were generated and a Fisher's Exact Test for count data was performed. To test scoring results for age dependence Spearman's rank correlation coefficients were calculated. Results were considered significant for *p*-values less than 0.05.

3. Results

3.1. Fresh Cadavers

1 cadaver demonstrated MSU deposits within the orbits (Figure 1), 1 cadaver showed MSU deposits within the thoracic aorta (Figure 2) and all cadavers showed MSU deposits within the foot tendons (AT, PT, FHL, TAT) (Figure 3). MSU deposits detected by DECT were histologically proven to be present by polarized light microscopy in a total of 10/10 biopsies (100%).

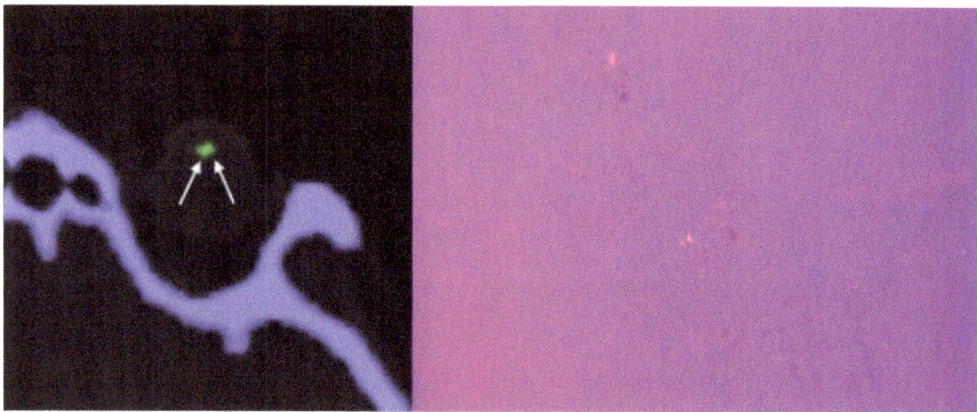

Figure 1. 80-year-old male cadaver. Axial DECT image showing Score 1 MSU deposit in the left lens (white arrows). Corresponding microscopic image taken from the lens, showing diffuse packed and patchy MSU deposits with strong negative birefringence (bluish structures).

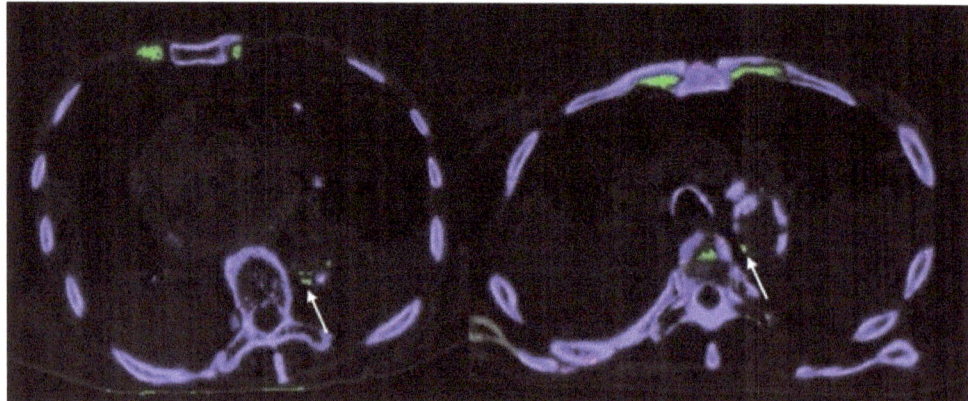

Figure 2. Axial DECT images showing histologically verified Score 1 MSU deposits in thoracic aorta (white arrows). Note: MSU deposits in anterior costochondral cartilage and intervertebral disc.

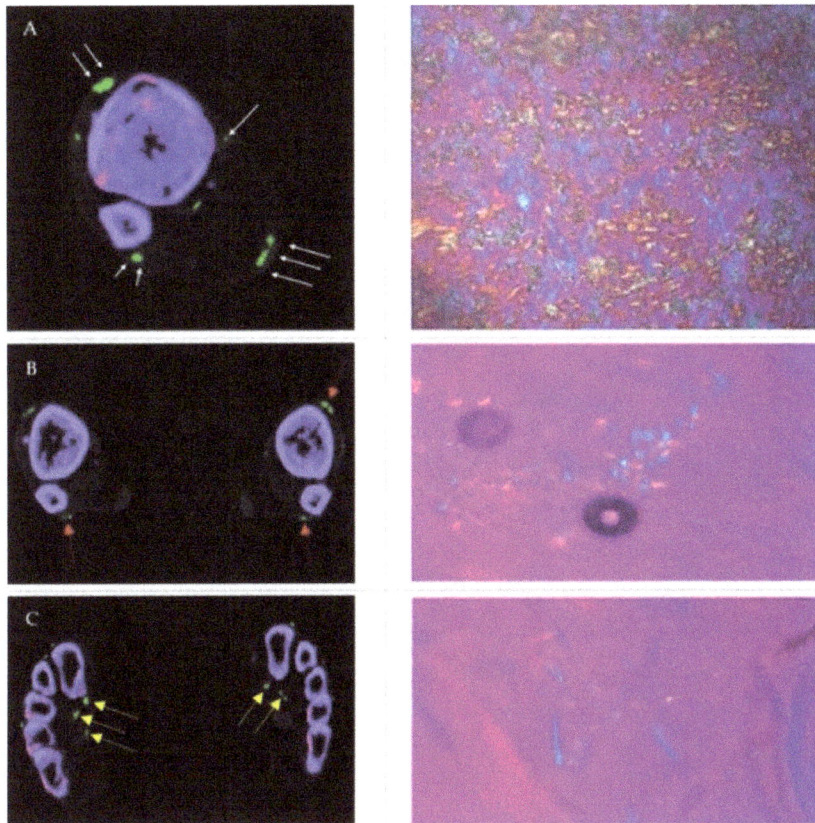

Figure 3. (**A**) Axial DECT image showing MSU deposits within the TAT, PT, AT, and TPT (white arrows) with corresponding microscopic image taken from the AT, showing large diffuse packed and patchy MSU crystals with strong negative birefringence (bluish structures). (**B**) Axial DECT image demonstrating MSU deposits within the TAT and PT (red arrows) with corresponding microscopic image taken from the PT. (**C**) Axial DECT image showing MSU deposits within the FHL and flexor digitorum longum tendon (yellow arrows) with corresponding microscopic image taken from the FHL.

3.2. Embalmed Cadavers

In the head, 4/41 (9.8%) cadavers showed MSU deposits within the lens and 40/41 (97.6%) of the cadavers demonstrated MSU deposition within the ear cartilage. No MSU deposits were detected within the neurocranium and intracerebral vessels. 30/41 cadavers (73.2%) showed MSU deposits within the thoracic aorta and all cadavers demonstrated calcified aortic wall plaques (Table 1). Only 1/41 cadavers (2.4%) showed MSU deposits within the abdominal aorta.

Table 1. Localization and scoring of calcified plaque (first line) and MSU deposits (second line) in embalmed cadavers.

Anatomical Location	Score 0	Score 1	Score 2	Score 3
Aorta				
root	6/41 (14.6%) 31/41 (75.6%)	0/41 (0%) 10/41 (24%)	11/41 (26.9%) 0/41 (0%)	24/41 (58.5%) 0/41 (0%)
ascending	13/41 (31.7%) 34/41 (82.9%)	0/41 (0%) 7/41 (17.1%)	7/41 (17.1%) 0/41 (0%)	21/41 (51.2%) 0/41 (0%)
arch	1/41 (2.4%) 31/41 (75.6%)	0/41 (0%) 10/41 (24%)	3/41 (7.3%) 0/41 (0%)	37/41 (90.2%) 0/41 (0%)
descending	2/41 (4.9%) 13/41 (31.7%)	0/41 (0%) 22/41 (53.7%)	3/41 (7.3%) 2/41 (4.9%)	36/41 (87.9%) 4/41 (9.8%)
abdominal	0/41 (0%) 40/41 (97.6%)	2/41 (4.9%) 1/41 (2.4%)	0/41 (0%) 0/41 (0%)	39/41 (95.1%) 0/41 (0%)
Supraaortal vessels	2/41 (4.9%) 28/41 (68.3%)	0/41 (0%) 12/41 (29.3%)	6/41 (14.6%) 1/41 (2.4%)	33/41 (80.5%) 0/41 (0%)
Iliac vessels	0/41 (0%) 36/41 (87.8%)	2/41 (4.9%) 5/41 (12.2%)	0/41 (0%) 0/41 (0%)	39/41 (95.1) 0/41 (0%)
Valves				
tricuspid	41/41 (100%) 41/41 (100%)	0/41 (0%) 0/41 (0%)	0/41 (0%) 0/41 (0%)	0/41 (0%) 0/41 (0%)
mitral	41/41 (100%) 41/41 (100%)	0/41 (0%) 0/41 (0%)	0/41 (0%) 0/41 (0%)	0/41 (0%) 0/41 (0%)
Coronary arteries				
LAD	2/41 (4.9%) 41/41 (100%)	0/41 (0% 0/41 (0%)	3/41 (7.3%) 0/41 (0%)	36/41 (87.9%) 0/41 (0%)
LM	11/41 (26.8%) 41/41 (100%)	0/41 (0% 0/41 (0%)	3/41 (7.3%) 0/41 (0%)	27/41 (65.9%) 0/41 (0%)
RCA	8/41 (19.5%) 41/41 (100%)	0/41 (0% 0/41 (0%)	5/41 (12.2%) 0/41 (0%)	28/41 (68.3%) 0/41 (0%)
CX	8/41 (19.5%) 41/41 (100%)	0/41 (0% 0/41 (0%)	4/41 (9.8%) 0/41 (0%)	29/41 (70.7%) 0/41 (0%)

Note: Score 0 = absent, score 1 = 5 or fewer foci, score 2 = 6–8 foci, >3 section, score 3 ≥9 foci, >3 sections. LAD = left anterior descending artery, LM = left main artery, RCA = right coronary artery, CX = circumflex artery.

For the ascending aorta, Fisher's Exact Test showed a significant association between MSU deposits and calcified plaques ($p = 0.02$). Spearman's rank correlation showed a weak but significant positive dependence on age for calcified plaques (rho = 0.332, $p = 0.034$); however, no dependence on age was demonstrated for MSU deposits (rho = -0.07, $p = 0.68$). All other vessels or regions in the body trunk demonstrated no significant association or age dependence for calcified plaques or MSU deposits.

None of the cadavers were positive for MSU deposits in the coronary arteries and valves (Table 1). Only calcified plaques within the LAD showed a weak but significant positive dependence on age (rho = 0.387, $p = 0.012$); all other coronary arteries showed no dependence on age. In all 41 cadavers (100%) MSU deposits were detected in costochondral cartilages (Figures 2 and 4), and 3/41 (7.3%) showed MSU deposits within kidney stones (Figure 4).

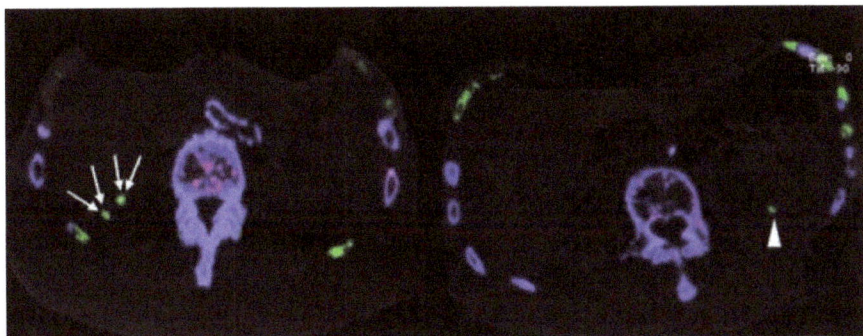

Figure 4. Axial DECT images showing MSU deposits in kidney stones (white arrows) and MSU deposit in renal calyx (arrowhead).

11/41 (26.8%) cadavers showed MSU deposits within the MTP joints (Table 2). The first MTP joint was the most commonly involved joint in 6/11 MTP positive cadavers (54.5%) (Table 2).

Table 2. Scoring of MSU deposits in foot joints of embalmed cadavers.

Anatomical Location	Positive Joints	Score 0	Score 1	Score 2	Score 3
MTP joints	11/41 (26.8%)	30/41 (73.2%)	2/41 (4.9%)	6/41 (14.6%)	3/41 (7.3%)
MTP I	6/11 (54.5%)		1/6 (16.7%)	3/6 (50%)	2/6 (33.3%)
MTP I – V	4/11 (36.4%)		0/4 (0%)	3/4 (75%)	1/4 (25%)
MTP I + V	1/11 (10%)		1/1 (100%)	0/1 (0%)	0/1 (0%)
Interphalangeal joint	0/41 (0%)				
Ankle	0/41 (0%)				
Tarsus	0/41 (0%)				

Note: Score 0 = absent, score 1 = 5 or fewer foci, score 2 = 6–8 foci, >3 section, score 3 ≥ 9 foci, >3 sections. MTP = metatarsophalangeal.

46.3% of cadavers demonstrated MSU deposits within foot tendons, larger than 5 mm (Table 3). The most common Score 3 MSU deposition site was the AT at 31.7%, followed by TAT at 19.5% (Table 3).

Table 3. Scoring of MSU deposits in foot tendons of embalmed cadavers.

Anatomical Location	Score 0	Score 1	Score 2	Score 3
EHL	1/41 (2.4%)	24/41 (58.5%)	11/41 (27.5%)	5/41 (12.2)
FHL	1/41 (2.4%)	31/41 (75.6%)	8/41 (19.5%)	1/41 (2.4%)
TAT	1/41 (2.4%)	13/41 (31.7%)	19/41 (46.3%)	8/41 (19.5%)
TPT	1/41 (2.4%)	31/41 (75.6)	8/41 (19.5%)	1/41 (2.4%)
PT	1/41 (2.4%)	19/41 (46.3%)	18/41 (43.9%)	3/41 (7.3%)
AT	1/41 (2.4%)	22/41 (53.6%)	5/41 (12.2.%)	13/41 (31.7%)

Note: Score 0 = absent, Score 1 = MSU deposits < 5 mm, Score 2 = MSU deposits between 5–10 mm, Score 3 = MSU deposits ≥ 10 mm. EHL = extensor hallucis longus, FHL = flexor hallucis longus, TAT = tibialis anterior tendon, TPT = tibialis posterior tendon, PT = peroneal tendons, AT = achilles tendon.

4. Discussion

DECT screening for gout deposits in cadavers shows a high prevalence. Histological correlation in fresh cadavers could confirm these positive DECT findings as MSU deposits (and not artefacts). MSU deposits are predominantly seen within vessel walls in calcified plaques (however not in the brain), in rib cartilage, and in foot tendons.

In hyperuricemia, supersaturation leads to the precipitation of urate crystals in the plasma and within joints. Additionally, all other interstitial fluids will be supersaturated as well and may drive crystal-induced inflammation. Tophi can present in unexpected anatomical locations; therefore vigilance is required when unusual symptoms or signs occur in a patient suspected to have gout [22].

DECT has emerged as a useful diagnostic imaging modality for the diagnosis of gout, by offering the advantage of directly assessing MSU deposits as well as displaying the anatomic extent of the disease [2,5]. DECT can be used to monitor response to drug therapy and maximize clinical management, thus optimizing patient outcomes [23]. It has been impacted in patients to urate lowering therapy [24].

DECT detects MSU deposits in peripheral joints with sensitivities of 78 to 100% and specificities of 78 to 100% [25–27]. MTP 1 joint is the most affected joint in gouty arthritis [28], consistent with our findings in 6/11 (54.5%) MTP positive embalmed cadavers. Pascart et al. [29] showed that the extent of the MSU burden in peripheral joints (knee joint and feet joints) measured with DECT predicted the risk of flares.

However, in the last 30 years, only one study evaluated cadaveric MTP 1 joints [30] and reported that 12/70 (17.1%) consecutive autopsies showed MSU crystal deposits in polarizing light microscopy. 2/12 (16.7%) subjects had a history of podagra or gouty arthritis pre-mortem in this study. This suggests a possible post-mortem crystallization since the level of serum uric acid necessary for supersaturation decreases with a reduction in body temperature from 6.8 mg% at 37° to 2.4 mg% at 30° as previously reported by Loeb et al. [31]. Post-mortem crystallization could therefore also explain higher numbers of positive MTP 1 joints (6/11 positive MTP joints) in our DECT study.

Tendon involvement in patients with gout is frequent and affects joint stability and flexibility. Racide et al. [32] postulated that tendons rupture at the sites of MSU crystal deposits because the urate crystals lead to a reduction in the tensile strength of the tendon. Tendon rupture due to tophus infiltration has been described in patients with chronic gout, although this is an uncommon event [33].

In a study by Dalbeth et al. [34] in 92 patients, MSU deposits in tendons occurred in tophaceous gout. The most commonly involved tendon in the foot was the AT (39.1%), followed by the PT (18.1%). The TAT and the extensor tendons were involved less commonly in 7.6–10.3%. These findings are in line with our study, where the most commonly involved Score 3 MSU deposition site was the AT at 31.7%, followed by TAT at 19.5%.

Yuan et al. [35] also reported tendons as the most frequent anatomical location of MSU deposits, in up to 41.4%, consistent with our findings. It is unknown if small MSU deposits (Score 1 and 2) in tendons are of clinical importance; this should be investigated in future studies. Furthermore, postprocessing seems to take an important role, to increase sensitivity for MSU deposits not only in joints but especially in tendons, as seen in previous studies [16,36], which should also be assessed in further investigations.

The gouty infiltration of tendons and soft tissues should hence also be considered a rare differential diagnosis for nonspecific soft tissue masses, even in asymptomatic patients with unknown hyperuricemia prior to their first tophaceous manifestation [37].

Previous studies have shown a high incidence of uric acid kidney stones with the highest prevalence in the middle east and in Europe [38]. DECT is useful in discriminating uric acid stones and other stone types with 92–100% accuracy, a positive predictive value of 100%, and a negative predictive value of 98.5% [39]. In a recent study by Li et al. [40] nephrolithiasis was reported in 27/84 (32.1%) patients with gout, with a high incidence of pure uric acid (UA) kidney stones in 17/27 (63%). DECT imaging may permit patients with UA stones to benefit from conservative treatment and avoid interventional procedures. We detected a low number of 3/41 (7.3%) UA stones in our cadaveric study.

Confirmed urate crystals in the eyes have been rarely reported in the past 40 years [41]. The majority of gout patients' ocular abnormalities are asymptomatic [42]. Precipitation of urate crystal has been described in eyelids, tarsal plates, conjunctiva, cornea, sclera, tendons of extraocular muscles, orbit, and lens. It has been reported that tophi can be deposited in the iris or in the anterior chamber, causing anterior uveitis or glaucoma [43]. Lin et al. [42], found uric acid crystals on the ocular surface in 3/380 (0.79%) consecutive gout patients. They further reported that patients with UA crystals in their ocular surface also showed many tophi in both ears, finger roots, feet, and kidneys, but this was not confirmed by DECT. In our study 1/4 lens positive embalmed cadavers also showed UA kidney stones, 2/4 MSU deposits in MTP joints, and all of them (4/4) showed MSU deposits in rib cartilages and were positive for MSU deposits in foot tendons. A possible correlation should be investigated in further studies.

In general, we demonstrated MSU deposits in the lens in 4/41 embalmed cadavers (9.8%), which was proven by polarizing light microscopy in fresh cadavers. Ferry et al. [44] reported in 69 severe gout patients that the most common abnormality was bilateral ocular redness caused by hyperemia of conjunctival and episcleral vessels. When evaluating a patient with bilateral chronic conjunctival redness, the clinician should consider MSU deposits in the differential diagnosis. A statistically significant difference in subconjunctival hemorrhage in gout patients and other groups was reported, whereas the subconjunctival hemorrhage in gout patients was not absorbed after three months. This underscores the importance of early detection of ocular MSU deposits [42].

Only one DECT study by Carr et al. [45] evaluated extensive MSU deposits in rib cartilage, in 19/20 gout patients (95%) without any difference between patients and controls indicating that it is not a disease-specific finding but instead represents a physiologic process. This is consistent with our findings, where all cadavers (100%) were positive for MSU deposits in rib cartilages. Further studies should prove whether physiologic MSU deposits in rib cartilage occur. MSU deposits in ear cartilage have only been scarcely reported in a few case reports. We found a high frequency of MSU deposits in ear cartilage in 40/41 cadavers (97.6%). Tophi in the external middle ear or ear helix should be considered in the differential diagnosis of ear masses alongside common pathologies [46].

Kumral et al. demonstrated that high uric acid levels are strongly associated with CAD and that elevated uric acid might be injurious for large cerebral arteries [47]. To our knowledge, this is the first study performing DECT imaging of the neurocranium and intracerebral vessels in cadavers. Interestingly MSU deposits in intracerebral vessels could not be detected in our study and also have not been reported to date. Karagiannis et al. [48] showed that serum UA is an independent predictor for early death after acute stroke and UA lowering therapy improved outcomes in stroke patients receiving intravenous thrombolysis followed by thrombectomy. McFarland et al. [49] reported an inverse association between urate levels and Parkinson Disease, Lewy body dementia, and possibly Alzheimer's disease.

Among patients with gout, characteristic gout severity factors are associated with cardiovascular disease (CVD). Disveld et al. [50] showed that crystal-proven gout is strongly associated with an increased prevalence of CVD. This underscores the importance of early detection of cardiovascular MSU deposits. Andres et al. [51] reported a significant increase in coronary calcification and MSU deposits in the knees and MTP 1 joints in patients with asymptomatic hyperuricemia. However, these calcifications were not evaluated in terms of cardiovascular MSU deposits, as assessed in our study. In contrast, Pascart et al. [52] found that the extent of MSU burden in knees and feet detected by DECT and ultrasound did not increase the estimated risk of a cardiovascular event in 42 gout patients.

Only a paucity of gouty tophi in the mitral valve, aortic valve, and pulmonal valve has been previously reported [53]. In our study, mitral and tricuspid valves were evaluated and did not show any MSU deposits. Our preliminary findings can support the hypothesis of an association between calcified plaques and cardiovascular deposition of MSU in the ascending aorta in 30/41 cadavers (73.2%), but not in coronary arteries, supraaortal vessels, and valves, which has recently been described in assessing gout patients using DECT [7,54]. Several studies reflect the suboptimal care received by gout patients and suggest an urgent need to optimize treatment and prevent adverse outcomes. As previously reported, DECT provides the option of quantifying the MSU burden [55] and hence can be used to monitor the response of patients during MSU lowering therapy [56]. In future studies, it may be interesting to characterize and volumetrize the deposits, especially in the vessel walls. Artificial intelligence sofware could also be used to facilitate the analysis, which has already been successfully applied in other regions [57–59].

Limitations

Prior medical history of the cadavers was not available.

Volume rendering imaging of MSU deposits was not performed and should be investigated in further clinical studies to quantify gouty burden.

This study is limited by the small sample size for cardiovascular studies and therefore larger cohorts are stringent necessary in order to define the prognostic value of MSU deposits for CVD outcomes.

5. Conclusions

DECT can be used to detect MSU deposits in both fresh and embalmed cadavers. DECT showed MSU deposits within the lens, thoracic aorta, and foot tendons of our cadavers, whereas no MSU deposits could be detected in neurocranium/intracerebral vessels and coronary arteries. Findings were confirmed with microscopy. In addition to detecting MSU deposits within the peripheral joints and tendons, DECT offers the potential to image MSU deposits in the other body parts and organ systems and thus may be feasible as a screening tool to detect MSU deposits and to measure total uric acid burden in the whole body.

The clinical impact of this cadaver study should be further investigated.

Author Contributions: Conceptualization, A.S.K., S.S., C.S., G.F., J.H., M.T., J.S.W. and H.S.; Data curation, A.S.K., C.S., W.K., B.M., J.H. and H.S.; Formal analysis, A.S.K., S.S., C.S., W.K., M.T. and M.R.; Investigation, A.S.K., S.S., C.S., G.F., B.M., J.H., M.R. and H.S.; Methodology, A.S.K., S.S., C.S., W.K., G.F., J.S.W. and H.S.; Project administration, A.S.K. and E.R.G.; Resources, E.R.G.; Software, C.S.; Supervision, A.S.K., G.F., M.T. and M.R.; Validation, B.M., M.T. and J.S.W.; Visualization, W.K. and H.S.; Writing—original draft, A.S.K., S.S. and C.S.; Writing—review & editing, A.S.K., C.S., J.S.W., M.R. and E.R.G. All authors have read and agreed to the published version of the manuscript.

Funding: This research received no external funding.

Institutional Review Board Statement: Not applicable.

Informed Consent Statement: Not applicable.

Data Availability Statement: Data supporting reported results may be provided upon reasonable request.

Conflicts of Interest: The authors declare no conflict of interest.

References

1. Harris, M.D.; Siegel, L.B.; Alloway, J.A. Gout and hyperuricemia. *Am. Fam. Phys.* **1999**, *59*, 925–934.
2. Neogi, T.; Jansen, T.L.; Dalbeth, N.; Fransen, J.; Schumacher, H.R.; Berendsen, D.; Brown, M.; Choi, H.; Edwards, N.L.; Janssens, H.J.E.M.; et al. 2015 Gout classification criteria: An American College of Rheumatology/European League Against Rheumatism collaborative initiative. *Ann. Rheum. Dis.* **2015**, *74*, 1789–1798. [CrossRef]
3. Richette, P.; Doherty, M.; Pascual, E.; Barskova, V.; Becce, F.; Castaneda, J.; Coyfish, M.; Guillo, S.; Jansen, T.; Janssens, H.; et al. 2018 updated European League Against Rheumatism evidence-based recommendations for the diagnosis of gout. *Ann. Rheum. Dis.* **2020**, *79*, 31–38. [CrossRef]
4. Hu, H.J.; Liao, M.Y.; Xu, L.Y. Clinical utility of dual-energy CT for gout diagnosis. *Clin. Imaging* **2015**, *39*, 880–885. [CrossRef]
5. Schwabl, C.; Taljanovic, M.; Widmann, G.; Teh, J.; Klauser, A.S. Ultrasonography and dual-energy computed tomography: Impact for the detection of gouty deposits. *Ultrasonography* **2021**, *40*, 197–206. [CrossRef]
6. Chhana, A.; Doyle, A.; Sevao, A.; Amirapu, S.; Riordan, P.; Dray, M.; McGlashan, S.; Cornish, J.; Dalbeth, N. Advanced imaging assessment of gout: Comparison of dual-energy CT and MRI with anatomical pathology. *Ann. Rheum. Dis.* **2018**, *77*, 629–630. [CrossRef]
7. Klauser, A.S.; Halpern, E.J.; Strobl, S.; Gruber, J.; Feuchtner, G.; Bellmann-Weiler, R.; Weiss, G.; Stofferin, H.; Jaschke, W. Dual-Energy Computed Tomography Detection of Cardiovascular Monosodium Urate Deposits in Patients With Gout. *JAMA Cardiol.* **2019**, *4*, 1019–1028. [CrossRef]
8. Barazani, S.H.; Chi, W.W.; Pyzik, R.; Chang, H.; Jacobi, A.; O'Donnell, T.; Fayad, Z.A.; Ali, Y.; Mani, V. Quantification of uric acid in vasculature of patients with gout using dual-energy computed tomography. *World J. Radiol.* **2020**, *12*, 184–194. [CrossRef]
9. Khanna, P.; Johnson, R.J.; Marder, B.; LaMoreaux, B.; Kumar, A. Systemic Urate Deposition: An Unrecognized Complication of Gout? *J. Clin. Med.* **2020**, *9*, 3204. [CrossRef]

10. Pascart, T.; Carpentier, P.; Choi, H.K.; Norberciak, L.; Ducoulombier, V.; Luraschi, H.; Houvenagel, E.; Legrand, J.; Verclytte, S.; Becce, F.; et al. Identification and characterization of peripheral vascular color-coded DECT lesions in gout and non-gout patients: The VASCURATE study. *Semin. Arthritis Rheum.* **2021**, *51*, 895–902. [CrossRef]
11. Wang, P.; Smith, S.E.; Garg, R.; Lu, F.; Wohlfahrt, A.; Campos, A.; Vanni, K.; Yu, Z.; Solomon, D.H.; Kim, S.C. Identification of monosodium urate crystal deposits in patients with asymptomatic hyperuricemia using dual-energy CT. *RMD Open* **2018**, *4*, e000593. [CrossRef]
12. Dalbeth, N.; Becce, F.; Botson, J.K.; Zhao, L.; Kumar, A. Dual-energy CT assessment of rapid monosodium urate depletion and bone erosion remodelling during pegloticase plus methotrexate co-therapy. *Rheumatology* **2022**, *Online ahead of print*. [CrossRef]
13. Pascart, T.; Budzik, J.F. Dual-energy computed tomography in crystalline arthritis: Knowns and unknowns. *Curr. Opin. Rheumatol.* **2022**, *34*, 103–110. [CrossRef]
14. Tse, J.J.; Kondro, D.A.; Kuczynski, M.T.; Pauchard, Y.; Veljkovic, A.; Holdsworth, D.W.; Frasson, V.; Manske, S.L.; MacMullan, P.; Salat, P. Assessing the Sensitivity of Dual-Energy Computed Tomography 3-Material Decomposition for the Detection of Gout. *Investig. Radiol.* **2022**. *Online ahead of print*. [CrossRef]
15. Ahn, S.J.; Zhang, D.; Levine, B.D.; Dalbeth, N.; Pool, B.; Ranganath, V.K.; Benhaim, P.; Nelson, S.D.; Hsieh, S.S.; FitzGerald, J.D. Limitations of dual-energy CT in the detection of monosodium urate deposition in dense liquid tophi and calcified tophi. *Skelet. Radiol.* **2021**, *50*, 1667–1675. [CrossRef]
16. Dubief, B.; Avril, J.; Pascart, T.; Schmitt, M.; Loffroy, R.; Maillefert, J.F.; Ornetti, P.; Ramon, A. Optimization of dual energy computed tomography post-processing to reduce lower limb artifacts in gout. *Quant. Imaging Med. Surg.* **2022**, *12*, 539–549. [CrossRef]
17. Park, E.H.; Yoo, W.H.; Song, Y.S.; Byon, J.H.; Pak, J.; Choi, Y. Not All Green Is Tophi: The Importance of Optimizing Minimum Attenuation and Using a Tin Filter to Minimize Clumpy Artifacts on Foot and Ankle Dual-Energy CT. *Am. J. Roentgenol.* **2020**, *214*, 1335–1342. [CrossRef]
18. Mallinson, P.I.; Coupal, T.; Reisinger, C.; Chou, H.; Munk, P.L.; Nicolaou, S.; Ouellette, H. Artifacts in dual-energy CT gout protocol: A review of 50 suspected cases with an artifact identification guide. *Am. J. Roentgenol.* **2014**, *203*, W103–W109. [CrossRef]
19. Chou, H.; Chin, T.Y.; Peh, W.C. Dual-energy CT in gout–A review of current concepts and applications. *J. Med. Radiat. Sci.* **2017**, *64*, 41–51. [CrossRef]
20. Károlyi, M.; Szilveszter, B.; Kolossváry, M.; Takx, R.A.; Celeng, C.; Bartykowszki, A.; Jermendy, Á.L.; Panajotu, A.; Karády, J.; Raaijmakers, R.; et al. Iterative model reconstruction reduces calcified plaque volume in coronary CT angiography. *Eur. J. Radiol.* **2017**, *87*, 83–89. [CrossRef]
21. Gondrie, M.J.; van der Graaf, Y.; Jacobs, P.C.; Oen, A.L.; Mali, W.P. The association of incidentally detected heart valve calcification with future cardiovascular events. *Eur. Radiol.* **2011**, *21*, 963–973. [CrossRef]
22. Forbess, L.J.; Fields, T.R. The broad spectrum of urate crystal deposition: Unusual presentations of gouty tophi. *Semin. Arthritis Rheum.* **2012**, *42*, 146–154. [CrossRef]
23. Weaver, J.S.; Vina, E.R.; Munk, P.L.; Klauser, A.S.; Elifritz, J.M.; Taljanovic, M.S. Gouty Arthropathy: Review of Clinical Manifestations and Treatment, with Emphasis on Imaging. *J. Clin. Med.* **2021**, *11*, 166. [CrossRef]
24. Gamala, M.; Linn-Rasker, S.P.; Nix, M.; Heggelman, B.G.F.; van Laar, J.M.; Pasker-de Jong, P.C.M.; Jacobs, J.W.G.; Klaasen, R. Gouty arthritis: Decision-making following dual-energy CT scan in clinical practice, a retrospective analysis. *Clin. Rheumatol.* **2018**, *37*, 1879–1884. [CrossRef]
25. Choi, H.K.; Burns, L.C.; Shojania, K.; Koenig, N.; Reid, G.; Abufayyah, M.; Law, G.; Kydd, A.S.; Ouellette, H.; Nicolaou, S. Dual energy CT in gout: A prospective validation study. *Ann. Rheum. Dis.* **2012**, *71*, 1466–1471. [CrossRef]
26. Strobl, S.; Halpern, E.J.; Ellah, M.A.; Kremser, C.; Gruber, J.; Bellmann-Weiler, R.; Deml, C.; Schmalzl, A.; Rauch, S.; Klauser, A.S. Acute Gouty Knee Arthritis: Ultrasound Findings Compared With Dual-Energy CT Findings. *Am. J. Roentgenol.* **2018**, *210*, 1323–1329. [CrossRef]
27. Klauser, A.S.; Halpern, E.J.; Strobl, S.; Abd Ellah, M.M.H.; Gruber, J.; Bellmann-Weiler, R.; Auer, T.; Feuchtner, G.; Jaschke, W. Gout of hand and wrist: The value of US as compared with DECT. *Eur. Radiol.* **2018**, *28*, 4174–4181. [CrossRef]
28. Stewart, S.; Dalbeth, N.; Vandal, A.C.; Rome, K. The first metatarsophalangeal joint in gout: A systematic review and meta-analysis. *BMC Musculoskelet. Disord.* **2016**, *17*, 69. [CrossRef]
29. Pascart, T.; Grandjean, A.; Capon, B.; Legrand, J.; Namane, N.; Ducoulombier, V.; Motte, M.; Vandecandelaere, M.; Luraschi, H.; Godart, C.; et al. Monosodium urate burden assessed with dual-energy computed tomography predicts the risk of flares in gout: A 12-month observational study: MSU burden and risk of gout flare. *Arthritis Res. Ther.* **2018**, *20*, 210. [CrossRef]
30. Wall, B.; Agudelo, C.A.; Tesser, J.R.; Mountz, J.; Holt, D.; Turner, R.A. An autopsy study of the prevalence of monosodium urate and calcium pyrophosphate dihydrate crystal deposition in first metatarsophalangeal joints. *Arthritis Rheum.* **1983**, *26*, 1522–1524. [CrossRef]
31. Loeb, J.N. The influence of temperature on the solubility of monosodium urate. *Arthritis Rheum.* **1972**, *15*, 189–192. [CrossRef]
32. Radice, F.; Monckeberg, J.E.; Carcuro, G. Longitudinal tears of peroneus longus and brevis tendons: A gouty infiltration. *J. Foot Ankle Surg.* **2011**, *50*, 751–753. [CrossRef]
33. Mahoney, P.G.; James, P.D.; Howell, C.J.; Swannell, A.J. Spontaneous rupture of the Achilles tendon in a patient with gout. *Ann. Rheum. Dis.* **1981**, *40*, 416–418. [CrossRef]

34. Dalbeth, N.; Kalluru, R.; Aati, O.; Horne, A.; Doyle, A.J.; McQueen, F.M. Tendon involvement in the feet of patients with gout: A dual-energy CT study. *Ann. Rheum. Dis.* **2013**, *72*, 1545–1548. [CrossRef]
35. Yuan, Y.; Liu, C.; Xiang, X.; Yuan, T.L.; Qiu, L.; Liu, Y.; Luo, Y.B.; Zhao, Y. Ultrasound scans and dual energy CT identify tendons as preferred anatomical location of MSU crystal depositions in gouty joints. *Rheumatol. Int.* **2018**, *38*, 801–811. [CrossRef]
36. Strobl, S.; Kremser, C.; Taljanovic, M.; Gruber, J.; Stofferin, H.; Bellmann-Weiler, R.; Klauser, A.S. Impact of Dual-Energy CT Postprocessing Protocol for the Detection of Gouty Arthritis and Quantification of Tophi in Patients Presenting With Podagra: Comparison With Ultrasound. *Am. J. Roentgenol.* **2019**, *213*, 1315–1323. [CrossRef]
37. Anagnostakos, K.; Thiery, A.; Meyer, C.; Tapos, O. An Untypical Case of Gouty Infiltration of Both Peroneal Tendons and a Longitudinal Lesion of the Peroneus Brevis Tendon Mimicking Synovial Sarcoma. *Case Rep. Orthop.* **2018**, *2018*, 8790916. [CrossRef]
38. Sakhaee, K. Epidemiology and clinical pathophysiology of uric acid kidney stones. *J. Nephrol.* **2014**, *27*, 241–245. [CrossRef]
39. Nestler, T.; Nestler, K.; Neisius, A.; Isbarn, H.; Netsch, C.; Waldeck, S.; Schmelz, H.U.; Ruf, C. Diagnostic accuracy of third-generation dual-source dual-energy CT: A prospective trial and protocol for clinical implementation. *World J. Urol.* **2019**, *37*, 735–741. [CrossRef]
40. Li, Z.X.; Jiao, G.L.; Zhou, S.M.; Cheng, Z.Y.; Bashir, S.; Zhou, Y. Evaluation of the chemical composition of nephrolithiasis using dual-energy CT in Southern Chinese gout patients. *BMC Nephrol.* **2019**, *20*, 273. [CrossRef]
41. Sharon, Y.; Schlesinger, N. Beyond Joints: A Review of Ocular Abnormalities in Gout and Hyperuricemia. *Curr. Rheumatol. Rep.* **2016**, *18*, 37. [CrossRef]
42. Lin, J.; Zhao, G.Q.; Che, C.Y.; Yang, S.S.; Wang, Q.; Li, C.G. Characteristics of ocular abnormalities in gout patients. *Int. J. Ophthalmol.* **2013**, *6*, 307–311.
43. Yourish, N. Conjunctival tophi associated with gout. *AMA Arch. Ophthalmol.* **1953**, *50*, 370–371. [CrossRef] [PubMed]
44. Ferry, A.P.; Safir, A.; Melikian, H.E. Ocular abnormalities in patients with gout. *Ann. Ophthalmol.* **1985**, *17*, 632–635. [PubMed]
45. Carr, A.; Doyle, A.J.; Dalbeth, N.; Aati, O.; McQueen, F.M. Dual-Energy CT of Urate Deposits in Costal Cartilage and Intervertebral Disks of Patients With Tophaceous Gout and Age-Matched Controls. *AJR Am. J. Roentgenol.* **2016**, *206*, 1063–1067. [CrossRef] [PubMed]
46. Chabra, I.; Singh, R. Gouty tophi on the ear: A review. *Cutis* **2013**, *92*, 190–192.
47. Kumral, E.; Karaman, B.; Orman, M.; Kabaroglu, C. Association of uric acid and carotid artery disease in patients with ischemic stroke. *Acta. Neurol. Scand.* **2014**, *130*, 11–17. [CrossRef]
48. Karagiannis, A.; Mikhailidis, D.P.; Tziomalos, K.; Sileli, M.; Savvatianos, S.; Kakafika, A.; Gossios, T.; Krikis, N.; Moschou, I.; Xochellis, M.; et al. Serum uric acid as an independent predictor of early death after acute stroke. *Circ. J.* **2007**, *71*, 1120–1127. [CrossRef]
49. McFarland, N.R.; Burdett, T.; Desjardins, C.A.; Frosch, M.P.; Schwarzschild, M.A. Postmortem brain levels of urate and precursors in Parkinson's disease and related disorders. *Neurodegener. Dis.* **2013**, *12*, 189–198. [CrossRef]
50. Disveld, I.J.M.; Fransen, J.; Rongen, G.A.; Kienhorst, L.B.E.; Zoakman, S.; Janssens, H.; Janssen, M. Crystal-proven Gout and Characteristic Gout Severity Factors Are Associated with Cardiovascular Disease. *J. Rheumatol.* **2018**, *45*, 858–863. [CrossRef]
51. Andrés, M.; Quintanilla, M.A.; Sivera, F.; Sánchez-Payá, J.; Pascual, E.; Vela, P.; Ruiz-Nodar, J.M. Silent Monosodium Urate Crystal Deposits Are Associated With Severe Coronary Calcification in Asymptomatic Hyperuricemia: An Exploratory Study. *Arthritis Rheumatol.* **2016**, *68*, 1531–1539. [CrossRef]
52. Pascart, T.; Capon, B.; Grandjean, A.; Legrand, J.; Namane, N.; Ducoulombier, V.; Motte, M.; Vandecandelaere, M.; Luraschi, H.; Godart, C.; et al. The lack of association between the burden of monosodium urate crystals assessed with dual-energy computed tomography or ultrasonography with cardiovascular risk in the commonly high-risk gout patient. *Arthritis Res. Ther.* **2018**, *20*, 97. [CrossRef]
53. Iacobellis, G. A rare and asymptomatic case of mitral valve tophus associated with severe gouty tophaceous arthritis. *J. Endocrinol. Investig.* **2004**, *27*, 965–966. [CrossRef] [PubMed]
54. Feuchtner, G.M.; Plank, F.; Beyer, C.; Schwabl, C.; Held, J.; Bellmann-Weiler, R.; Weiss, G.; Gruber, J.; Widmann, G.; Klauser, A.S. Monosodium Urate Crystal Deposition in Coronary Artery Plaque by 128-Slice Dual-Energy Computed Tomography: An Ex Vivo Phantom and In Vivo Study. *J. Comput. Assist. Tomogr.* **2021**, *45*, 856–862. [CrossRef] [PubMed]
55. Neogi, T. Clinical practice. Gout. *N. Engl. J. Med.* **2011**, *364*, 443–452. [CrossRef] [PubMed]
56. Zhang, Z.; Zhang, X.; Sun, Y.; Chen, H.; Kong, X.; Zhou, J.; Ma, L.; Jiang, L. New urate depositions on dual-energy computed tomography in gouty arthritis during urate-lowering therapy. *Rheumatol. Int.* **2017**, *37*, 1365–1372. [CrossRef]
57. Mushtaq, M.; Akram, M.U.; Alghamdi, N.S.; Fatima, J.; Masood, R.F. Localization and Edge-Based Segmentation of Lumbar Spine Vertebrae to Identify the Deformities Using Deep Learning Models. *Sensors* **2022**, *22*, 1547. [CrossRef]
58. Sirshar, M.; Hassan, T.; Akram, M.U.; Khan, S.A. An incremental learning approach to automatically recognize pulmonary diseases from the multi-vendor chest radiographs. *Comput. Biol. Med.* **2021**, *134*, 104435. [CrossRef]
59. Akbar, S.; Sharif, M.; Akram, M.U.; Saba, T.; Mahmood, T.; Kolivand, M. Automated techniques for blood vessels segmentation through fundus retinal images: A review. *Microsc. Res. Tech.* **2019**, *82*, 153–170. [CrossRef]

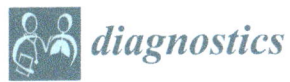

Review

Imaging of the Temporomandibular Joint

Seyed Mohammad Gharavi *, Yujie Qiao, Armaghan Faghihimehr and Josephina Vossen *

Department of Radiology, West Hospital, VCU School of Medicine, Virginia Commonwealth University, 1200 East Broad Street, North Wing, Box 980470, Richmond, VA 23298-0470, USA; yujie.qiao@vcuhealth.org (Y.Q.); armaghan.faghihimehr@vcuhealth.org (A.F.)
* Correspondence: seyedmohammad.gharavi@vcuhealth.org (S.M.G.); josephina.vossen@vcuhealth.org (J.V.)

Abstract: Temporomandibular disorder (TMD) is a common musculoskeletal condition that causes pain and disability for patients and imposes a high financial burden on the healthcare system. The most common cause of TMD is internal derangement, mainly secondary to articular disc displacement. Multiple other pathologies such as inflammatory arthritis, infection, and neoplasm can mimic internal derangement. MRI is the modality of choice for evaluation of the TMJ. Radiologists need to be familiar with the normal anatomy and function of the TMJ and MR imaging of the internal derangement and other less common pathologies of the TMJ.

Keywords: TMJ; temporomandibular joint; imaging; temporomandibular disorder; radiologist; internal derangement; arthritis; neoplasm

1. Introduction

The temporomandibular joint (TMJ) plays a crucial role in mastication, jaw mobility, verbal, and emotional expression. The prevalence of chronic TMJ pain ranges from 5 to 31%, and the incidence of first-time pain is 4% per year [1,2]. Temporomandibular disorder (TMD) is a term used to describe several pathologies that involve the TMJ and surrounding bone and soft tissues. TMD is the second most common musculoskeletal condition after back pain to cause pain and disability with an annual cost of $4 billion in the United States [3]. The incidence of TMD peaks in the second to the fourth decade of life with a higher prevalence among women [4,5]. While internal derangement is the most common TMJ pathology, radiologists should not overlook other less common pathologies such as inflammatory arthritis, infection, trauma, and neoplasm.

We aim to review normal TMJ anatomy and function, most common TMDs, and their imaging presentations.

2. Normal Anatomy

Interpreting TMJ imaging requires an understanding of the normal anatomy of the joint. TMJ is a synovial joint between the glenoid fossa of the temporal bone and the mandibular condyle. The central anatomic structure of the TMJ is the articular disc or meniscus. The disc is an oval-shaped fibrocartilaginous structure composed of anterior and posterior articular bands and a thinner center, called the intermediate zone. The intermediate zone gives the disc a biconcave appearance on the sagittal view. The posterior band is usually thicker than the anterior band, and both bands are wider in the transverse dimension than in the anteroposterior dimension. The retrodiscal tissue or bilaminar zone is a rich neurovascular tissue that serves as a posterior disc attachment, blending the disc with the joint capsule and temporal bone. The lateral aspect of the disc connects with the joint capsule and inserts into the condylar neck. Anteriorly, the attachments of the disc are variable and called the "disc-capsular complex". The lateral pterygoid muscle fibers and tendons attach the anterior band of the disc to this complex. The position of the disc is evaluated by the location of the posterior band and intermediate zone in relation to the

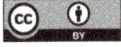

mandibular condyle. In the closed-mouth position, the posterior band should lie near the 12 o'clock position on the sagittal projection. The intermediate zone should be located between the condyle and the temporal bone. The medial and lateral corners of the disc align with the condylar borders and do not bulge medially or laterally [6].

TMJ has two compartments that function as two small joints within a same capsule. This allows for a greater range of motion with respect to the joint's size. The superior compartment separates the glenoid fossa of the temporal bone from the disc, while the inferior compartment separates the disc from the mandibular condyle. In the initial phase of mouth opening, the condyle rotates in the lower joint compartment. Subsequently, it translates anteriorly in the upper compartment [6]. The lateral pterygoid muscle contributes to jaw opening, and the medial pterygoid, masseter, and temporalis muscles facilitate jaw closure. As the condyle translates anteriorly, the disc should move between the condyle and the articular eminence. A normal disc does not move in the coronal plane during mouth opening (Figures 1 and 2).

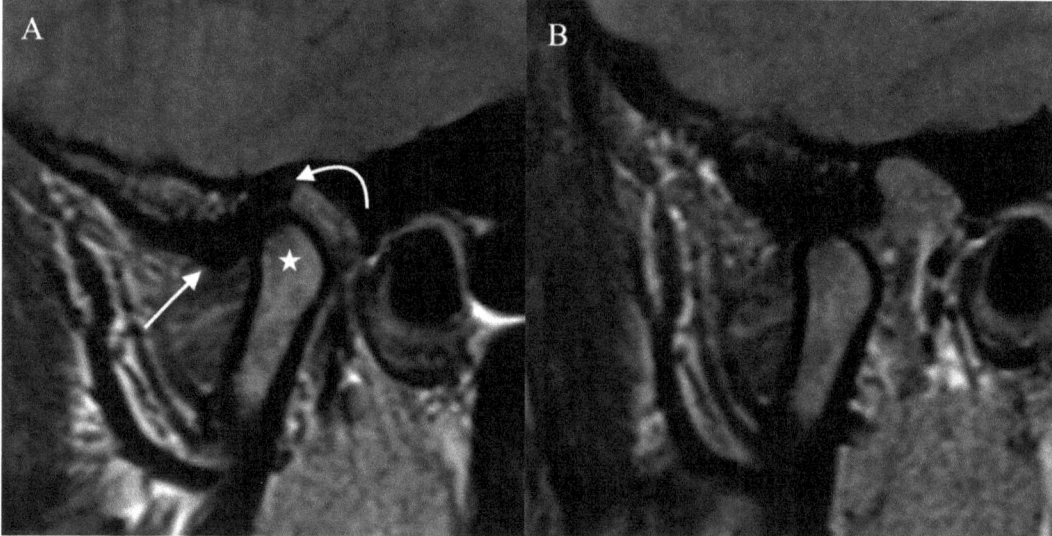

Figure 1. Normal Temporomandibular joint MRI. Proton density sagittal image of the TMJ in closed mouth (**A**) position shows normal location and bow-tie appearance of the articular disc with anterior (straight arrow) and posterior bands (curved arrow). The mandibular condyle (star) is in an anatomic location within the mandibular fossa. On open mouth images (**B**), normal condylar rotation and anterior translation are noted.

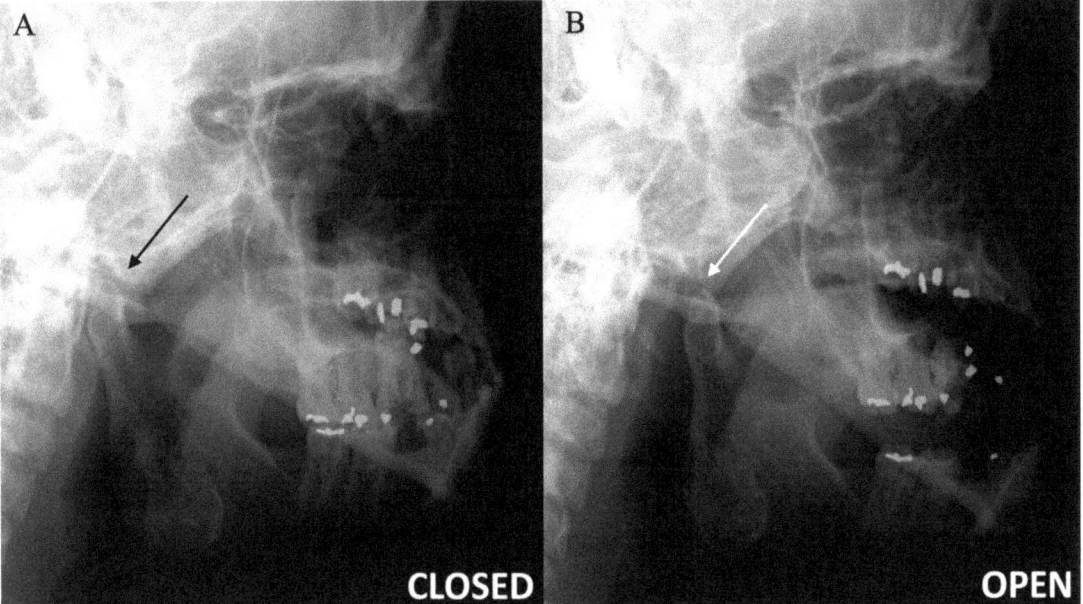

Figure 2. Temporomandibular joint radiographs. Axiolateral TMJ views in the closed mouth (**A**) and open mouth (**B**) positions demonstrate the normal location of the mandibular condyle within the mandibular fossa (black arrow) and normal condylar rotation and anterior translation (white arrow), respectively.

3. Imaging

TMJ radiographic examinations include transcranial (oblique lateral view), trans maxillary (modified AP view), trans pharyngeal (oblique lateral view), and submental vertex radiographs. Cross-sectional imaging is usually indicated in cases where malocclusion or intra-articular abnormalities are suspected.

With its ability to evaluate the bones, CT is the mainstay imaging modality in the setting of trauma. CT is also particularly valuable in assessing surgical reconstruction, detecting calcified loose bodies, and in some cases of inflammatory, infectious, and neoplastic disease. Cone-beam computed tomography (CBCT) has shown comparable osseous detail to CT, with the advantage of decreased radiation dose.

MRI is the best modality for the evaluation of intra-articular processes. Given the high MRI contrast resolution of the soft tissues, it is currently the gold standard for diagnosing disc disorders. The standard MR imaging protocol consists of oblique sagittal and coronal proton density-weighted (PDWI) sequences in closed- and open-mouth positions. Images are acquired perpendicular or parallel to the long axis of the mandibular condyle to optimize the visualization of the disc and the osseous structures. In addition, T2WI is useful for detecting degenerative periarticular changes and the presence of a joint effusion. Gadolinium contrast is not used routinely but would be indicated in cases where infection, inflammatory arthropathy, or neoplasm is suspected.

Cine gradient echo (GRE) images depict disc movement and can be used to evaluate condylar translation. Newer dynamic techniques, such as a half-Fourier acquired single-shot turbo spin-echo (HASTE) or balanced steady-state free precession sequence (SSFP), can contribute to the evaluation of the disc movement. Due to higher signal-to-noise ratios, 3 T MRI magnets have the advantage of depicting improved anatomic and pathologic details of the TMJ compared with 1.5 T.

Ultrasound can be considered a non-invasive, readily available, and less expensive technique for the evaluation of the TMJ. The sonographer should perform a high-resolution ultrasound (12–20 MHz high-frequency linear transducer) by placing the probe perpendicular to the zygomatic arch and parallel to the mandibular condyle. The operator should acquire transverse and longitudinal images in closed-mouth and open-mouth positions. Adjusting and tilting the probe during the exam will help to optimize the visualization of the disc, condylar changes, and joint effusion [7,8]. Ultrasound evaluation is limited when evaluating deeper structures and/or any osseous abnormalities. On ultrasound, the normal articular disc appears as a hypoechoic, inverted c-shape structure, situated superior to the hyperechoic condylar cortex (Figure 3).

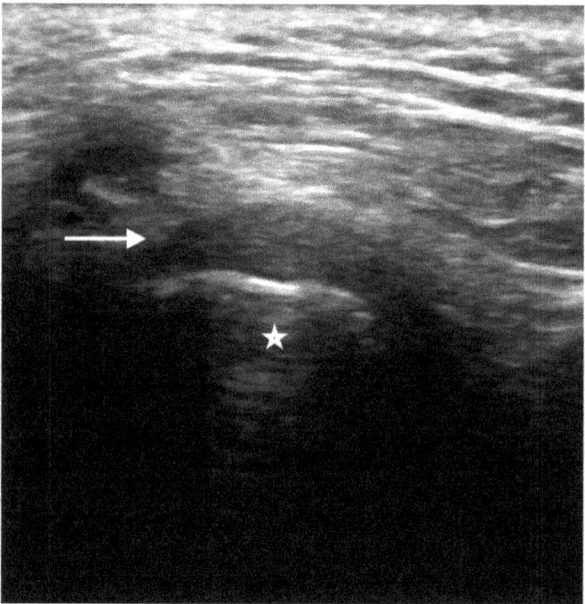

Figure 3. Normal ultrasound of the articular disc. Sonographic images of the TMJ with the probe longitudinal to the articular disc on closed mouth views demonstrate the normal hypoechoic appearance of the mandibular condyle (star), with a rim of the hyperechoic cortex. The articular disc (straight arrow) demonstrates the normal inverted c-shaped morphology and hypoechogenicity, situated just superior to the condylar cortex.

4. Pathology

4.1. Internal Derangement

The most common TMD is internal derangement (ID), which implies a mechanical interference of the smooth joint movement. ID peaks in the second to the fourth decade of life with a female-to-male ratio of 3:1 and most commonly presents with jaw pain, clicking, or locking [9,10]. The most common cause of ID is the displacement of the articular disc.

MRI is the standard imaging modality for assessing ID in TMJ [11]. Several key features should be evaluated while interpreting the MRI of TMJ derangement, including the position and morphology of the disc, the morphology and signal of the mandibular condyle, the presence of joint effusion, and condylar translation with dynamic imaging.

In a closed mouth position on an oblique sagittal plane, the posterior band of the disc should lie superior to the condylar head at the 12 o'clock position. The disc is anteriorly displaced if the posterior band lies more than 30 degrees anterior to the vertical line through the condylar head, at around 10 to 11 o'clock [12]. The condyle and disc both translate anteriorly as the mouth opens, and the disc stays between the articular eminence and mandibular condyle.

In the earliest stage of internal derangement, the disc has a normal biconcave morphology but is anteriorly displaced in the closed mouth position (Figure 4). However, the disc returns to the normal anatomical position or recaptures as the condyle translates anteriorly during mouth opening. In the intermediate stage, the disc still has a normal morphology, is displaced in a closed-mouth position, and does not recapture with mouth opening. In the later stages, the disc is chronically displaced and has an abnormal morphology, e.g., it is perforated or the posterior attachment to the bilaminar zone is disrupted. Imaging features of degenerative joint disease such as flattening of the condyle, osteophytes, joint effusion, or the abnormal T1 and T2 signal of the condyle can also be seen in more advanced stages [9,13–15]. A commonly used classification of TMJ disc displacement using clinical and imaging findings was described by Wilkes [16].

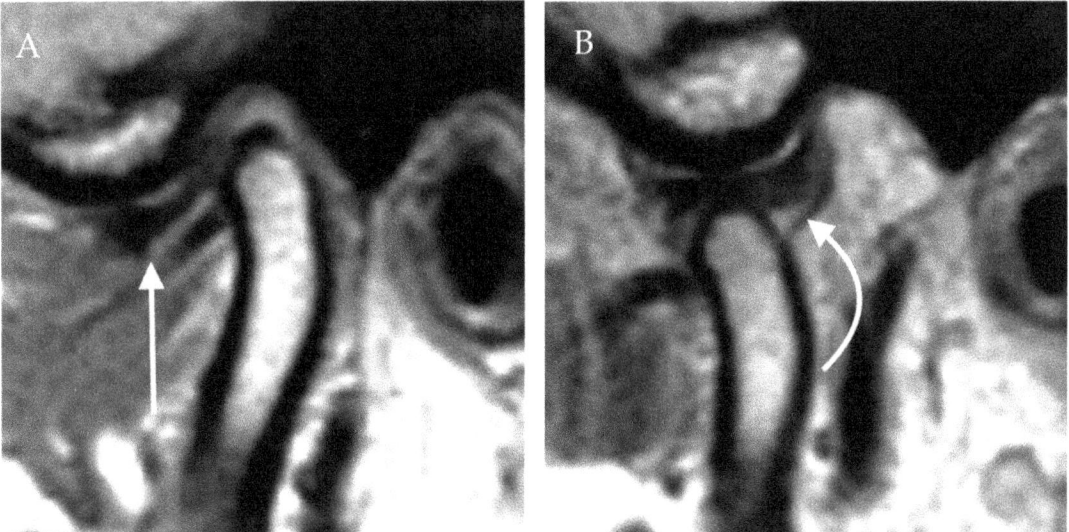

Figure 4. Anterior disc displacement with recapture. Proton density sagittal image of the TMJ in closed mouth (**A**) position shows anterior displacement of the articular disc with otherwise normal bow-tie appearance (straight arrow). The mandibular condyle is situated in an anatomic location within the mandibular fossa. On open mouth images (**B**), normal condylar rotation and anterior translation are noted. Note the recapture of the articular disc, which is now in the normal position (curved arrow). The bow-tie appearance of the articular disc is preserved.

Ultrasound can be used as an alternative modality for evaluating ID, particularly for disc displacement and joint effusion. However, this modality is considered less useful in detecting bone abnormalities in condyle [8,17].

4.2. Osteoarthritis

Osteoarthritis (OA) is related to the breakdown of joint cartilage and underlying subchondral bone. Primary OA is more common in older patients. On the other hand, secondary OA can be seen in younger patients with ID, prior trauma, or other TMJ arthropathies [18]. The commonly seen imaging findings on CT or MRI are flattening of the condyles, osteophytes, bone erosions, joint space narrowing, subchondral sclerosis, and marrow signal abnormality [19]. Signs and symptoms of OA in TMJ are pain, movement limitations, and crepitus.

4.3. Avascular Necrosis

Avascular necrosis is the result of impaired blood flow to the condyle. It can be seen in the context of different etiologies such as trauma, sickle cell anemia, or systemic lupus erythematosus. On CT, the condyle of the mandible is deformed with significant subchondral sclerosis. On MR, the marrow is dark on T1WI and shows a mixed signal on T2WI [20].

4.4. Idiopathic Condylar Resorption

Idiopathic condylar resorption or "cheerleader syndrome" is a poorly understood disease that is most commonly occurs in adolescents and young women. This aggressive form of degenerative disease of the TMJ has been attributed to an exaggerated response to minor traumatic injury induced by excess estrogen receptors [9,21,22]. Imaging demonstrates loss of condylar bone mass and flattening of the anterior or superior aspect of the condyle (Figure 5).

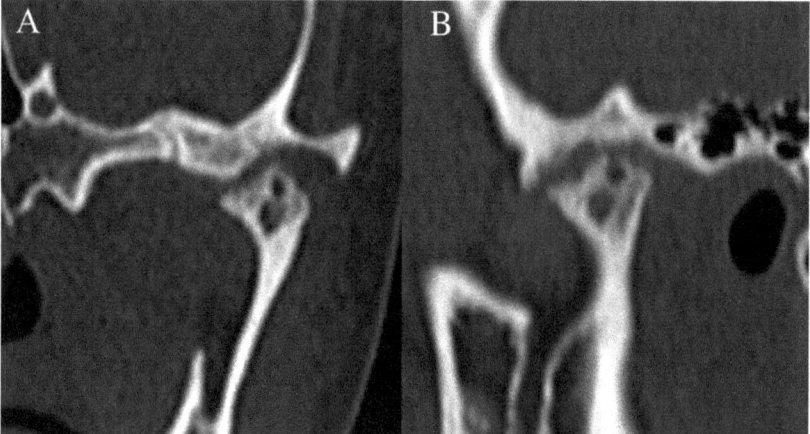

Figure 5. Idiopathic condylar resorption. Sagittal (**A**) and coronal (**B**) images through the TMJ in bone windows demonstrate extensive loss of the mandibular condyle and additional erosive changes of the underlying mandibular fossa and articular eminence.

4.5. Inflammatory Arthropathies

4.5.1. Rheumatoid Arthritis

Rheumatoid arthritis (RA) is the most common inflammatory arthritis in adults that can affect the TMJ [23]. TMJ symptoms are seen in approximately 50% of patients with RA. However, TMJ involvement is not a classic finding of RA [24]. For most patients, the diagnosis of RA is made before the development of TMJ symptoms. The most common symptoms are pain, joint swelling, and limited jaw motion [25]. More severe involvement can lead to trismus, facial deformity, and chronic loss of function [26].

Contrast-enhanced MRI and CT are commonly used for the evaluation of inflammatory arthritis such as RA in the TMJ. Synovial proliferation, joint space narrowing, articular erosion, flattening of the condyle, disc deformity, shorter condylar height, and abnormal condylar motion are common imaging findings that are seen with RA [23,27–29]. Unlike OA, in RA articular disc displacement occurs later in the course of disease and the disc can remain in a normal position despite substantial changes to the underlying condylar bone [30]. In patients with long-standing RA, disc displacement occurs more often due to the lack of bony support by the underlying osseous structures, not morphologic changes of the disc itself [30].

While no definite radiologic classification has been established to evaluate the severity of RA in the TMJ, Mohamed et al. showed that in patients with moderate to severe disease activity, the condyle has a smaller AP dimension. They also showed that disease activity had a statistically significant direct correlation with all osteoarthritic changes except for the glenoid and condylar erosions [29].

4.5.2. Juvenile Idiopathic Arthritis

Juvenile idiopathic arthritis (JIA) is the most common rheumatologic disease of childhood and adolescents. The rate of TMJ involvement in JIA differs based on the subtypes, ranging from 40% to 70% [13,31]. Longer disease duration, early age at onset, polyarticular or systemic course, and lack of HLA-B27 are risk factors for TMJ involvement [28]. The early diagnosis and management of TMJ involvement in JIA patients are essential because a delay in diagnosis can damage the mandibular growth plate and compromise normal facial growth. Clinical diagnosis is complicated because the patient may be asymptomatic until a relatively late stage of the disease [30].

Contrast-enhanced MRI is the preferred imaging modality and shows both the acute findings and secondary degenerative arthritis. Synovial enhancement, joint effusion, and synovial thickening are the most common findings early in the disease process. As inflammation and joint destruction continue, chronic secondary arthritic changes such as pannus formation, bone erosions, and disc destruction become more prevalent, eventually leading to condylar flattening and deformity (Figure 6) [32].

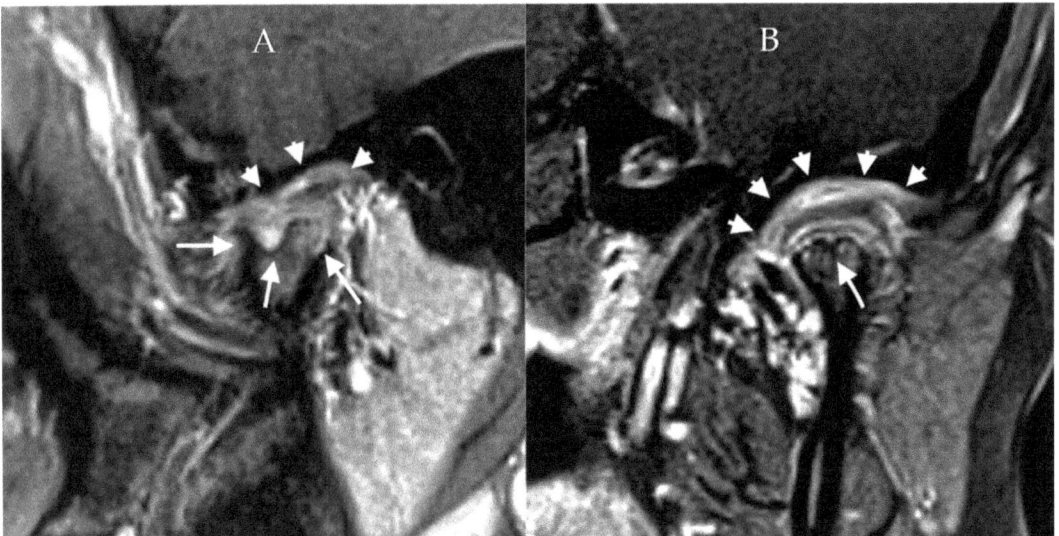

Figure 6. Juvenile idiopathic arthritis. Post-contrast T1W fat-saturated sagittal (A) and coronal (B) images of the TMJ demonstrate flattening and irregularity of the condyle with erosions (long tail arrows), resulting in an irregular foreshortened appearance from chronic inflammation. Joint effusion is noted with surrounding synovial enhancement (short tail arrows), consistent with an acute JIA flair.

Several scoring systems have been proposed for radiological grading of inflammation and damage of the temporomandibular joint in JIA patients based on the presence or degree of MRI findings such as bone marrow edema and enhancement, joint effusion, synovial thickening or enhancement, condylar flattening or erosion, and abnormal disc morphology [32,33].

4.5.3. Calcium Pyrophosphate Deposition Disease

Calcium pyrophosphate deposition disease (CPPD) is a noninfectious inflammatory arthropathy characterized by crystal deposits in the articular and periarticular soft tissues [34]. Two primary forms of CPPD have been described, common and tumoral, with the tumoral type affecting the TMJ [35]. CPPD of the TMJ is rare overall, and only a few case reports have been published in the literature [36–38].

The definitive diagnosis of CPPD is made by joint aspiration and fluid analysis showing the presence of calcium pyrophosphate crystals, but the radiologic evaluation is critical for evaluating the extent of underlying osseous destruction, secondary osteoarthritis, the presence of joint fluid, and to exclude other etiologies. CT is the best imaging modality for this disease and generally shows a calcified mass in the joint with secondary destructive and degenerative changes [35]. Therefore, MRI is rarely used as the initial imaging modality if CPPD is suspected. However, MRI is still often performed since common symptoms of TMJ CPPD disease such as pain, joint swelling, and limited range of motion are also symptoms in other TMD, for which MRI is indicated as standard practice. Notable MRI features are periarticular T2 hypointense signals with heterogeneous enhancement, which can mimic more concerning diseases such as chondrosarcoma [35]. Treatment ranges from medical management to surgical debridement of the joint with or without possible resection of the involved condyle [37,39].

4.5.4. Septic Arthritis

TMJ septic arthritis is rare but is associated with high morbidity and significant long-term disability [40]. The most common organism cultured is Staphylococcus aureus, which infects the joint either from direct inoculation or hematogenous spread [41].

Imaging findings of TMJ septic arthritis are similar to those of infections in other joints, namely synovial enhancement, joint effusion, surrounding soft tissue, and bone marrow edema. These findings are best visualized on MRI (Figure 7). Differentiation of septic arthritis from other inflammatory diseases is predominately based on the clinical presentation and the acuity of the symptoms. In septic arthritis, severe pain often occurs suddenly, with extreme tenderness on palpation, and is usually accompanied by other general symptoms such as malaise, fevers, or nausea/vomiting [41].

4.6. Trauma

Trauma to the jaw can cause a condylar fracture, glenoid fossa fracture, or TMJ dislocation. Condylar fracture accounts for 25–50% of mandibular fractures and is classified as the condylar head (intra- or extra-articular) or neck fracture [23].

In patients with a condylar fracture, the unopposed force of the lateral pterygoid muscle usually causes inferior and anteromedial dislocation of the condylar head and the lateral displacement and telescoping of the ramus (Figure 8). Multidetector CT is the modality of choice for evaluating facial and mandibular fractures in the acute setting. Most condylar fractures will show functionally favorable outcomes after closed reduction. However, traumatic dislocation of the disc or injury to the retrodiscal soft tissue can lead to joint ankylosis, a devastating complication. Studies have shown a correlation between the severity and pattern of condylar fractures on CT and risk of soft tissue injuries. However, MRI is the modality of choice to evaluate retrodiscal tissue injury and disc dislocation [42,43].

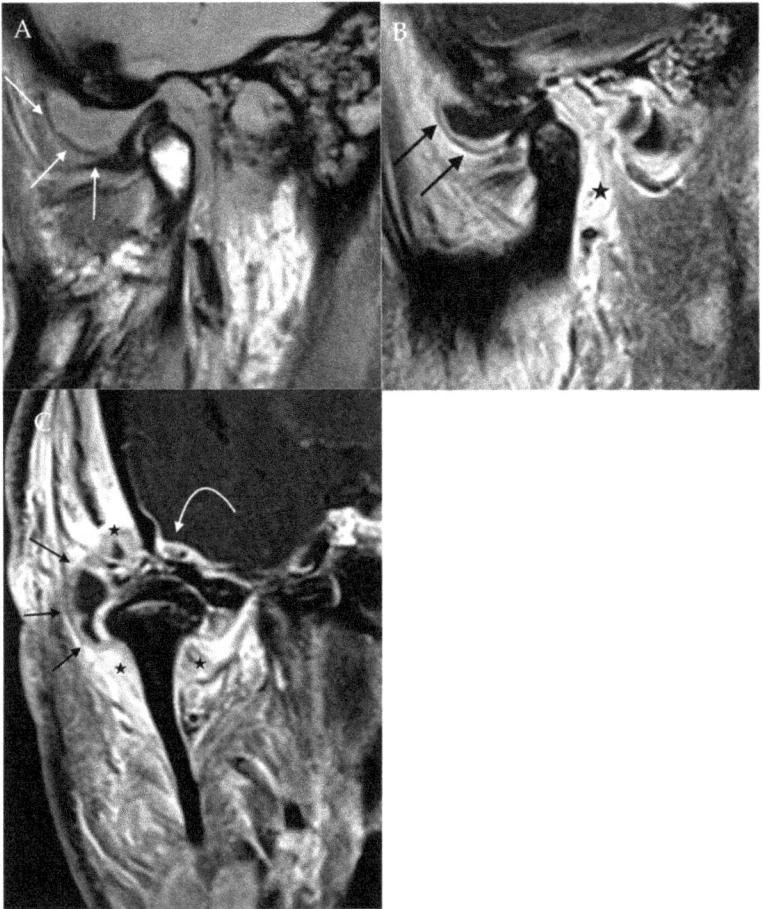

Figure 7. Septic arthritis. Proton density sagittal image of the TMJ (**A**) demonstrates a large joint effusion expanding the space between the articular disc and articular tubercle (straight white arrow). Post-contrast T1Wfat-saturated sagittal (**B**) and coronal (**C**) images demonstrate extensive surrounding synovial enhancement (black arrows) and soft tissue enhancement (star). Also noted is enhancement along the dura of the right temporal lobe (curved arrow), indicating the intracranial extension of infection.

4.7. Tumor and Tumor-like Lesions

4.7.1. Osteochondroma

Osteochondroma is a benign bone lesion that can arise from the mandibular condyle or glenoid fossa. It is considered to be the most common benign tumor of the TMJ [9]. On CT, it often appears as a pedunculated osseous mass, usually arising from the anterior surface of the condyle and at the insertion of the lateral pterygoid muscle (Figure 9). Continuity with the parent bone without cortical interruption is an essential characteristic feature. When small, it is challenging to differentiate osteochondroma from an osteophyte. Larger lesions can cause condylar displacement with associated pain or malocclusion [14,44]. Based on the growth pattern on CT, Chen et al. classified osteochondromas into two main types: type 1, which protrudes from the condyle and involves less than two-thirds of the surface of the condyle, and type 2, which is causing global expansion of the condyle [44].

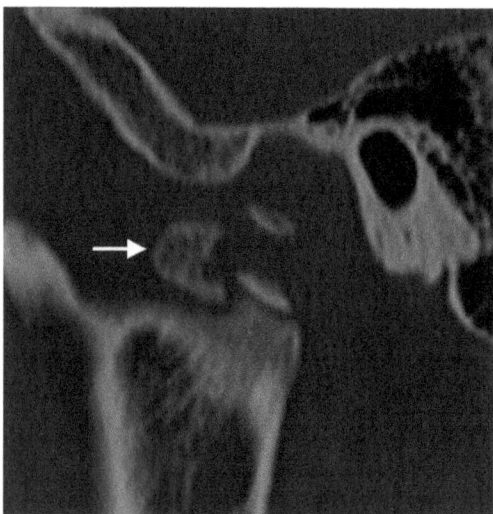

Figure 8. Trauma. Sagittal CT image of the TMJ demonstrates comminuted fracture of the condylar neck with a displacement of the fracture fragments. Mild sclerosis around the fracture lines suggests a component of interval healing. The tip of the mandibular condyle (arrow) is displaced antero-inferiorly.

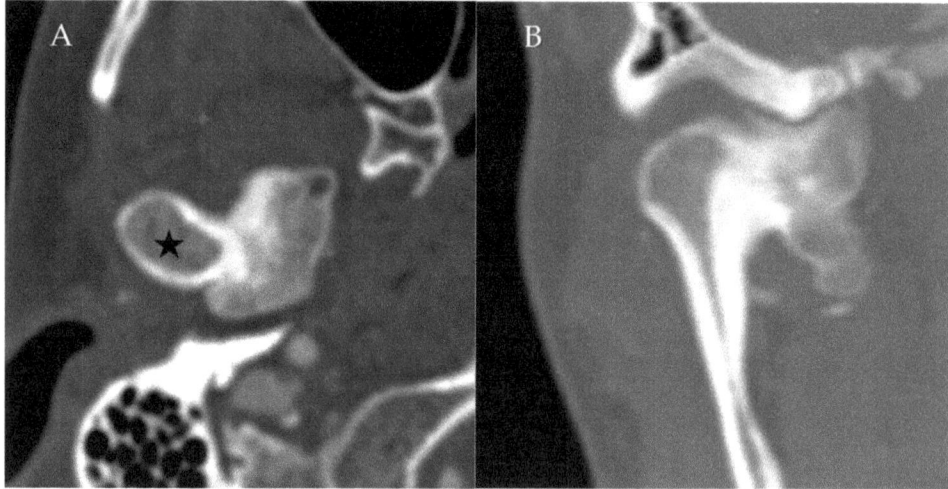

Figure 9. Condylar Osteochondroma. Axial (**A**) CT in bone windows and reformatted coronal (**B**) image demonstrates a prominent bony mass arising along the medial aspect of the mandibular condyle (star), with a well-corticated appearance and no aggressive features.

MRI shows a predominantly low T1 signal exophytic mass with a T2-hyperintense cartilage cap. The size of the cartilage cap is directly related to the risk of malignant transformation to or harboring chondrosarcoma [45].

4.7.2. Pigmented Villonodular Synovitis

Pigmented Villonodular Synovitis (PVNS) is a benign synovial proliferation process of uncertain origin, most commonly involving larger joints and uncommonly affecting the TMJ. Malignant PVNS is extremely rare but has been reported in the TMJ [46]. The CT depicts a soft tissue mass arising from the joint with areas of hyper attenuation which enhances after contrast injection. The adjacent bone might demonstrate erosions and sclerosis. MRI is the modality of choice for the diagnosis of PVNS, showing an intra-articular mass with areas of hemosiderin deposition depicted as low signal intensity on T1WI and T2WI and blooming artifact on GRE sequences [3].

4.7.3. Synovial Chondromatosis

Synovial chondromatosis (SC) is a rare, benign synovial proliferative disease characterized by the growth of cartilaginous nodules in the synovium that eventually calcify and detach from the joint. As a result, SC usually presents with joint effusion and multiple loose bodies (Figure 10). Unlike PVNS, which never calcifies, the loose bodies in SC are typically calcified. Therefore, a CT can help differentiate the two entities [3,9].

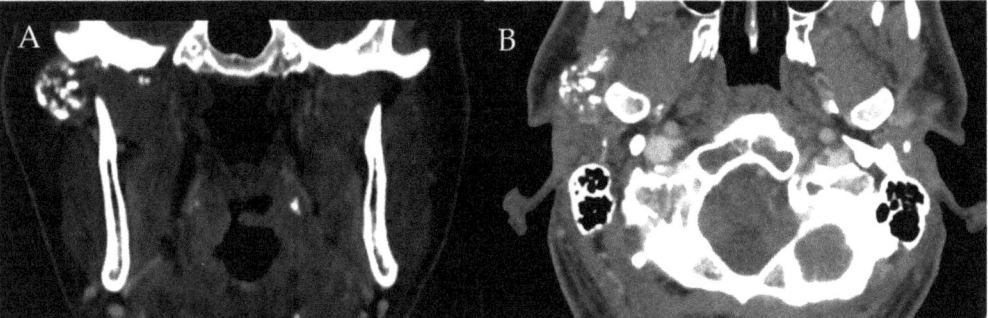

Figure 10. Synovial Chondromatosis. Coronal (**A**) and axial (**B**) CT shows multiple calcified loose bodies in the right TMJ consistent with synovial chondromatosis.

4.7.4. Chondrosarcoma

Chondrosarcoma is a malignant tumor that arises from embryogenic cartilaginous cells and is characterized by the production of a cartilaginous matrix. Chondrosarcoma can be primary—without pre-existent benign lesion—or secondary—arising from pre-existent benign lesions such as enchondroma or osteochondroma. Chondrosarcoma of the TMJ is extremely rare, with only 50 cases reported in the literature. The mean age of patients is 45.5 years with a female predominance (F:M = 1.4:1) [47]. The primary symptom of TMJ chondrosarcoma is preauricular swelling, followed by preauricular pain and trismus. Other findings, such as pain with mastication, obstruction of the external auditory canal, hearing loss, and limited jaw opening are commonly seen with all TMDs.

On CT, chondrosarcoma appears as a soft tissue mass with flocculent calcifications in the joint with or without bone erosion. A few cases with erosion of the glenoid fossa and intracranial invasion have been reported. On MRI, chondrosarcoma appears as an intermediate-to-low T1 and high T2 signal mass with foci of low T1 and T2 signal due to calcification. It shows heterogeneous enhancement on post-contrast images [47,48].

4.7.5. Osteosarcoma

Osteosarcoma is a malignant bone tumor arising from the osteogenic mesenchymal matrix and producing osteoid, fibrous, cartilaginous, and osseous tissue. It usually involves the long bones but rarely involves the jaw and is called gnathic osteosarcoma. Jaw osteosarcoma is not as aggressive as osteosarcoma in the long bones, with the mean age of patients being 35 years–10 years younger than long bone osteosarcoma. In addition, there is a male predilection, with the male-to-female ratio of 2:1 [14,49]. Radiographically, osteosarcoma can have a lytic, sclerotic, or mixed appearance with malignant periosteal reaction. On MRI, osteosarcoma resembles chondrosarcoma, presenting as a heterogeneously enhancing, intermediate T1 and high T2 signal mass (Figure 11). However, on CT or radiographs, osteosarcoma usually does not show typical ring-and-arc or whorl shape calcifications.

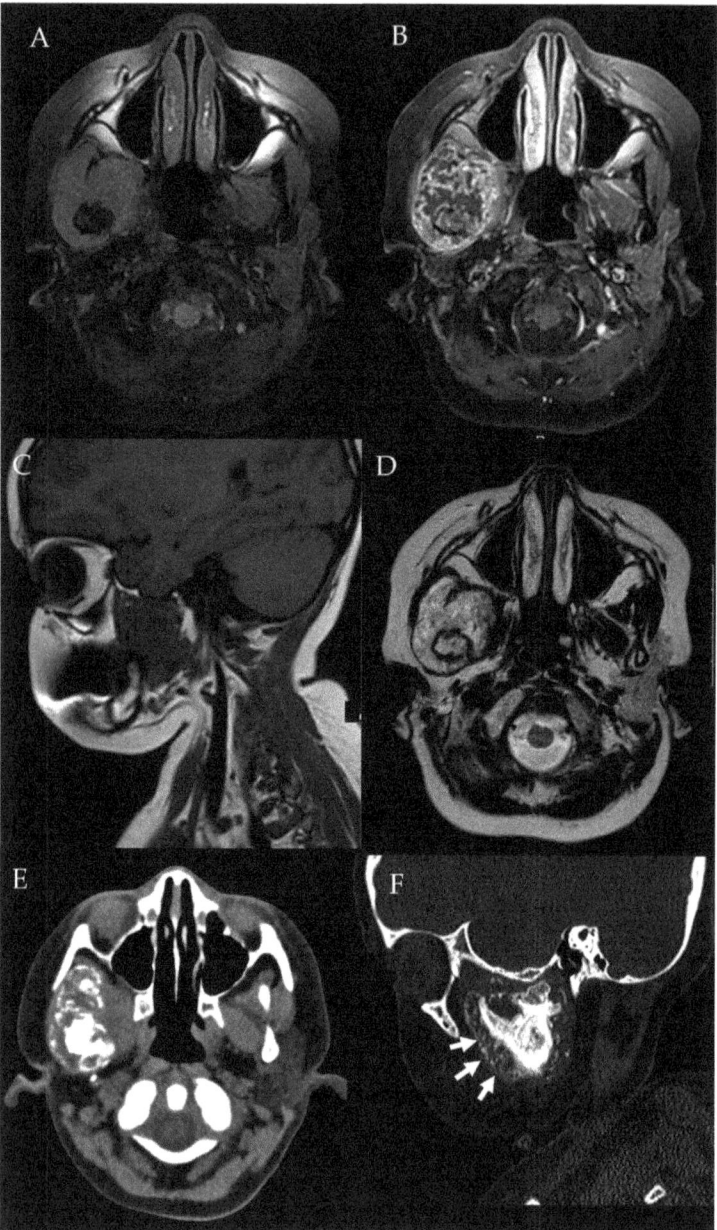

Figure 11. Condylar chondroblastic osteosarcoma. Axial pre-contrast (**A**) and post-contrast T1W (**B**), sagittal pre-contrast T1W (**C**), and axial T2W (**D**) images demonstrate a heterogeneously enhancing and T2-hyperintense right condylar mass in a nine-year-old patient. Axial (**E**) and sagittal (**F**) CT images show a soft tissue mass with mineralized matrix and aggressive periosteal reaction (small arrows) at the TMJ. Biopsy confirmed chondroblastic osteosarcoma.

4.7.6. Metastatic Disease

Most metastases involve the mandibular body and not the condyle; therefore, metastatic disease to TMJ is rare [12]. Metastatic lesions in the TMJ most commonly originate from the breast, lung, prostate, kidney, and thyroid [50,51]. Metastases with different origins, such as melanoma, pancreatic, hepatocellular, and rectal cancer, have been reported in the literature [52–54]. The signs and symptoms of TMJ metastatic disease are nonspecific and similar to other TMDs, including pain, restricted motion, clicking, trismus, and malocclusion [54–56].

On CT, TMJ metastases present as lytic and destructive bone lesions, but sclerotic or mixed lesions can also be seen with lesions from prostate, lung, and breast origin [57]. TMJ metastases can present with a soft tissue mass with adjacent bone erosion. On MRI, T2 hyperintense and enhancing lesions with adjacent marrow edema may be seen.

Other malignant processes such as lymphoma, multiple myeloma, and malignant synovial sarcoma of the TMJ have been reported [58].

5. Summary

Internal derangement is the most common TMJ pathology which can be best evaluated by MRI. The key imaging finding on MR is disc displacement with or without recapture. Other important but less frequent TMJ pathologies are osteoarthritis, idiopathic condylar resorption, inflammatory arthropathies, trauma-related conditions, and tumor and tumor-like lesions.

Author Contributions: Writing—original draft preparation, S.M.G., Y.Q., A.F. and J.V.; writing—review and editing, S.M.G., Y.Q., A.F. and J.V.; supervision, S.M.G., Y.Q. and J.V. All authors have read and agreed to the published version of the manuscript.

Funding: This research received no external funding.

Institutional Review Board Statement: Not applicable.

Informed Consent Statement: Not applicable.

Data Availability Statement: Not applicable.

Conflicts of Interest: The authors declare that they have no conflict of interest.

References

1. Valesan, L.F.; Da-Cas, C.D.; Réus, J.C.; Denardin, A.C.S.; Garanhani, R.R.; Bonotto, D.; Januzzi, E.; de Souza, B.D.M. Prevalence of Temporomandibular Joint Disorders: A Systematic Review and Meta-Analysis. *Clin. Oral Investig.* **2021**, *25*, 441–453. [CrossRef]
2. Slade, G.D.; Fillingim, R.B.; Sanders, A.E.; Bair, E.; Greenspan, J.D.; Ohrbach, R.; Dubner, R.; Diatchenko, L.; Smith, S.B.; Knott, C.; et al. Summary of Findings from the OPPERA Prospective Cohort Study of Incidence of First-Onset Temporomandibular Disorder: Implications and Future Directions. *J. Pain* **2013**, *14*, T116–T124. [CrossRef]
3. Morales, H.; Cornelius, R. Imaging Approach to Temporomandibular Joint Disorders. *Clin. Neuroradiol.* **2016**, *26*, 5–22. [CrossRef]
4. Bagis, B.; Ayaz, E.A.; Turgut, S.; Durkan, R.; Özcan, M. Gender Difference in Prevalence of Signs and Symptoms of Temporomandibular Joint Disorders: A Retrospective Study on 243 Consecutive Patients. *Int. J. Med. Sci.* **2012**, *9*, 539–544. [CrossRef]
5. Manfredini, D.; Chiappe, G.; Bosco, M. Research Diagnostic Criteria for Temporomandibular Disorders (RDC/TMD) Axis I Diagnoses in an Italian Patient Population. *J. Oral Rehabil.* **2006**, *33*, 551–558. [CrossRef]
6. Som, P.M.; Curtin, H.D. *Head and Neck Imaging—2 Volume Set*; Expert Consult—Online and Print; Mosby Elsevier: Maryland Heights, MO, USA, 2011; ISBN 9780323053556.
7. Talmaceanu, D.; Lenghel, L.M.; Bolog, N.; Buduru, S.; Leucuta, D.; Rotar, H. High-Resolution Ultrasound Imaging Compared to Magnetic Resonance Imaging for Temporomandibular Joint Disorders: An In Vivo Study. *Eur. J. Radiol.* **2020**, *132*, 109291. [CrossRef]
8. Klatkiewicz, T.; Gawriołek, K.; Pobudek Radzikowska, M.; Czajka-Jakubowska, A. Ultrasonography in the Diagnosis of Temporomandibular Disorders: A Meta-Analysis. *Med. Sci. Monit.* **2018**, *24*, 812–817. [CrossRef]
9. Aiken, A.; Bouloux, G.; Hudgins, P. MR Imaging of the Temporomandibular Joint. *Magn. Reson. Imaging Clin. N. Am.* **2012**, *20*, 397–412. [CrossRef]
10. Manevska, N.; Makazlieva, T.; Stojanoski, S.; Vela, I.; Komina, S. Solitary Metastatic Deposit in the Mandible from Follicular Thyroid Carcinoma. *World J. Nucl. Med.* **2020**, *19*, 291–295. [CrossRef]

11. Helms, C.A.; Kaplan, P. Diagnostic Imaging of the Temporomandibular Joint: Recommendations for Use of the Various Techniques. *AJR Am. J. Roentgenol.* **1990**, *154*, 319–322. [CrossRef]
12. Rammelsberg, P.; Pospiech, P.R.; Jäger, L.; Pho Duc, J.M.; Böhm, A.O.; Gernet, W. Variability of Disk Position in Asymptomatic Volunteers and Patients with Internal Derangements of the TMJ. *Oral Surg. Oral Med. Oral Pathol. Oral Radiol. Endod.* **1997**, *83*, 393–399. [CrossRef]
13. Larheim, T.A.; Hol, C.; Ottersen, M.K.; Mork-Knutsen, B.B.; Arvidsson, L.Z. The Role of Imaging in the Diagnosis of Temporomandibular Joint Pathology. *Oral Maxillofac. Surg. Clin. N. Am.* **2018**, *30*, 239–249. [CrossRef] [PubMed]
14. Tamimi, D.; Kocasarac, H.D.; Mardini, S. Imaging of the Temporomandibular Joint. *Semin. Roentgenol.* **2019**, *54*, 282–301. [CrossRef] [PubMed]
15. Tamimi, D.; Jalali, E.; Hatcher, D. Temporomandibular Joint Imaging. *Radiol. Clin. N. Am.* **2018**, *56*, 157–175. [CrossRef] [PubMed]
16. Wilkes, C.H. Internal Derangements of the Temporomandibular Joint. Pathological Variations. *Arch. Otolaryngol. Head Neck Surg.* **1989**, *115*, 469–477. [CrossRef]
17. Manfredini, D.; Guarda-Nardini, L. Ultrasonography of the Temporomandibular Joint: A Literature Review. *Int. J. Oral Maxillofac. Surg.* **2009**, *38*, 1229–1236. [CrossRef]
18. Kalladka, M.; Quek, S.; Heir, G.; Eliav, E.; Mupparapu, M.; Viswanath, A. Temporomandibular Joint Osteoarthritis: Diagnosis and Long-Term Conservative Management: A Topic Review. *J. Indian Prosthodont. Soc.* **2014**, *14*, 6–15. [CrossRef]
19. Ahmad, M.; Hollender, L.; Anderson, Q.; Kartha, K.; Ohrbach, R.; Truelove, E.L.; John, M.T.; Schiffman, E.L. Research Diagnostic Criteria for Temporomandibular Disorders (RDC/TMD): Development of Image Analysis Criteria and Examiner Reliability for Image Analysis. *Oral Surg. Oral Med. Oral Pathol. Oral Radiol. Endod.* **2009**, *107*, 844–860. [CrossRef]
20. Fu, K.-Y.; Li, Y.-W.; Zhang, Z.-K.; Ma, X.-C. Osteonecrosis of the Mandibular Condyle as a Precursor to Osteoarthrosis: A Case Report. *Oral Surg. Oral Med. Oral Pathol. Oral Radiol. Endod.* **2009**, *107*, e34–e38. [CrossRef]
21. Mitsimponas, K.; Mehmet, S.; Kennedy, R.; Shakib, K. Idiopathic Condylar Resorption. *Br. J. Oral Maxillofac. Surg.* **2018**, *56*, 249–255. [CrossRef]
22. Tanimoto, K.; Awada, T.; Onishi, A.; Kubo, N.; Asakawa, Y.; Kunimatsu, R.; Hirose, N. Characteristics of the Maxillofacial Morphology in Patients with Idiopathic Mandibular Condylar Resorption. *J. Clin. Med. Res.* **2022**, *11*, 952. [CrossRef]
23. Petscavage-Thomas, J.M.; Walker, E.A. Unlocking the Jaw: Advanced Imaging of the Temporomandibular Joint. *AJR Am. J. Roentgenol.* **2014**, *203*, 1047–1058. [CrossRef]
24. Sodhi, A.; Naik, S.; Pai, A.; Anuradha, A. Rheumatoid Arthritis Affecting Temporomandibular Joint. *Contemp. Clin. Dent.* **2015**, *6*, 124–127.
25. Ruparelia, P.B.; Shah, D.S.; Ruparelia, K.; Sutaria, S.P.; Pathak, D. Bilateral TMJ Involvement in Rheumatoid Arthritis. *Case Rep. Dent.* **2014**, *2014*, 262430. [CrossRef]
26. Okeson, J.P. The Classification of Orofacial Pains. *Oral Maxillofac. Surg. Clin. N. Am.* **2008**, *20*, 133–144. [CrossRef]
27. Kretapirom, K.; Okochi, K.; Nakamura, S.; Tetsumura, A.; Ohbayashi, N.; Yoshino, N.; Kurabayashi, T. MRI Characteristics of Rheumatoid Arthritis in the Temporomandibular Joint. *Dentomaxillofac. Radiol.* **2013**, *42*, 31627230. [CrossRef]
28. Suenaga, S.; Ogura, T.; Matsuda, T.; Noikura, T. Severity of Synovium and Bone Marrow Abnormalities of the Temporomandibular Joint in Early Rheumatoid Arthritis: Role of Gadolinium-Enhanced Fat-Suppressed T1-Weighted Spin Echo MRI. *J. Comput. Assist. Tomogr.* **2000**, *24*, 461–465. [CrossRef]
29. Youssef Mohamed, M.M.; Dahaba, M.M.; Farid, M.M.; Ali Elsayed, A.M. Radiographic Changes in TMJ in Relation to Serology and Disease Activity in RA Patients. *Dentomaxillofac. Radiol.* **2020**, *49*, 20190186. [CrossRef]
30. Ahmad, M.; Schiffman, E.L. Temporomandibular Joint Disorders and Orofacial Pain. *Dent. Clin. N. Am.* **2016**, *60*, 105–124. [CrossRef]
31. Cannizzaro, E.; Schroeder, S.; Müller, L.M.; Kellenberger, C.J.; Saurenmann, R.K. Temporomandibular Joint Involvement in Children with Juvenile Idiopathic Arthritis. *J. Rheumatol.* **2011**, *38*, 510–515. [CrossRef]
32. Vaid, Y.N.; Dunnavant, F.D.; Royal, S.A.; Beukelman, T.; Stoll, M.L.; Cron, R.Q. Imaging of the Temporomandibular Joint in Juvenile Idiopathic Arthritis. *Arthritis Care Res.* **2014**, *66*, 47–54. [CrossRef] [PubMed]
33. Kellenberger, C.J.; Junhasavasdikul, T.; Tolend, M.; Doria, A.S. Temporomandibular Joint Atlas for Detection and Grading of Juvenile Idiopathic Arthritis Involvement by Magnetic Resonance Imaging. *Pediatr. Radiol.* **2018**, *48*, 411–426. [CrossRef] [PubMed]
34. Rosales-Alexander, J.L.; Balsalobre Aznar, J.; Magro-Checa, C. Calcium Pyrophosphate Crystal Deposition Disease: Diagnosis and Treatment. *Open Access Rheumatol.* **2014**, *6*, 39–47. [CrossRef] [PubMed]
35. Naqvi, A.H.; Abraham, J.L.; Kellman, R.M.; Khurana, K.K. Calcium Pyrophosphate Dihydrate Deposition Disease (CPPD)/Pseudogout of the Temporomandibular Joint—FNA Findings and Microanalysis. *Cytojournal* **2008**, *5*, 8. [CrossRef] [PubMed]
36. Brontoladi, S.; Sembronio, S.; Tel, A.; Lazzarotto, A.; Robiony, M. A Case Report of Chondrocalcinosis of the Temporomandibular Joint: Surgical Management and Literature Review. *Oral Maxillofac. Surg. Cases* **2020**, *6*, 100180. [CrossRef]
37. Garip, M.; Verhelst, P.-J.; Van der Cruyssen, F.; Sciot, R.; Luyten, F.P.; Bila, M.; Coropciuc, R.; Politis, C. Periarticular Chondrocalcinosis of the Left Temporomandibular Joint: A Case Report. *Oral Maxillofac. Surg. Cases* **2020**, *6*, 100145. [CrossRef]

38. Magarelli, N.; Amelia, R.; Melillo, N.; Nasuto, M.; Cantatore, F.; Guglielmi, G. Imaging of Chondrocalcinosis: Calcium Pyrophosphate Dihydrate (CPPD) Crystal Deposition Disease—Imaging of Common Sites of Involvement. *Clin. Exp. Rheumatol.* **2012**, *30*, 118–125.
39. Reynolds, J.L.; Matthew, I.R.; Chalmers, A. Tophaceous Calcium Pyrophosphate Dihydrate Deposition Disease of the Temporomandibular Joint. *J. Rheumatol.* **2008**, *35*, 717–721.
40. Gayle, E.A.; Young, S.M.; McKenna, S.J.; McNaughton, C.D. Septic Arthritis of the Temporomandibular Joint: Case Reports and Review of the Literature. *J. Emerg. Med.* **2013**, *45*, 674–678. [CrossRef]
41. Leighty, S.M.; Spach, D.H.; Myall, R.W.; Burns, J.L. Septic Arthritis of the Temporomandibular Joint: Review of the Literature and Report of Two Cases in Children. *Int. J. Oral Maxillofac. Surg.* **1993**, *22*, 292–297. [CrossRef]
42. Dwivedi, A.N.D.; Tripathi, R.; Gupta, P.K.; Tripathi, S.; Garg, S. Magnetic Resonance Imaging Evaluation of Temporomandibular Joint and Associated Soft Tissue Changes Following Acute Condylar Injury. *J. Oral Maxillofac. Surg.* **2012**, *70*, 2829–2834. [CrossRef] [PubMed]
43. Dreizin, D.; Nam, A.J.; Tirada, N.; Levin, M.D.; Stein, D.M.; Bodanapally, U.K.; Mirvis, S.E.; Munera, F. Multidetector CT of Mandibular Fractures, Reductions, and Complications: A Clinically Relevant Primer for the Radiologist. *Radiographics* **2016**, *36*, 1539–1564. [CrossRef] [PubMed]
44. Chen, M.-J.; Yang, C.; Qiu, Y.-T.; Zhou, Q.; Huang, D.; Shi, H.-M. Osteochondroma of the Mandibular Condyle: A Classification System Based on Computed Tomographic Appearances. *J. Craniofac. Surg.* **2014**, *25*, 1703–1706. [CrossRef] [PubMed]
45. Murphey, M.D.; Choi, J.J.; Kransdorf, M.J.; Flemming, D.J.; Gannon, F.H. Imaging of Osteochondroma: Variants and Complications with Radiologic-Pathologic Correlation. *Radiographics* **2000**, *20*, 1407–1434. [CrossRef]
46. Yoon, H.-J.; Cho, Y.-A.; Lee, J.-I.; Hong, S.-P.; Hong, S.-D. Malignant Pigmented Villonodular Synovitis of the Temporomandibular Joint with Lung Metastasis: A Case Report and Review of the Literature. *Oral Surg. Oral Med. Oral Pathol. Oral Radiol. Endod.* **2011**, *111*, e30–e36. [CrossRef]
47. Faro, T.F.; Martins-de-Barros, A.V.; Lima, G.T.W.F.; Raposo, A.P.; Borges, M.d.A.; Araújo, F.A.d.C.; Carvalho, M.d.V.; Nogueira, E.F.d.C.; Laureano Filho, J.R. Chondrosarcoma of the Temporomandibular Joint: Systematic Review and Survival Analysis of Cases Reported to Date. *Head Neck Pathol.* **2021**, *15*, 923–934. [CrossRef]
48. Lee, K.; Kim, S.H.; Kim, S.-M.; Myoung, H. Temporomandibular Joint Chondrosarcoma: A Case Report and Literature Review. *J. Korean Assoc. Oral Maxillofac. Surg.* **2016**, *42*, 288–294. [CrossRef]
49. Uchiyama, Y.; Matsumoto, K.; Murakami, S.; Kanesaki, T.; Matsumoto, A.; Kishino, M.; Furukawa, S. MRI in a Case of Osteosarcoma in the Temporomandibular Joint. *Dentomaxillofac. Radiol.* **2014**, *43*, 20130280. [CrossRef]
50. Pretzl, C.; Lübbers, H.-T.; Grätz, K.W.; Kruse, A.L. Metastases in the temporomandibular joint: A review from 1954 to 2013. Rare causes for temporomandibular disorders. *Swiss Dent. J.* **2014**, *124*, 1067–1083.
51. Kruse, A.L.D.; Luebbers, H.-T.; Obwegeser, J.A.; Edelmann, L.; Graetz, K.W. Temporomandibular Disorders Associated with Metastases to the Temporomandibular Joint: A Review of the Literature and 3 Additional Cases. *Oral Surg. Oral Med. Oral Pathol. Oral Radiol. Endodontol.* **2010**, *110*, e21–e28. [CrossRef]
52. Matsuda, S.; Yoshimura, H.; Kondo, S.; Sano, K. Temporomandibular Dislocation Caused by Pancreatic Cancer Metastasis: A Case Report. *Oncol. Lett.* **2017**, *14*, 6053–6058. [CrossRef] [PubMed]
53. Nortjé, C.J.; van Rensburg, L.J.; Thompson, I.O. Case Report. Magnetic Resonance Features of Metastatic Melanoma of the Temporomandibular Joint and Mandible. *Dentomaxillofac. Radiol.* **1996**, *25*, 292–297. [CrossRef] [PubMed]
54. Scolozzi, P.; Becker, M.; Lombardi, T. Mandibular Condylar Metastasis Mimicking Acute Internal Derangement of the Temporomandibular Joint. *J. Can. Dent. Assoc.* **2012**, *78*, c77. [PubMed]
55. Menezes, A.V.; Lima, M.P.; Mendonca, J.E.d.F.; Haiter-Neto, F.; Kurita, L.M. Breast Adenocarcinoma Mimicking Temporomandibular Disorders: A Case Report. *J. Contemp. Dent. Pract.* **2008**, *9*, 100–106. [CrossRef] [PubMed]
56. Chang, V.K.O.; Thambar, S. TMJ Pain as a Presentation of Metastatic Breast Cancer to the Right Mandibular Condyle. *BMJ Case Rep.* **2021**, *14*, e241601. [CrossRef]
57. Patricia, A.; Kaba, S.P.; Trierveiler, M.M.; Shinohara, E.H. Osteoblastic Metastasis from Breast Affecting the Condyle Misinterpreted as Temporomandibular Joint Disorder. *Indian J. Cancer* **2011**, *48*, 252–253. [CrossRef]
58. Nomura, F.; Kishimoto, S. Synovial Sarcoma of the Temporomandibular Joint and Infratemporal Fossa. *Auris Nasus Larynx* **2014**, *41*, 572–575. [CrossRef]

Article

Lumbar Spine Computed Tomography to Magnetic Resonance Imaging Synthesis Using Generative Adversarial Network: Visual Turing Test

Ki-Taek Hong [1,†], Yongwon Cho [1,2,†], Chang Ho Kang [1,*], Kyung-Sik Ahn [1], Heegon Lee [1], Joohui Kim [1], Suk Joo Hong [3], Baek Hyun Kim [4] and Euddeum Shim [4]

1. Department of Radiology, Korea University College of Medicine, Korea University Anam Hospital, Seoul 02841, Korea; keytech2@naver.com (K.-T.H.); dragon1won@gmail.com (Y.C.); glassesik@gmail.com (K.-S.A.); cielo1462@gmail.com (H.L.); joohee8426@naver.com (J.K.)
2. AI Center, Korea University Anam Hospital, Seoul 02841, Korea
3. Korea University Guro Hospital, Seoul 02841, Korea; hongsj@korea.ac.kr
4. Korea University College of Medicine, Korea University Ansan Hospital, Seoul 02841, Korea; kimbaekh@hanmail.net (B.H.K.); edshim1213@gmail.com (E.S.)
* Correspondence: mallecot@gmail.com; Tel.: +82-29-206-540
† These authors contributed equally to this study.

Abstract: (1) Introduction: Computed tomography (CT) and magnetic resonance imaging (MRI) play an important role in the diagnosis and evaluation of spinal diseases, especially degenerative spinal diseases. MRI is mainly used to diagnose most spinal diseases because it shows a higher resolution than CT to distinguish lesions of the spinal canals and intervertebral discs. When it is inevitable for CT to be selected instead of MR in evaluating spinal disease, evaluation of spinal disease may be limited. In these cases, it is very helpful to diagnose spinal disease with MR images synthesized with CT images. (2) Objective: To create synthetic lumbar magnetic resonance (MR) images from computed tomography (CT) scans using generative adversarial network (GAN) models and assess how closely the synthetic images resembled the true images using visual Turing tests (VTTs). (3) Material and Methods: Overall, 285 patients aged ≥ 40 years who underwent lumbar CT and MRI were enrolled. Based on axial CT and T2-weighted axial MR images from 285 patients, an image synthesis model using a GAN was trained using three algorithms (unsupervised, semi-supervised, and supervised methods). Furthermore, VTT to determine how similar the synthetic lumbar MR images generated from lumbar CT axial images were to the true lumbar MR axial images were conducted with 59 patients who were not included in the model training. For the VTT, we designed an evaluation form comprising 600 randomly distributed axial images (150 true and 450 synthetic images from unsupervised, semi-supervised, and supervised methods). Four readers judged the authenticity of each image and chose their first- and second-choice candidates for the true image. In addition, for the three models, structural similarities (SSIM) were evaluated and the peak signal to noise ratio (PSNR) was compared among the three methods. (4) Results: The mean accuracy for the selection of true images for all four readers for their first choice was 52.0% (312/600). The accuracies of determining the true image for each reader's first and first + second choices, respectively, were as follows: reader 1, 51.3% and 78.0%; reader 2, 38.7% and 62.0%, reader 3, 69.3% and 84.0%, and reader 4, 48.7% and 70.7%. In the case of synthetic images chosen as first and second choices, supervised algorithm-derived images were the most often selected (supervised, 118/600 first and 164/600 second; semi-supervised, 90/600 and 144/600; and unsupervised, 80/600 and 114/600). For image quality, the supervised algorithm received the best score (PSNR: 15.987 ± 1.039, SSIM: 0.518 ± 0.042). (5) Conclusion: This was the pilot study to apply GAN to synthesize lumbar spine MR images from CT images and compare training algorithms of the GAN. Based on VTT, the axial MR images synthesized from lumbar CT using GAN were fairly realistic and the supervised training algorithm was found to provide the closest image to true images.

Citation: Hong, K.-T.; Cho, Y.; Kang, C.H.; Ahn, K.-S.; Lee, H.; Kim, J.; Hong, S.J.; Kim, B.H.; Shim, E. Lumbar Spine Computed Tomography to Magnetic Resonance Imaging Synthesis Using Generative Adversarial Network: Visual Turing Test. *Diagnostics* **2022**, *12*, 530. https://doi.org/10.3390/diagnostics12020530

Academic Editor: Majid Chalian

Received: 10 January 2022
Accepted: 16 February 2022
Published: 18 February 2022

Publisher's Note: MDPI stays neutral with regard to jurisdictional claims in published maps and institutional affiliations.

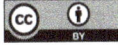

Copyright: © 2022 by the authors. Licensee MDPI, Basel, Switzerland. This article is an open access article distributed under the terms and conditions of the Creative Commons Attribution (CC BY) license (https:// creativecommons.org/licenses/by/ 4.0/).

Keywords: convolution neural network; deep learning; GAN; spine; synthetic image

1. Introduction

The generative adversarial network (GAN) is a breakthrough deep learning technology that synthesize realistic images that are almost similar to true images. GAN generates new images that did not exist in the past by receiving input of various noises from an artificial neural network and has recently received a lot of attention and has been actively studied. Existing deep learning technology, such as CNN (convolutional neural network), used one multi-layered artificial neural network, but GAN interacts with two artificial neural networks, finally creating a realistic image that is difficult to distinguish. GAN was frequently used to synthesize a new image or change an image, but recently the scope of use has been expanding.

Recent deep learning has allowed its application in medical imaging [1]. The generative adversarial network (GAN) model, which has attracted attention in the field of deep learning, can generate and transform images using two adversarial artificial neural networks, unlike conventional convolutional neural network (CNN) models. GANs can be trained using two adversarial networks, producing realistic images that are almost indistinguishable from real images [2]. The direction of deep learning is opposite to the generative neural network and the discriminative neural network. The generative neural network should make the discriminative neural network think that the realistic image synthesized by the generative neural network is a true image. Conversely, learning should be conducted to determine that the image synthesized by the generative neural network is a fake image by the discriminative neural network.

In medical imaging research, GANs have been used to synthesize positron emission tomography (PET) images from CT images and CT images from MR images [3,4]. In addition, GANs based on unsupervised learning were used to translate CT to MRI images in musculoskeletal images [5].

Computed tomography (CT) and magnetic resonance imaging (MRI) are important for the diagnosis and evaluation of spinal diseases, particularly degenerative spinal diseases. MRI is usually used to diagnose most degenerative spinal diseases because it shows higher resolution than CT in distinguishing lesions of the spinal canals, intervertebral discs, and soft tissues. However, MRI requires significant time for image acquisition, the cost of filming is higher than that of CT, and patients with claustrophobia or MR-incompatible devices sometimes have difficulties with MR examination so that the examination needs careful accommodations, such as requiring special equipment or putting patients in sleep [1]. In addition, if patients cannot afford the cost of MRI, CT is instead used to evaluate spinal disease. In these cases, the evaluation of spinal disease may be limited. However, synthesizing MR images from CT images may allow more accurate and efficient spinal disease diagnosis and evaluation.

Therefore, the purpose of this study was to develop a lumbar spine CT to MRI synthesis AI model using GAN and to validate the performance of realistic synthesis of the model with VTT and qulitive analysis based on GAN.

2. Material and Methods
2.1. Ethics Statement

This study was approved by the Institutional Review Board and Ethics Committee of Korea University Anam Hospital. The requirement for informed consent was waived because the data were collected retrospectively and analyzed anonymously. The study complied with the ethical principles of the 1964 Declaration of Helsinki revised by the World Medical Organization in Edinburgh in 2000.

2.2. Data Preparation for Training and Test

This study enrolled a total of 285 patients aged ≥ 40 years who visited the spine center of the Department of Neurosurgery, Orthopedic Surgery, Rehabilitation Medicine, and Anesthesia Pain Medicine at Korea University Anam Hospital and underwent both lumbar CT and lumbar MRI within 6 months between April 2018 and April 2020. CT scans and MR images were acquired using various models of multidetector CT scanners (IQon Spectral, Philips, Amsterdam, The Netherlands; Ingenuity Core, Philips, Amsterdam, The Netherlands; Somatom Definition Flash, Siemens, Erlangen, Germany; Somatom Definition AS, Siemens, Erlangen, Germany) and 3.0-T MR scanners (Achieva, Philips, Amsterdam, The Netherlands; Magnetom Skyra, Siemens. Erlangen, Germany; Magnetom Prisma Fit; Siemens, Erlangen, Germany).

In the PACS registry, lumbar CT and lumbar MR images satisfying the inclusion criteria for a given period (between April 2018 and April 2020) were obtained. Among the lumbar CT images, images passing through the disc parallel to the vertebral end plate at each level were selected. The lumbar MR images matched with these lumbar CT images were found and stored. The unsupervised and semi-supervised methods started learning with these lumbar CT and MR images. The lumbar CT and MR images were cropped first, and the supervised method started learning with these cropped lumbar CT and MR images. In this way the 285 patients' data were learned divided into unsupervised, semi-supervised, and supervised methods. For the visual Turing test, 59 additional patients' data were selected and stored in the way mentioned above. Lumbar MR images were synthesized with the already learned unsupervised, semi-supervised, and supervised methods from the lumbar CT images of 59 patients.

One radiologist with 15 years of experience obtained and reviewed the lumbar CT and MR images for the inclusion criteria in the picture archiving and communication system registry. The inclusion criteria for the study were as follows. First, the dates between CT and MRI did not exceed 6 months. Patients with metallic implants and severe procedures or surgeries that could deform the structure of the lumbar spine were excluded. In most cases, CT was performed for a more accurate evaluation of the bony structure or calcified or ossified lesions after or before the MR examination. Second, patients over 40 years of age were included because our goal was to validate synthetic images in the context of degenerative spinal disease. Third, the patients had no diseases that destroyed the vertebral body or spinal canal, such as spondylitis and malignant tumors; however, patients with mild compression fractures of the vertebral body without spinal canal or disc space involvement were included. Axial CT and T2-weighted MR image data were used. Because this was a preliminary study to confirm the feasibility of the GAN, only one type of MR sequence was selected; namely axial T2-weighted MR images parallel to the endplate of the vertebral body and passing through the middle of the intervertebral disc. CT and MR image pairs with different axes were excluded. A computer scientist (15 years of experience) performed deep learning based on GAN to convert from CT to MR images on the selected dataset.

Cropping of a specific area for the supervised learning of the third algorithm was bounded by the abdominal aorta and IVC at the front, the facet joints at the sides, and the spinous process and paravertebral muscles at the back. The first and second were unsupervised and semi-supervised learning, with lumbar CT totaling 40,173 from L1–2 to the L5–S1 levels and lumbar MRI totaling 9622 from the same level. The third was supervised learning, which is different from the first and second because the image was cropped and matched around the spinal canal at the same vertebra level and the same patient by one radiologist. A total of 4629 lumbar CTs (L1–2: 812, L2–3: 891, L3–4: 1048, L4–5: 1035, and L5–S1: 843), and 3566 lumbar MRIs (L1–2: 558, L2–3: 650, L3–4: 788, L4–5: 800, and L5–S1: 770) were used for supervised learning (Table 1).

Table 1. Demographic characteristics of the study population by group.

		Training (with Tuning)		Test (VTT)
Patients		285		59
CT slices	Unsupervised training Semi-supervised training Supervised training	40,173 4629		150 CT axial images
Level-L1–2		812		32
Level-L2–3		891		33
Level-L3–4		1048		33
Level-L4–5		1035		31
Level-L5–S1		843		21
MRI slices	Unsupervised training Semi-supervised training Supervised training	9622 3566		150 true and 450 synthetic MR axial images
Level-L1–2		558		32 + 96
Level-L2–3		650		33 + 99
Level-L3–4		788		33 + 99
Level-L4–5		800		31 + 93
Level-L5–S1		770		21 + 63
Age (years)				
Male		63.18 ± 16.47		68.56 ± 4.24
Female		68.08 ± 15.46		69.66 ± 7.07
Sex				
Male		129		18
Female		156		41

Note: The number of levels was used for training in the third method (matching of level and patients). There were no demographic differences between the training and test groups ($p = 0.1163$ for age and $p = 0.$ for sex in the datasets). CT, computed tomography; MRI, magnetic resonance imaging; VTT, visual Turing test.

2.3. Training the GAN to Generate Lumbar MR Images from CT Images

The GAN applied in this study used unsupervised generative attentional networks with adaptive layer-instance normalization (AdaLIN) to translate image (U-GAT-IT) [6], which is an image translation method to create synthetic images. The advantage of this model is that it allows the learning of shape and texture to be learned asymmetrically compared to conventional methods. Loss functions are used, such as adversarial loss, cycle loss, identity loss, and CAM loss. For deep learning, Ubuntu 18.04 was used on a GPU server with three 24 GB memory Titan RTXs, as well as a CUDA toolkit (440.82), and cuDNN 10.2 (NVIDIA Cooperation, Santa Clara, CA, USA). The software environment used for learning was Pytorch 3.xx or higher.

3. Deep Learning Framework

The proposed deep learning architecture for generating synthetic lumbar MRI from real lumbar CT is illustrated in Figure 1. We used the UGAIT [7] integrated attention module to design two generators, $G_{s \to t}$ and $G_{t \to s}$, and two discriminators, D_s and D_t, using lumbar CT and MRI extracted from each domain to convert the real lumbar CT to their corresponding lumbar MRI. The attention module of the generator focuses on specific regions that can be distinguished from other domains. This model was trained by feeding lumbar CT slices with the corresponding real lumbar MRI from each training subject slice by slice (first, unsupervised second, semi-supervised, and supervised learning). Once the deep learning model is trained, it can be used on a new lumbar CT to generate synthetic lumbar MRIs. We customized this framework (UGAIT [7]) to enhance the image generation for synthetic lumbar MRI.

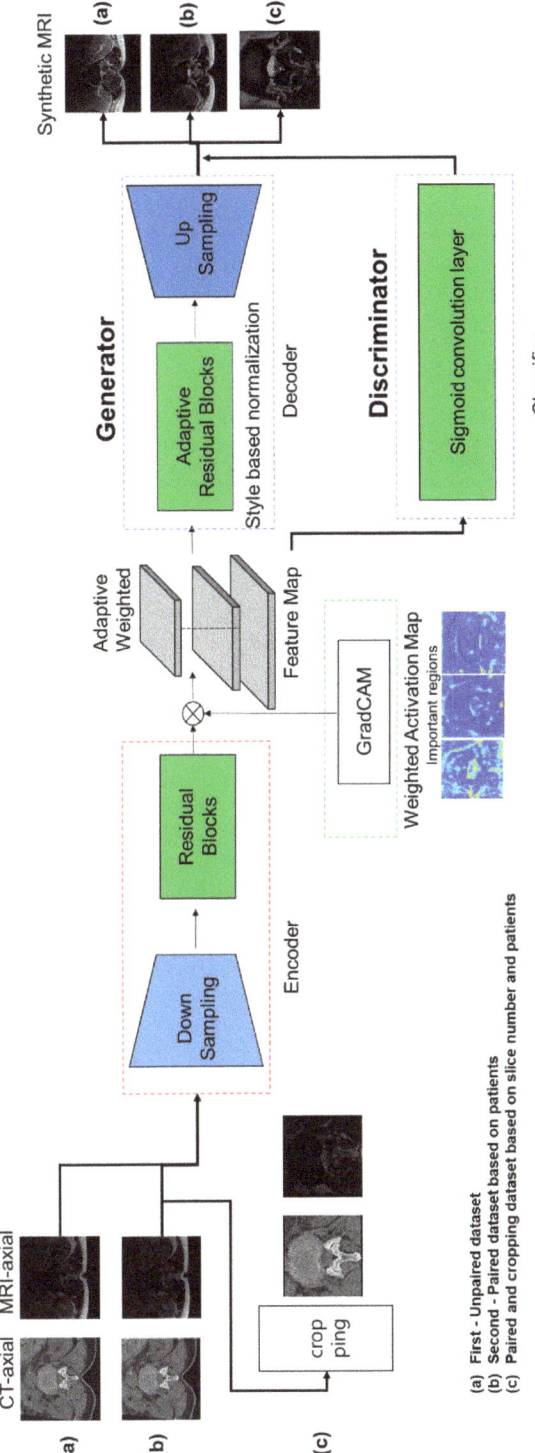

Figure 1. Model architecture for generating synthetic lumbar MRI from real lumbar axial CT images. The detailed explanation is described in the general architecture. MRI, magnetic resonance imaging; CT, computed tomography.

Three different training methods were used to develop the synthesis models in Figure 1. The first (Figure 1a) was an unsupervised learning method that randomly matched lumbar CT and MR images. The synthetic MR images from lumbar CT and the true MR images were randomly compared using this unsupervised method. The second (Figure 1b) was a semi-supervised method that matched lumbar CT and MR images from the same patient. The synthetic and true MR images of the same patient were compared using this method rather than random comparisons. The third (Figure 1c) was the supervised method, in which a specific area was cropped from the same spinal level image of the same patient and then lumbar CT and MR images were matched. At the same level as the lumbar CT image of the same patient, we compared the synthetic MR images in which only a specific part around the vertebral body containing the spinal canal was cropped, to true MR images. Image cropping was performed around the vertebral body and spinal canal. The crop was bounded by the abdominal aorta and inferior vena cava at the front, the facet joints at the sides, and the spinous process and paravertebral muscles at the back.

4. General Architecture

For image-to-image translation, we modified UGAIT, which consists of the following steps: a convolution layer, rectified linear unit activation, and instance normalization. The convolution layer included a 3 × 3 kernel, stride-2, and upsampling with the nearest neighbor. In the first step, the number of convolution filters was set to 64 and doubled with every step, reaching 1024 in the last step. Moreover, to concentrate on more important regions and ignore trivial areas for generating images differing between lumbar CT and MRI, this network included the attention map extracted from the auxiliary classifier. These attention maps were integrated into the generator and discriminator to focus on semantically important regions for transforming the shape of the images. While the attention map of the generator induces interesting regions to specifically distinguish between different domains, the attention map of the discriminator can be helpful for fine-tuning to distinguish between real and synthetic images in the target domain. Furthermore, to enhance the style transfer or image translation with different amounts of change in shape and texture, this network consists of AdaLIN by adaptively selecting a proper ratio between layer normalization and instance normalization in residual blocks in Figure 2. However, the disadvantage of this network is that it does not generate regions, such as canals in the spine. To enhance the reconstruction of the synthetic lumbar MR images, we customized the residual block and residual adain block in a single generator. First, the residual block included batch normalization instead of instance normalization and the style-based recalibration module layer for style pooling as a powerful component for image generation. Second, the residual adain block included image processing for blurring at the upsampling bottleneck. We demonstrated these fundamental issues using image translation, which can be learned bidirectionally. This results in many advantages that may address the limitations of the existing cycle GAN or CUT [8,9], as well as U-GAT-IT [7].

The discriminator had a structure similar to that of PatchGAN [10]. The architecture of the discriminator is illustrated in Figure 3. The first four convolution layers applied stride-2 and the remaining convolution layers applied stride-1. The first convolution layer inputted 1-channel images and outputted 64-channel feature maps. Subsequently, each time the feature map passed through the convolution layer, the number of channels was doubled. The output was obtained by converting the number of channels to number in the last layer. The discriminator loss, $l_{disc}(G, F, D_x, D_y)$, consisted of the LSGAN losses [11]. Loss Equation (1) was calculated using the output, as follows:

$$l_{disc}(G, F, D_x, D_y) = \mathbb{E}_{y \sim P_y}[||D_Y(y)||_1] + \mathbb{E}_{x \sim P_x}[||1 - D_Y(G(x; F(c)))||_1] + \mathbb{E}_{x \sim P_x}[||D_X(x)||_1] + \mathbb{E}_{y \sim P_y}[||1 - D_X(G(y; C_x))||_1] \quad (1)$$

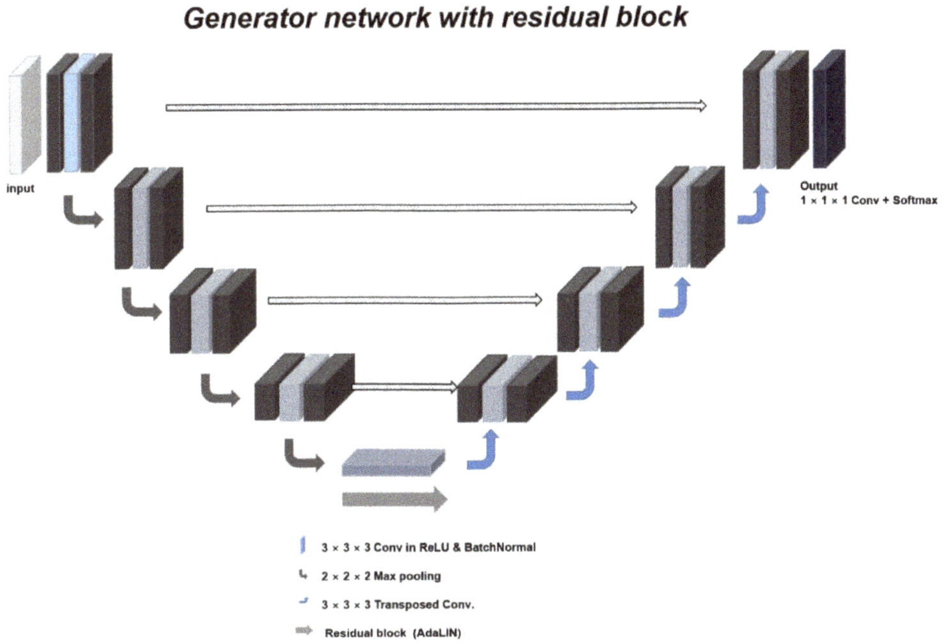

Figure 2. Model architecture of the image generator including residual blocks for upsampling. This network has a ResNet structure. The AdaLin includes fully connected layers and LeakyReLu activation layers. ResNet, residual neural network; AdaLin, adaptive layer-instance normalization; LeakyReLu, leaky rectified linear unit.

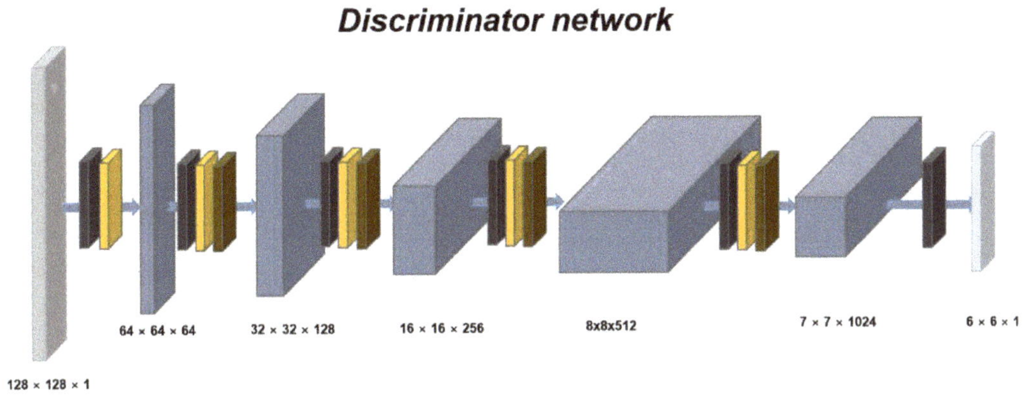

Figure 3. Model architecture of the discriminator for generating synthetic MR images from lumbar spine CT. The generator used a PatchGAN discriminator. Each number of the feature maps is the width, height, and channels of the feature map. The layers for networks were constructed by the color boxes. MR, magnetic resonance; CT, computed tomography.

5. Visual Turing Test

The VTT, which determined how similar the synthetic lumbar MR axial images generated from lumbar CT axial images were to the true lumbar MR axial images, was conducted with 59 patients who were not used in the training data. The method was executed by selecting a set of lumbar MR images composed of one true and three synthetic MR images with reference to the lumbar CT image. For VTT, we designed an evaluation form (Figure 4) comprising 600 axial images (150 true and 450 synthetic images from the unsupervised, semi-supervised, and supervised algorithms) that were randomly distributed.

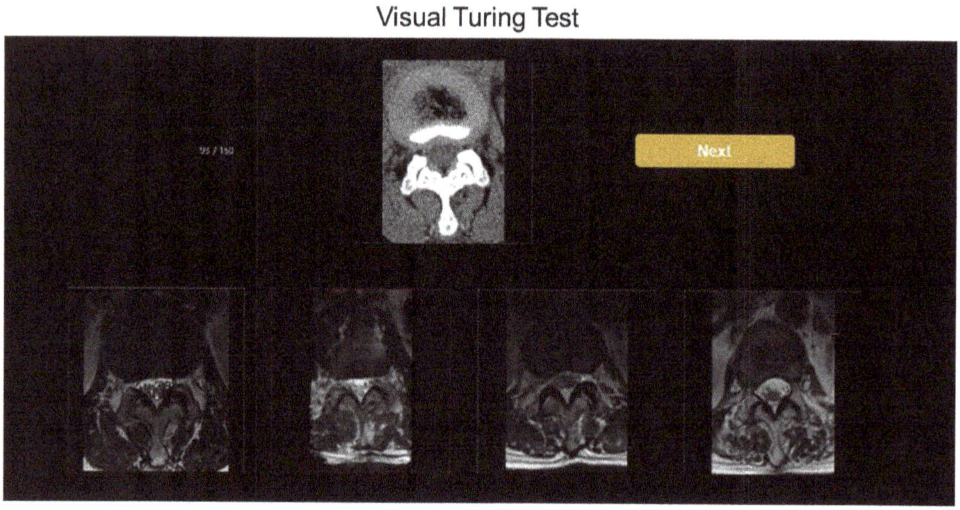

Figure 4. The validation set comprised 150 true and 450 synthetic images developed by 3 algorithms. The true and synthetic images were randomly mixed and displayed on the web solution. Four readers independently determined which MR image best reflected the axial CT image at the disc level and for real. The yellow and red frames of the MR images indicated the first and second choices, respectively. MR, magnetic resonance; CT, computed tomography.

Two board-certified radiologists (a general radiologist and a musculoskeletal [MSK] radiologist with 15 and 20 years of experience, respectively) and two radiology residents participated in the VTT. We used a program that showed five images (one CT, one true MR, and three synthetic MRI images) on a single screen in random order. The participants were asked to select two MR images that they considered the most accurate among the four lumbar MR images with reference to the CT image (Figure 4). The four radiologists were blinded to each other's evaluation of the VTT and were not shown the true or synthetic images before the VTT. The number of choices totaled 300, each with a 40-s time limit. The four participants judged the authenticity of each image and chose the first and second candidates for the true image.

The demographics of the 59 patients and the tested spinal levels are shown in Table 1. The VTT excluded 64 levels where CT and MRI were difficult to perform in VTT (8 L1–2, 4 L2–3, 4 L3–4, 13 L4–5, and 35 L5–S1 levels). The reasons for exclusion included mismatching CT and MRI scan directions, which made image comparison difficult, and cases without CT or MRI findings at that level. Finally, 150 CT, 150 true MRI, and 450 synthetic MRI images were selected for the VTT.

6. Statistical Analyses

The accuracies of each reader in identifying the true MR image were compared using paired t-tests (R software version 3.5.1; R Foundation for Statistical Computing, Vienna, Austria). The statistical differences in visual comparisons according to each spinal level and the three learning methods were also compared using paired t-tests. Statistical significance was set at $p < 0.05$.

To analyze the inter-rater reliability for identifying the true images, we calculated the percent positive agreement (PPA) Equation (2), Chamberlain's percent positive agreement

(CPPA) Equation (3) [12,13], and Cohen's kappa coefficient (K) Equation (4) [14]. These evaluation metrics are commonly used to evaluate the agreement of readers using VTT.

$$\text{PPA} = 100 \times \frac{2a}{2a+b+c} \qquad (2)$$

$$\text{CPPA} = 100 \times \frac{a}{a+b+c} \qquad (3)$$

$$K = \frac{p_o - p_e}{1 - p_e} \qquad (4)$$

$$p_o = \frac{a+d}{a+b+c+d}, \quad p_e = \left(\frac{a+b}{a+b+c+d} \times \frac{a+c}{a+b+c+d}\right) + \left(\frac{c+d}{a+b+c+d} \times \frac{b+d}{a+b+c+d}\right)$$

where a is the number of cases in which two readers equally found true images, and b and c are the numbers of cases in which one of the two readers only found true images. d indicates the number of cases in which the two readers did not find true images equally. Figure 5a shows an example of a confusion matrix for measuring the PPA, CPPA, and K.

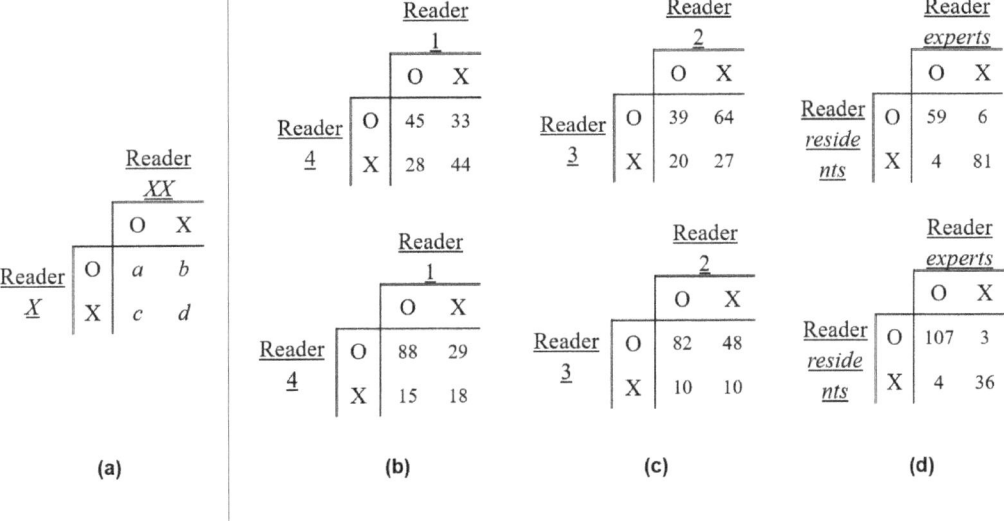

Figure 5. (a) An example confusion matrix for identifying real images (b) between two expert radiologists; top: priority-first, bottom: priority-first + second, (c) between two residents; top: priority-first, bottom: priority-first + second, and (d) between experts and resident radiologists; top: priority-first, bottom: priority-first + second.

To quantitatively evaluate the three methods of synthetic image quality, Peak SNR (PSNR) and the structural similarity index measurement (SSIM) between the true and synthetic images were used as performance metrics for the developed model as follows:

$$\text{PSNR}(x, y) = 20 \log_{10} \frac{MAX_x}{||x-y||_2} \qquad (5)$$

$$\text{SSIM}(x, y) = \frac{(2\mu_x \mu_y + C_1)(2\sigma_{xy} + C_2)}{\left(\mu_x^2 + \mu_y^2 + C_1\right)\left(\sigma_x^2 + \sigma_y^2 + C_2\right)} \qquad (6)$$

where $C_1 = (K_1L)^2$ and $C_2 = (K_2L)^2$. We used $K_1 = 0.01$ and $K_2 = 0.03$, as in the original paper [11].

7. Results

7.1. Accuracy of Identifying the True Images

Regarding the first choice of true images, the mean accuracy for all four readers was 52.0% (312/600). The accuracies of identifying the true images for the first and first + second choices, respectively, for each reader were as follows (Table 2); reader 1, 51.3% (77/150) and 78.0% (117/150); reader 2, 38.7% (58/150) and 62.0% (93/150); reader 3, 69.3% (104/150) and 84.0% (130/150); and reader 4, 48.7% (73/150) and 70.7% (114/150).

Table 2. Assessment of the choice of true lumbar MR images through the VTT by the four readers.

		Visual Turing Test						p-Value
		Total	Level 1–2	Level 2–3	Level 3–4	Level 4–5	Level 5–S1	
Reader 1	first	51.3% (77/150)	40.6% (13/32)	51.5% (17/33)	66.7% (22/33)	58.1% (18/31)	33.3% (7/21)	reference
	first + second	78.0% (117/150)	81.3% (26/32)	75.8% (25/33)	87.9% (29/33)	77.4% (24/31)	61.9% (13/21)	reference
Reader 2	first	38.7% (58/150)	46.9% (15/32)	39.4% (13/33)	42.4% (14/33)	32.3% (10/31)	28.6% (6/21)	0.2497
	first + second	62.0% (93/150)	78.1% (25/32)	60.6% (20/33)	69.7% (23/33)	58.1% (18/31)	41.6% (10/21)	0.2178
Reader 3	first	69.3% (104/150)	59.4% (19/32)	66.7% (22/33)	78.8% (26/33)	67.7% (21/31)	76.2% (16/21)	0.1190
	first + second	84.0% (130/150)	81.3% (26/32)	81.8% (27/33)	87.9% (29/33)	90.3% (28/31)	95.2% (20.21)	0.4396
Reader 4	first	48.7% (73/150)	65.6% (21/32)	51.5% (17/33)	39.4% (13/33)	41.9% (13/31)	42.9% (9/21)	0.8125
	first + second	70.7% (114/150)	81.3% (26/32)	78.8% (26/33)	60.6% (20/33)	67.7% (21/31)	61.9% (13/21)	0.9671
Total	first	52.0% (312/600)	53.1% (68/128)	52.3% (69/132)	56.8% (75/132)	50.0% (62/124)	45.2% (38/84)	-
	first + second	74.3% (446/600)	78.1% (100/128)	74.2% (98/132)	76.5% (101/132)	73.4% (91/124)	66.7% (56/84)	-

Note: Readers 1 and 4 are expert radiologists and readers 2 and 3 are resident radiologists. MR, magnetic resonance; VTT, visual Turing test.

7.2. Comparisons of Training Methods for Generating Synthetic MR Images

For synthetic images selected as first or second choices, supervised algorithm-derived images were the most frequently selected (118/600 first and 280/600 first + second), followed by semi-supervised (90/600 and 254/600), and unsupervised (80/600 and 220/600) in Table 3. Readers 1 and 3 mainly selected the synthetic lumbar MR images from supervised learning as the true images (reader 1: 38/150 first and 72/150 first + second and reader 3: 32/150 and 92/150). Readers 2 and 4, however, mainly chose synthetic lumbar MR images from unsupervised learning as true images (reader 2: 38/150 first and 77/150 first + second and reader 4: 31/150 and 72/150).

Table 3. Comparisons of the selected proportions of the three deep learning algorithms.

		Deep Learning Algorithm		
		Unsupervised	Semi-Supervised	Supervised
Reader 1	first	10	25	38
	first + second	45	66	72
Reader 2	first	38	28	26
	first + second	77	72	58
Reader 3	first	1	13	32
	first + second	26	52	92
Reader 4	first	31	24	22
	first + second	72	64	58
Total	first	80/600 (13.3%)	90/600 (15.0%)	118/600 (19.7%)
	first + second	220/600 (36.7%)	254/600 (42.3%)	280/600 (46.7%)

The highest levels of true image selection accuracy among the five spinal levels for readers 1–4 were 66.7% (22/33) for level L3–4, 46.9% (15/32) for level L1–2, 78.8% (26/33) for level L3–4, and 65.6% (21/32) for level L1–2 (Table 2). The mean accuracies of the levels were 53.1% (68/128) for L1–2, 52.3% (69/132) for L2–3, 56.8% (75/132) for L3–4, 50.0% (62/124) for L4–5, and 45.2% (38/841) for level L5–S1. The differences in accuracy between these four readers were not significant ($p > 0.05$).

7.3. Evaluations between the Expert and Resident Reader Groups

Our analysis of the inter-rater reliability for identifying true images showed PPA, CPPA, and K (Figure 5 and Table 4) values for the two expert readers of 59.6%, 42.5%, and 0.187 (first), and 80.0%, 66.7%, and 0.258 (first + second), respectively. The values for the two resident readers were 48.15%, 31.7%, −0.389 (first) and 66.7%, 58.6%, 0.072 (first + second), respectively. The PPAs, CPPAs, and Ks for all readers were 92.2%, 85.5%, and 0.845 (first), and 96.8%, 93.9%, and 0.880 (first + second), respectively (Table 4).

Table 4. Three inter-reader agreements for identifying the true MR images for each reader, including the expert and resident radiologists.

		PPA (%)	CPPA (%)	K
Two expert radiologists	first	59.6	42.5	0.187
	first + second	80.0	66.7	0.258
Two resident radiologists	first	48.2	31.7	−0.389
	first + second	66.1	58.6	0.072
Expert radiologists versus Resident radiologists	first	92.2	85.5	0.845
	first + second	96.8	93.9	0.880

PPA, percent positive agreement; CPPA, Chamberlain's percent positive agreement; K, Cohen's kappa coefficient; first, first selection of each reader; second, second selection of each reader.

7.4. Evaluations of PSNR and SSIM among the Three Algorithms

The results for quantitative image quality among the three algorithms (unsupervised, semi-supervised, and supervised training) are shown in Table 5. The PSNRs of each slice among the 59 patients of the test datasets were 15.278 ± 0.830 (unsupervised), 15.319 ± 1.037 (semi-supervised), and 15.987 ± 1.039 (supervised), respectively. The SSIMs of each slice among the 59 patients of the test datasets were 0.490 ± 0.051 (unsupervised), 0.479 ± 0.048 (semi-supervised), and 0.518 ± 0.042 (supervised), respectively.

Table 5. Overall statistics for two measures of model quality for three algorithms (unsupervised, semi-supervised, and supervised): PSNR and SSIM. The average and standard deviation for each measure about from axial slices of the 5 spine levels among the 59 subjects in our test datasets.

		PSNR	SSIM
First method: Unsupervised learning	Level 1–2	16.062 ± 1.347	0.538 ± 0.060
	Level 2–3	15.678 ± 1.647	0.526 ± 0.067
	Level 3–4	15.772 ± 1.352	0.507 ± 0.062
	Level 4–5	14.844 ± 1.350	0.465 ± 0.068
	Level 5–S1	14.033 ± 1.258	0.412 ± 0.064
	Total	15.278 ± 0.830	0.490 ± 0.051
Second method: Semi-supervised learning	Level 1–2	16.234 ± 1.964	0.529 ± 0.069
	Level 2–3	16.149 ± 2.020	0.515 ± 0.073
	Level 3–4	15.708 ± 1.824	0.492 ± 0.069
	Level 4–5	14.670 ± 1.729	0.448 ± 0.075
	Level 5–S1	13.836 ± 1.865	0.398 ± 0.079
	Total	15.319 ± 1.037	0.479 ± 0.048
Second method: Semi-supervised learning	Level 1–2	16.554 ± 1.203	0.557 ± 0.094
	Level 2–3	16.732 ± 1.395	0.553 ± 0.102
	Level 3–4	16.560 ± 1.116	0.544 ± 0.084
	Level 4–5	15.863 ± 1.449	0.521 ± 0.087
	Level 5–S1	14.228 ± 1.341	0.455 ± 0.076
	Total	15.987 ± 1.039	0.518 ± 0.042

Note: bold is the best score.

8. Discussion

8.1. The Research of Other Algorithms and GAN

GAN is a learning technique that has recently been a focus of deep learning using AI, which is used to generate or transform images using adversarial generative neural networks to create artificial but realistic-looking images [6,15]. While conventional CNN models have utilized a method to train one multilayer artificial neural network, GAN differs in progressing learning by the interaction of two artificial neural networks. In the presence of generative and discriminative neural networks, generative neural networks are trained such that their images can be truly distinguished in discriminative neural networks, and discriminative neural networks are trained to discriminate images made in generative neural networks as fake images. Through the adversarial learning process of these two neural networks, a GAN can generate synthetic images that are difficult to distinguish from real images [3].

Recently, researchers have searched for methods to replace MRI with CT scans when planning radiation therapy [16–18]. However, CT-based MRI construction has received little attention. It is challenging to generate an MR image directly from a CT image using a linear model because it is difficult to generate high-level image domains based on low-level images. In response, we proposed a synthesis method based on CNNs [19] with adversarial training [20] to generate a lumbar spine MR image from a CT scan. A 2019 study synthesized MR images from brain CT images using GAN [21], and studies published in 2017 reported the process of converting brain MR images to CT using GAN [22]. In addition, studies have reported on the conversion of images from one modality into images from another using GAN. Lee et al. reported the synthesis of spine MR images from spine CT images using GAN, with a mean overall similarity of synthetic MR T2-weighted images evaluated by radiologists of 80.2% [23]. They concluded that the synthetic MR images from spine CT images using GANs would improve the diagnostic usefulness of CT.

This is a preliminary step in determining whether lumbar synthetic MR images generated from lumbar CTs by applying GAN are clinically applicable. We first assessed whether the synthetic images generated from lumbar CT scans were distinguishable from the true MR images. If radiologists with various experiences find it difficult to distinguish between true and synthetic MRIs via VTT, the MR images synthesized through GAN may be sufficiently similar to true MRIs [24] and warrant testing in the clinical setting. The first study on lumbar spine MR image synthesis from CT was published in 2020 [25]. Using a small dataset, the authors generated synthetic lumbar spine MR images using GAN and determined the similarities between the synthesized and true MR images. In contrast to this work, we did not perform quantitative comparisons using the mean absolute error and peak signal-to-noise ratio or qualitative comparisons of each structure of the spine, including the discs, facet joints, spinal canals, and thecal sacs.

In medical imaging, computer-based vision evaluation methods are largely used to measure detection and segmentation accuracy, emphasizing the classification of regions according to anatomy from a predefined library. As an alternative, motivated by the ability of humans to provide far richer descriptions, we constructed a VTT that used binary questions to probe a model's ability to distinguish fake images from true images. In our VTT, the probability of finding a true image was 52%; in other words, the ability to distinguish between real and fake images was half of the time. This probability is the same as in the situation in which a coin is thrown to predict which side will land facing upward. The results of VTT indicated that the GAN model developed in this study made synthetic lumbar MR images that were difficult to distinguish from real images.

A previous study applied a VTT to determine how synthetic lung nodules generated by GAN compared to the original lung nodules on CT [24]. Two radiologists participated in the VTT; the authors concluded that it was difficult for radiologists to distinguish between the generated and real nodules. A neuroimaging study also using a VTT [25] generated synthetic brain MR images using GANs and compared them to true brain MR images by VTT by an expert physician looking at 50 synthetic and 50 true MR images in random order and determining whether they were true or synthetic. The authors concluded that it was difficult for the expert physician to accurately distinguish between synthetic and true brain images. Synthetic high-resolution body CT images with progressive growing GAN (PGGAN) were also indistinguishable from real images in VTT [6].

8.2. The Present Study for Conversion from CT and MR Images

The present study utilized GAN trained with unsupervised, semi-supervised, and supervised methods and compared their fake image synthesis performance through VTTs. Supervised learning uses aligned training datasets in which the output image corresponds to each input image. By disconnecting the aligned data into an input and output set to train, medical synthesis becomes an unsupervised learning-based synthetic task. A semi-supervised learning can be configured to utilize both supervised and unsupervised learning. A highly supervised training typically requires a large volume of labeled datasets [26]. However, acquiring those from expert radiologists at a sufficient scale can be prohibitive; thus, we anticipated unsupervised training, which meant the unpairing of the CT and MR data, although our results showed that supervised training-derived images were selected most often as the first and second choices. In other words, the images produced using the supervised method were the most realistic images.

In contrast to our results, brain MRI to CT synthesis research showed that unpaired data-derived images were more realistic and contained fewer artifacts and less blurred images in comparisons of the conversion between unpaired and paired data using mean absolute error (MAE) values and peak-signal-to-noise ratio (PSNR) in true and synthesized CT [22]. Another study on transforming brain CT into MRI using GAN reported that the combination of paired and unpaired data showed more realistic images in MAE and PSNR than using paired or unpaired data individually [21]. The authors also reported that this combination solved the context-misalignment problem of unpaired training and alleviated the rigid registration task and blurred results of paired training. First, an unsupervised method of learning by randomly matching lumbar CT and MR images was used to convert CT into MRI; however, the main part of the synthetic MR images was converted differently from the real MR images in some synthetic MR images. To solve this problem of the first method, a learning method was performed with CT and MR image pairs for each patient. Finally, although the image conversion of CT to MR is more difficult than that of MR to CT, the use of paired data and cropped information can be more helpful for generating synthetic MR images. The above two studies were evaluated through measurements such as MAE and PSNR, but we attempted to evaluate the images through a VTT. Therefore, it is difficult to compare our results to those of previous studies. We also observed no difference in the accuracy of separating synthetic from true MRIs and in the inter-reader agreements among four expert and resident radiologists, providing indirect evidence that synthetic MRIs and true MRIs had comparable image fidelity, although the selection criteria between readers were likely to be subjective and differ according to experience.

The results of VTTs according to lumbar spine levels showed the highest rate of true image selection for the L3–4 level (56.8%), followed by the L1–2 level (53.1%). The L5–S1 level showed the lowest rate (45.2%), likely because the anatomical shape that changes from the lumbar spine to the sacrum differs from the other lumbar levels, making it more difficult to determine true or synthetic MR images than other lumbar levels based on the reference CT. However, the choice between lumbar levels did not differ significantly. For image quality, the supervised algorithm received the best score (PSNR: 15.987, SSIM: 0.518 ± 0.042, respectively in Table 5).

8.3. The Limitations of Our Study

This study has several limitations. The first is the limitation of the VTT. This test was used to assess how intuitively similar the synthetic MR images were to the true MR images and not to evaluate how well the synthetic MR images replicated the individual structures of true MR images. Our future goal is to determine whether MR images synthesized using GAN from lumbar CT images have clinical significance compared to true MRIs through structural analysis of the disc, spinal canal, and paraspinal muscles of the lumbar spine. The second limitation was that the L5–S1 levels were excluded from the study. In some CT examinations, continuous scans were performed from the superior end plate of L1 through the S1 level without adjusting the horizontal direction of the disc level. Therefore, the axial levels of CT often have different directions from those of MRI, which is strictly scanned around the intervertebral disc, making it difficult to compare images. Therefore, this study excluded 35 cases with L5–S1 images (L1–2: 8 cases, L2–3: 4 cases, L3–4: 4 cases, and L4–5: 13 cases). The third limitation was caused by image cropping in deep learning using the supervised method. In axial lumbar CT and MR images, the same part cannot be cropped around the vertebral body. Fourth, the training dataset of our study was small. We used 285 CT scans in deep learning with GAN, while other studies used 11,755 body CT scans during PGGAN training and 1018 lung cancer screening thoracic CT scans during DC-GAN training. The fourth limitation is related to the low number of patients and different CT scanners. A total of 285 patients' CT images were used for deep learning and 59 patients' CT images were used for the VTT that were not included in deep learning. Although five levels of CT images were used per patient, the limitation of this study was that a large number of CT images were not included in the deep learning, and another limitation of this study is that all patients could not be taken with the same type of CT equipment.

9. Conclusions

We developed three methods of a GAN model to convert from lumbar CT to MR images, which were evaluated with a VTT. Based on the VTT, the axial MR images synthesized from lumbar CT using GAN were fairly realistic and the supervised training algorithm was found to provide the closest image to true images.

If future research validates the clinical usefulness of replacing true lumbar spine MR images with synthetic images in particular cases, the lumbar spine CT to MR synthesis using GAN could expand the role of CT, which is traditionally narrowed in the diagnosis of degenerative spinal disease, and could also increase the diagnostic value of CT with additional reference information.

Author Contributions: K.-T.H. and Y.C. mainly contributed to the data collection and analysis, literature search, and manuscript writing, while C.H.K. mainly contributed to the study design and concepts. H.L. and J.K. analyzed and recorded the data. K.-S.A., S.J.H., B.H.K. and E.S. reviewed and edited the manuscript. All authors have read and agreed to the published version of the manuscript.

Funding: This research received no external funding.

Institutional Review Board Statement: Ethic Committee Name: Korea University Anam Hospital Clinical Trial Center (2022AN0032).

Informed Consent Statement: Not applicable.

Data Availability Statement: The datasets used and/or analyzed during the current study are available from the corresponding author upon reasonable request.

Acknowledgments: This research was technically supported by the Advanced Medical Imaging Institute of Korea University Anam Hospital.

Conflicts of Interest: The authors declare that they have no competing interest.

References

1. Chartrand, G.; Cheng, P.M.; Vorontsov, E.; Drozdzal, M.; Turcotte, S.; Pal, C.J.; Kadoury, S.; Tang, A. Deep Learning: A Primer for Radiologists. *RadioGraphics* **2017**, *37*, 2113–2131. [CrossRef] [PubMed]
2. Jo, Y.J.; Bae, K.M.; Park, J.Y. Research trends of generative adversarial networks and image generation and translation. *Electron. Telecommun. Trends* **2020**, *35*, 91–102.
3. Bi, L.; Kim, J.; Kumar, A.; Feng, D.; Fulham, M. Synthesis of positron emission tomography (PET) images via multi-channel generative adversarial networks (GANs). In *Molecular Imaging, Reconstruction and Analysis of Moving Body Organs, and Stroke imaging and Treatment*; Cardoso, M.J., Arbel, T., Eds.; Springer: Berlin/Heidelberg, Germany, 2017; pp. 43–51.
4. Nie, D.; Trullo, R.; Lian, J.; Petitjean, C.; Ruan, S.; Wang, Q.; Shen, D. Medical Image Synthesis with Context-Aware Generative Adversarial Networks. In *International Conference on Medical Image Computing and Computer-Assisted Intervention*; Springer: Cham, Switzerland, 2017; Volume 10435, pp. 417–425.
5. Jin, C.-B.; Kim, H.; Liu, M.; Han, I.H.; Lee, J.I.; Lee, J.H.; Joo, S.; Park, E.; Ahn, Y.S.; Cui, X. DC2Anet: Generating Lumbar Spine MR Images from CT Scan Data Based on Semi-Supervised Learning. *Appl. Sci.* **2019**, *9*, 2521. [CrossRef]
6. Park, H.Y.; Bae, H.-J.; Hong, G.-S.; Kim, M.; Yun, J.; Park, S.; Chung, W.J.; Kim, N. Realistic High-Resolution Body Computed Tomography Image Synthesis by Using Progressive Growing Generative Adversarial Network: Visual Turing Test. *JMIR Med. Inform.* **2021**, *9*, e23328. [CrossRef] [PubMed]
7. Kim, J.; Kim, M.; Kang, H.; Lee, K. U-gat-it: Unsupervised generative attentional networks with adaptive layer-instance normalization for image-to-image translation. *arXiv* **2019**, arXiv:1907.10830.
8. Zhu, J.Y.; Park, T.; Isola, P.; Efros, A.A. Unpaired image-to-image translation using cycle-consistent adversarial networks. In Proceedings of the 16th IEEE International Conference on Computer Vision, Venice, Italy, 22–29 October 2017; pp. 2242–2251.
9. Park, T.; Efros, A.A.; Zhang, R.; Zhu, J.-Y. Contrastive Learning for Unpaired Image-to-Image Translation. In *European Conference on Computer Vision*; Springer: Cham, Switzerland, 2020; pp. 319–345.
10. Isola, P.; Zhu, J.-Y.; Zhou, T.; Efros, A.A. Image-to-Image Translation with Conditional Adversarial Networks. In Proceedings of the 2017 IEEE Conference on Computer Vision and Pattern Recognition (CVPR), Honolulu, HI, USA, 21–26 July 2017; pp. 5967–5976.
11. Wang, Z.; Bovik, A.C.; Sheikh, H.R.; Simoncelli, E.P. Image quality assessment: From error visibility to structural similarity. *IEEE Trans. Image Process.* **2004**, *13*, 600–612. [CrossRef] [PubMed]
12. Bartlett, J.W.; Frost, C. Reliability, repeatability and reproducibility: Analysis of measurement errors in continuous variables. *Ultrasound Obstet. Gynecol.* **2008**, *31*, 466–475. [CrossRef] [PubMed]
13. Kong, K.A. Statistical Methods: Reliability Assessment and Method Comparison. *Ewha Med. J.* **2017**, *40*, 9–16. [CrossRef]
14. Cohen, J. A Coefficient of Agreement for Nominal Scales. *Educ. Psychol. Meas.* **1960**, *20*, 37–46. [CrossRef]
15. Kim, T.; Cha, M.; Kim, H.; Lee, J.K.; Kim, J. Learning to discover cross-domain relations with generative adversarial networks. In *International Conference on Machine Learning*; PMLR: London, UK, 2017; pp. 1857–1865.
16. Hsu, S.-H.; Cao, Y.; Huang, K.; Feng, M.; Balter, J.M. Investigation of a method for generating synthetic CT models from MRI scans of the head and neck for radiation therapy. *Phys. Med. Biol.* **2013**, *58*, 8419–8435. [CrossRef] [PubMed]
17. Zheng, W.; Kim, J.P.; Kadbi, M.; Movsas, B.; Chetty, I.J.; Glide-Hurst, C.K. Magnetic Resonance–Based Automatic Air Segmentation for Generation of Synthetic Computed Tomography Scans in the Head Region. *Int. J. Radiat. Oncol.* **2015**, *93*, 497–506. [CrossRef] [PubMed]
18. Kapanen, M.; Tenhunen, M. T1/T2*-weighted MRI provides clinically relevant pseudo-CT density data for the pelvic bones in MRI-only based radiotherapy treatment planning. *Acta Oncol.* **2013**, *52*, 612–618. [CrossRef] [PubMed]
19. Krizhevsky, A.; Sutskever, I.; Hinton, G.E. Imagenet classification with deep convolutional neural networks. In Proceedings of the Advances in Neural Information Processing Systems, Lake Tahoe, NV, USA, 3–8 December 2012; pp. 1097–1105.

20. Goodfellow, I.; Pouget-Abadie, J.; Mirza, M.; Xu, B.; Warde-Farley, D.; Ozair, S.; Courville, A.; Bengio, Y. Generative adversarial nets. In Proceedings of the Advances in Neural Information Processing Systems, Montreal, QC, Canada, 8–13 December 2014; pp. 2672–2680.
21. Jin, C.-B.; Kim, H.; Liu, M.; Jung, W.; Joo, S.; Park, E.; Ahn, Y.S.; Han, I.H.; Lee, J.I.; Cui, X. Deep CT to MR Synthesis Using Paired and Unpaired Data. *Sensors* **2019**, *19*, 2361. [CrossRef] [PubMed]
22. Wolterink, J.M.; Dinkla, A.M.; Savenije, M.H.; Seevinck, P.R.; van den Berg, C.A.; Išgum, I. Deep MR to CT synthesis using unpaired data. In *Simulation and Synthesis in Medical Imaging. SASHIMI 2017. Lecture Notes in Computer Science*; Tsaftaris, S., Gooya, A., Frangi, A., Prince, J., Eds.; Springer: Cham, Switzerland, 2017; Volume 10557, pp. 14–23.
23. Lee, J.H.; Han, I.H.; Kim, D.H.; Yu, S.; Lee, I.S.; Song, Y.S.; Joo, S.; Jin, C.-B.; Kim, H. Spine Computed Tomography to Magnetic Resonance Image Synthesis Using Generative Adversarial Networks: A Preliminary Study. *J. Korean Neurosurg. Soc.* **2020**, *63*, 386–396. [CrossRef] [PubMed]
24. Chuquicusma, M.J.M.; Hussein, S.; Burt, J.; Bagci, U. How to fool radiologists with generative adversarial networks? a visual turing test for lung cancer diagnosis. In Proceedings of the IEEE 15th International Symposium on Biomedical Imaging, Washington, DC, USA, 4–7 April 2018.
25. Han, C.; Hayashi, H.; Rundo, L.; Araki, R.; Shimoda, W.; Muramatsu, S.; Furukawa, Y.; Mauri, G.; Nakayama, H. GAN-based synthetic brain MR image generation. In Proceedings of the IEEE 15th International Symposium on Biomedical Imaging (ISBI 2018), Washington, DC, USA, 4–7 April 2018; pp. 734–738.
26. Gulshan, V.; Peng, L.; Coram, M.; Stumpe, M.C.; Wu, D.; Narayanaswamy, A.; Venugopalan, S.; Widner, K.; Madams, T.; Cuadros, J.; et al. Development and validation of a deep learning algorithm for detection of diabetic retinopathy in retinal fundus photographs. *JAMA* **2016**, *316*, 2402–2410. [CrossRef] [PubMed]

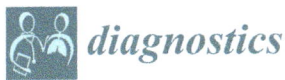

Article

Accuracy of Critical Shoulder Angle and Acromial Index for Predicting Supraspinatus Tendinopathy

Tzu-Herng Hsu [1,†], Che-Li Lin [2,3,†], Chin-Wen Wu [1,4], Yi-Wen Chen [1,4], Timporn Vitoonpong [5], Lien-Chieh Lin [1] and Shih-Wei Huang [1,4,*]

1. Department of Physical Medicine and Rehabilitation, Shuang Ho Hospital, Taipei Medical University, New Taipei City 23561, Taiwan; 17324@s.tmu.edu.tw (T.-H.H.); 09442@s.tmu.edu.tw (C.-W.W.); 17304@s.tmu.edu.tw (Y.-W.C.); 17483@s.tmu.edu.tw (L.-C.L.)
2. Department of Orthopedic Surgery, Shuang Ho Hospital, Taipei Medical University, New Taipei City 23561, Taiwan; 11010@s.tmu.edu.tw
3. Department of Orthopedics, School of Medicine, College of Medicine, Taipei Medical University, Taipei 11031, Taiwan
4. Department of Physical Medicine and Rehabilitation, School of Medicine, College of Medicine, Taipei Medical University, Taipei 11031, Taiwan
5. Rehabilitation Department, King Chulalongkorn Memorial Hospital, Bangkok 10330, Thailand; timpornvitoonpong@gmail.com
* Correspondence: 13001@s.tmu.edu.tw; Tel.: +886-222-490-088 (ext. 1602)
† These authors contributed equally to this work.

Abstract: Critical shoulder angle (CSA) is the angle between the superior and inferior bony margins of the glenoid and the most lateral border of the acromion. The acromial index (AI) is the distance from the glenoid plane to the acromial lateral border and is divided by the distance from the glenoid plane to the lateral aspect of the humeral head. Although both are used for predicting shoulder diseases, research on their accuracy in predicting supraspinatus tendinopathy in patients with shoulder pain is limited. Data were retrospectively collected from 308 patients with supraspinatus tendinopathy between January 2018 and December 2019. Simultaneously, we gathered the data of 300 patients with shoulder pain without supraspinatus tendinopathy, confirmed through ultrasound examination. Baseline demographic data, CSA, and AI were compared using the independent Student's t test and Mann–Whitney U test. Categorical variables were analyzed using the chi-square test. A receiver operating characteristic curve (ROC) analysis was performed to investigate the accuracy of CSA and AI for predicting supraspinatus tendinopathy, and the optimal cut-off point was determined using the Youden index. No statistical differences were observed for age, sex, body mass index, evaluated side (dominant), diabetes mellitus, and hyperlipidemia between the groups. The supraspinatus tendinopathy group showed higher CSAs ($p < 0.001$) than did the non-supraspinatus tendinopathy group. For predicting supraspinatus tendinopathy, the area under the curve (AUC) of ROC curve of the CSA was 76.8%, revealing acceptable discrimination. The AUC of AI was 46.9%, revealing no discrimination. Moreover, when patients with shoulder pain had a CSA > 38.11°, the specificity and sensitivity of CSA in predicting supraspinatus tendinopathy were 71.0% and 71.8%, respectively. CSA could be considered an objective assessment tool to predict supraspinatus tendinopathy in patients with shoulder pain. AI revealed no discrimination in predicting supraspinatus tendinopathy in patients with shoulder pain.

Keywords: shoulder; supraspinatus tendinopathy; critical shoulder angle; acromial index

Citation: Hsu, T.-H.; Lin, C.-L.; Wu, C.-W.; Chen, Y.-W.; Vitoonpong, T.; Lin, L.-C.; Huang, S.-W. Accuracy of Critical Shoulder Angle and Acromial Index for Predicting Supraspinatus Tendinopathy. *Diagnostics* 2022, 12, 283. https://doi.org/10.3390/diagnostics12020283

Academic Editors: Majid Chalian and Antonio Barile

Received: 23 November 2021
Accepted: 21 January 2022
Published: 22 January 2022

Publisher's Note: MDPI stays neutral with regard to jurisdictional claims in published maps and institutional affiliations.

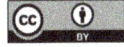

Copyright: © 2022 by the authors. Licensee MDPI, Basel, Switzerland. This article is an open access article distributed under the terms and conditions of the Creative Commons Attribution (CC BY) license (https://creativecommons.org/licenses/by/4.0/).

1. Introduction

Supraspinatus (SS) tendinopathy is a type of tendon disorder characterized by pain and impaired function. It is related to degeneration, irritation, overuse, and poor strain mechanics [1,2]. Shoulder impingement syndrome is also believed to lead to SS tendinopathy [3]. Moreover, the causes of SS tendinopathy are variable and can be divided into intrinsic and extrinsic factors [3]. Intrinsic factors include age, excessive weight, and impaired biomechanics, including malalignments and decreased flexibility, causing degenerative changes and reduced strength of the tendon [4–6]. Extrinsic factors can be divided into primary and secondary impingement, which result from increased subacromial loading and muscle overload/imbalance, respectively [3,7–10]. Studies have reported that SS tendinopathy leads to poor sleep quality, low quality of life, and work absenteeism [11–13].

Rotator cuff tendinopathy is the most common cause of shoulder disorders [14], and its prevalence rates range from 5–10%, 30–35%, and up to 80% in people aged <20 years, 60–80 years, and >80 years, respectively [15–17]. Despite their variable etiology, supraspinatus tendinopathy is the most common among rotator cuff diseases, affecting 61.9% of men and 38.1% of women [18]. Hsiao et al. reported that subacromial impingement occurred at 7.77 per 1000 person-years in the military and observed that those aged >40 years had an increased risk of subacromial impingement, thereby leading to an increased risk of SS tendinopathy [19].

"Critical shoulder angle" (CSA), proposed by Moor et al., representing the inclination of the lateral extension of the acromion and glenoid on an anteroposterior (AP) radiograph [20], was reported higher in patients with degenerative rotator cuff tear than in those with non-rotator cuff tears [21]. Recent studies have also used CSA to predict supraspinatus tendon tear [22] and the risk of supraspinatus retear after surgery [23]. Furthermore, CSA along with age was found to predict cuff tear arthropathy, osteoarthritis, rotator cuff impingement, and calcified tendinitis [24]. On the other hand, "Acromial index" (AI), introduced by Nyffeler et al., representing the lateral extension of the acromion above the humeral head [25], has been revealed as a predictor of rotator cuff tear [21,26]. However, the ability of AI to predict the postoperative outcomes of rotator cuff tears is conflicting [27,28]. As Neer reported, 95% of rotator cuff tears might arise from SS tendinopathy, which is caused by the predisposition to the conditions of anatomic impingement [7].

Despite many studies evaluating the outcomes of rotator cuff disorders by using CSA and AI, no study has investigated the relationship between CSA and AI with SS tendinopathy. Therefore, this study aims to establish the association between CSA, AI, and supraspinatus tendinopathy, comparing the accuracy of CSA and AI in predicting supraspinatus tendinopathy.

2. Materials and Methods

2.1. Study Design and Participants

This study was designed as a retrospective case–control cross-sectional investigation and performed in a medical university hospital between January 2018 and December 2019. All participants were recruited from orthopedic and rehabilitation outpatient departments, and the Institutional Review Board of Taipei Medical University (N202011086) approved the study protocol. We applied the following inclusion criteria: (1) age between 20 and 80 years, (2) having shoulder pain, and (3) undergoing shoulder X-ray and ultrasound evaluation. The following exclusion criteria were applied: (1) previously underwent shoulder surgery around the shoulder; (2) having glenohumeral osteoarthritis and acromioclavicular arthritis, which could affect CSA and AI measurements; and (3) poor quality of shoulder radiographic images. Based on the findings of the shoulder ultrasound and physical examination (both painful arc and empty can test positive), participants were divided into the SS tendinopathy group and non-SS tendinopathy group. Baseline demographic data, such as age, sex, affected side, body mass index (BMI), history of diabetes mellitus, and hyperlipidemia, were obtained from medical charts.

2.2. Radiographic Evaluation for CSA and AI

After demographic data collection, conventional AP shoulder radiographs were obtained on the day of the outpatient department visit. The image was taken with the patient in the upright standing position with a descending beam tilt of 20°. The shoulder AP image was obtained using a standardized protocol such that CSA could be measured accurately by clearly presenting the superior and inferior border of the glenoid fossa, and inferolateral border of the acromion. We adopted the CSA measurement protocol reported by Blonna et al. [29]. When the radiograph was not affected by rotation and overlapping of the anterior and posterior edges of the glenoid cavity, we defined it as having sufficient image quality for CSA assessment. Based on a previous study, the inter- and intra-observer reliability for measuring the CSA was excellent [30]. CSA was measured from the angle made by the superior and inferior bony margins of the glenoid and a line from the inferior bony margin of the glenoid to the most lateral border of the acromion (Figure 1A). As for AI, the GA was taken as the distance between the glenoid plane and lateral border of the acromion, and the GH was taken as the distance between the glenoid plane to the lateral aspect of the humeral head. AI was evaluated as the ratio of GA to GH (Figure 1B) [25].

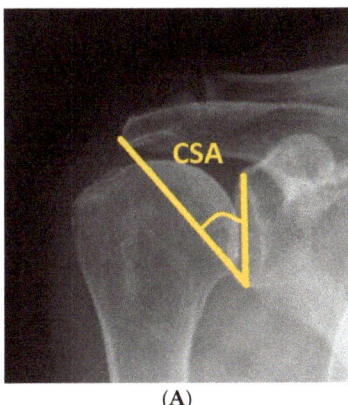
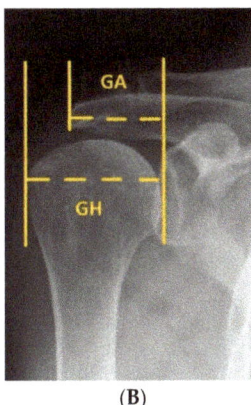

(A)   (B)

Figure 1. (**A**) The critical shoulder angle (CSA) is formed from a line connecting the inferior and superior borders of the glenoid fossa and another line connecting the inferior border of the glenoid with the inferolateral border of the acromion. (**B**) The acromial index is the ratio of the distance from the glenoid plane to the lateral border of the acromion (GA) to the distance from the glenoid plane to the most lateral aspect of the humeral head (GH). AI = GA / GH.

2.3. Ultrasound Evaluation with Physical Examination of SS Tendinopathy

SS tendinopathy was confirmed through ultrasound and physical examination after the radiographic evaluation. The ultrasound and physical examination were performed by different physiatrists in our department. An experienced physiatrist, who was blinded to the result of the radiographic study of the shoulder, performed the evaluation for SS tendinopathy. Patients with SS tendinopathy displayed shoulder pain when performing shoulder abduction between 60° and 120°, and patients did not have radiation of pain to the neck or down the arm [31,32]. In addition, the empty can test was performed as the provocation test [33]. For ultrasound examination, patients assumed the modified Crass position with the palm on the iliac crest and the elbow directed posteriorly [34]. Sonography revealed thickening (>8 mm), hypoechogenicity, and heterogeneity in cases of SS tendinopathy [35]. According to a review article, ultrasound demonstrated a sensitivity of 79% and a specificity of 94% for the detection of rotator cuff tendinopathy [36].

2.4. Sample Size Estimation

G-Power 3.1 was used to estimate the sample size required for an analysis of two groups of independent means in the study. We input the effect size dz was 0.15, an alpha of 0.05, with a power of 0.95. We determined that a minimum total sample size of 483 was required to identify differences between the study groups. Considering the probability of patients' data lacking and excluded due to the matching process, we enrolled more than 483 patients (653 patients) in our study to ensure adequate statistical power with an anticipated power of 0.95.

2.5. Statistical Analysis

Based on the ultrasound findings of SS tendinopathy, we divided all participants into the SS tendinopathy and non-SS tendinopathy groups. For reducing the influence of confounders, we match the demographic data such as age, sex, BMI, affected side, diabetes mellitus, and hyperlipidemia with a 1:1 ratio of both groups. The variables of age, sex, BMI, affected side, diabetes mellitus, hyperlipidemia, CSA, GA, GH, and AI are presented as the mean and number of patients. Continuous variables between the groups were compared using the independent Student's t-test after the Kolmogorov–Smirnov test was performed to confirm these were normal distribution. If the data were not a normal distribution, we performed the Mann–Whitney U test to compare the mean value between the groups. The chi-square test was used for comparing categorical variables between the groups. We performed receiver operating characteristic (ROC) curve analyses of CSA and AI to estimate their accuracy for predicting SS tendinopathy. The cut-off points of optimal sensitivity and specificity of CSA and AI were determined by the Youden index. All statistical analyses were performed using Statistical Package for the Social Sciences (version 19.0; IBM, Armonk, NY, USA), and $p < 0.05$ was considered statistically significant.

3. Results

In total, 806 participants with shoulder pain met the inclusion criteria. Of them, 34, 25, 61, and 33 were excluded because of osteoarthritis, fracture, supraspinatus tear, and poor image quality for CSA measurement, respectively. Finally, 653 patients were included in this study. Based on the findings of ultrasound and physical examination, 339 patients were diagnosed as having SS tendinopathy; 314 participants having shoulder pain without SS tendinopathy comprised the non-SS tendinopathy group. For controlling the bias of the retrospective study, we matched the baseline variables between these two groups. Finally, 308 (148 men and 160 women) and 300 (143 men and 157 women) participants were included in the SS tendinopathy and non-SS tendinopathy groups, respectively (Figure 2).

No statistical differences were observed in demographic variables, such as age, sex, dominant side, BMI, diabetes mellitus, and hyperlipidemia, between these two groups (Table 1). Among these supraspinatus tendinopathy patients, there were 103 (33.4%) with supraspinatus calcific tendonitis, 90 (29.2%) with partial thickness tear, 89 (28.9) with supraspinatus tendinosis, and 26 (8.4%) with full thickness tear.

Table 1. Demographic and characteristics of Supraspinatus tendinopathy (SS tendinopathy) and Non-Supraspinatus tendinopathy (non-SS tendinopathy) groups.

Variables	SS Tendinopathy (n = 308)	Non-SS Tendinopathy (n = 300)	p Value
Age, y	57.1 ± 12.3	57.2 ± 13.0	0.870
Sex, n (male)	148	143	0.935
Evaluated side, n (dominant)	178	169	0.743
BMI, kg/m^2	25.3 ± 3.5	25.2 ± 3.9	0.785
DM, n	59	65	0.481
Hyperlipidemia, n	28	32	0.587

Continuous data are shown as the mean ± standard deviation and categorical data as the number of patients; the p value was calculated using the Student's t test for continuous variables and the chi-square test for categorical; variables; BMI, body mass index; DM, diabetes mellitus; VAS, visual analog scale.

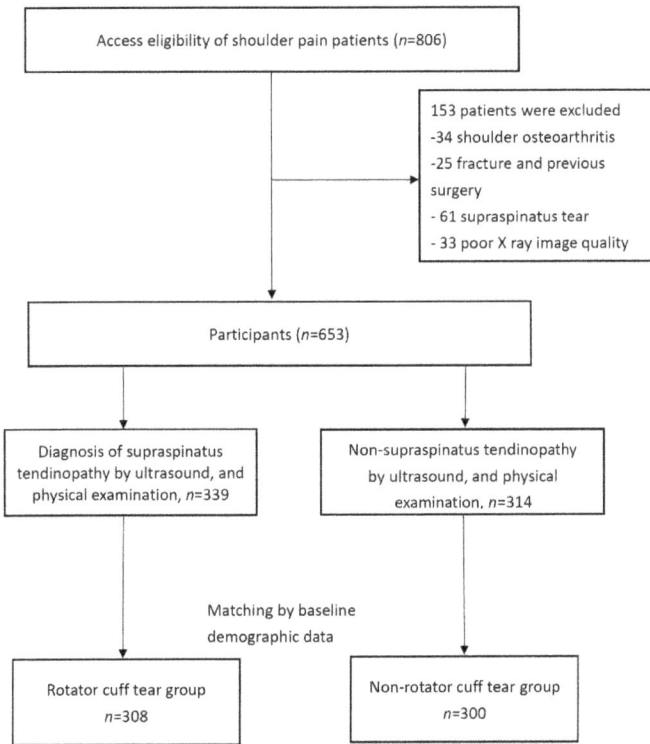

Figure 2. Flowchart of this study.

The results of the quantitative radiographic assessment presented in Table 2, demonstrated a significantly higher CSA in the SS tendinopathy group (40.29° ± 4.81°) than in the non-SS tendinopathy group (36.10° ± 3.55°; $p < 0.001$; 95% CI of difference: −4.9° to −3.5°). However, the GA, GH, and AI between the groups revealed no significant difference.

Table 2. Quantitative radiographic assessment of Supraspinatus tendinopathy (SS tendinopathy) and Non-Supraspinatus tendinopathy (non-SS tendinopathy) groups.

X-ray Index	SS Tendinopathy ($n = 308$)	Non-SS Tendinopathy ($n = 300$)	p Value
CSA	40.29 ± 4.81	36.10 ± 3.55	<0.001 *
GA	3.76 ± 0.40	3.78 ± 0.38	0.377
GH	4.96 ± 0.54	4.94 ± 0.54	0.733
AI	0.76 ± 0.08	0.77 ± 0.08	0.088

Data were presented as the mean ± standard deviation; CSA, critical shoulder angle; GA, glenoid plane to the lateral border of the acromion distance; GH, glenoid plane to the most lateral aspect of the humeral head (GH); AI, acromial index * $p < 0.05$ by Mann–Whitney U test.

The ROC curve shown in Figure 3 with the area under the curve (AUC) for CSA was 76.8%, showing acceptable discrimination for patients with SS tendinopathy. However, the AUC of AI was 46.9% for predicting patients with non-SS tendinopathy, which showed no discrimination. According to the Youden index, the cut-off point of CSA was 38.11° with a sensitivity of 71.8% and a specificity of 71.0% in predicting SS tendinopathy. (Figure 3).

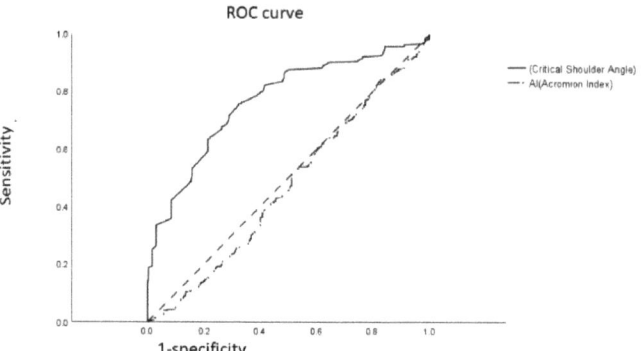

Figure 3. Receiver operating characteristic curve analysis of CSA degree and AI for predicting supraspinatus tendinopathy in patients with shoulder pain.

4. Discussion

To summarize, our results revealed that at a cut-off, CSA of 38.11° demonstrated acceptable discrimination for predicting SS tendinopathy in patients with shoulder pain. CSA showed a sensitivity of 71.8% and a specificity of 71.0%. However, AI revealed no discrimination for SS tendinopathy. This is the first study to investigate the diagnostic accuracy of SS tendinopathy in patients with shoulder pain by using CSA and AI on shoulder radiography.

Radiographic assessment is usually performed in clinics to evaluate patients with shoulder pain, with ultrasound possibly being required as a follow-up evaluation as determined by clinicians. Previous studies have revealed CSA as an objective assessment to predict rotator cuff tear, rotator cuff retear after surgery, shoulder impingement, calcified tendinitis, and glenohumeral osteoarthritis [23,24,37–39]. Our results first revealed CSA as a predictor of SS tendinopathy, which accounted for a proportion of patients with shoulder pain.

Immense stress is placed on the supraspinatus tendon, inserted under the acromion process, during shoulder abduction [7]. In addition, repetitive shoulder adduction places high loads on the supraspinatus tendon, thus causing SS tendinopathy [40,41]. Experimentally, increasing CSA would reduce the supero-inferior joint stability, leading to increased loads on the SS tendon to compensate for shoulder instability [40]. In addition, the workload of the rotator cuff increases in cases of high CSAs to counterbalance the ascending force of the deltoid, thus increasing mechanical burden and causing SS tendinopathy or tear [22]. SS tendinopathy can be a progressive disorder beginning with acute tendinitis, progressing to tendinosis with degeneration, and finally resulting in rotator cuff tear or rupture [7]. Numerous studies have demonstrated an association of CSA with rotator cuff tear or retear after surgery [23,25,39]. Theoretically, the mechanism detailed earlier could theoretically explain the relationship between CSA and SS tendinopathy.

Watanabe et al. and Heuberer et al. have reported a CSA of over 36.3° as a predictor of rotator cuff tear [24,42]. In addition, the more severe the rotator cuff tear is, the higher is CSA [43]. A recent systematic review by Zaid et al. demonstrated that several studies have reported significantly higher CSA in patients with rotator cuff tear compared to control groups [44]. Similarly, our results revealed significant differences in CSA between the SS tendinopathy and non-SS tendinopathy groups. This finding may be attributed to the same etiology that includes overload activity, muscle imbalance, shoulder impingement syndrome, and history of trauma [45,46]. In addition, SS tendinopathy is initially found before rotator cuff tear [7]; therefore, a high CSA could be a reasonable predictor of SS tendinopathy. Although SS tendinopathy may progress to supraspinatus tear, our study reported 38.11° as the cut-off of CSA for SS tendinopathy, which is higher than CSA in patients with rotator cuff tear (36° in earlier studies). This result may be attributed to the following reasons. First, our study included patients with shoulder pain, which increased the possibility of shoulder impingement caused by a high CSA; by contrast, previous studies were not limited to patients with shoulder pain [24,44]. Second, a study reported a higher CSA in degenerative rotator cuff tear than in traumatic rotator cuff tear (36.8° vs. 35.3°) [47]. Therefore, the difference in the proportion of the traumatic etiology of rotator cuff tear or SS tendinopathy may contribute to the difference in CSAs. Third, the different races may influence the type of build, which may cause different outcomes compared to previous studies.

In addition to CSA, a more lateral extension of the acromion is assumed to increase the force vector of the deltoid muscle, resulting in the subacromial abrasion of the rotator cuff tendon [25]. Based on this assumption, AI may be associated with rotator cuff tear or SS tendinopathy. Our results showed that AI is not suitable for predicting SS tendinopathy, although SS tendinopathy may potentially progress to rotator cuff tear. Miyazaki et al. reported that AI is associated with rotator cuff tear in Brazilians, but not in the Japanese population [48]; in addition, a different study revealed that AI may not be appropriate for predicting rotator cuff tear in the Taiwanese population [39]. Racial differences influencing unknown factors other than AI and impingement effect may be the reason for the conflicting results; thus, further investigation of such factors should be performed.

The strength of our study is using radiography to measure CSA for predicting SS tendinopathy in patients with shoulder pain, which was an objective assessment. CSA also demonstrated better accuracy than did AI in clinical applications for predicting SS tendinopathy. Nevertheless, our study has certain limitations. First, this was a retrospective study. To prevent heterogeneous data collection and bias of the radiographic image measurement, we controlled the demographic variables between the SS tendinopathy and non-SS tendinopathy groups by matching and standardizing the evaluation protocol of CSA and AI measurements. In addition, the assessor was blinded to the allocation of the group of patients with shoulder pain to reduce the evaluation bias. Second, morphologic parameters, such as low lateral acromion angles, anterior slope, and the shape of the acromion, were not analyzed in the study, which may affect rotator cuff pathologies [49–51]. Although these parameters of rotator cuff disease are debatable, the interaction among AI, CSA, and these parameters should be considered. Third, our study did not use MRI, which is considered a gold standard diagnostic tool, for detecting supraspinatus tendinopathy. However, considering cost, availability, safety, and efficiency of management, ultrasound is probably an option in most settings for the diagnosis of supraspinatus tendinopathy of daily practice. Finally, our study evaluated participants of a single race in Asia, and different races may affect results as previously mentioned. Finally, we evaluated only risk factors such as diabetes mellitus, hyperlipidemia, age, and BMI; factors such as biomechanical load in daily life and exercise should also be taken into account.

5. Conclusions

CSA could be used as an objective assessment tool to predict SS tendinopathy in patients with shoulder pain. Moreover, AI revealed no discrimination in predicting SS tendinopathy for patients with shoulder pain in our study. Although the AUC of CSA for predicting SS tendinopathy in patients with shoulder pain revealed acceptable discrimination, room for improvement remains. More extensive studies combined with other factors for predicting SS tendinopathy are required to strengthen the discrimination in the future.

Author Contributions: T.-H.H. and C.-L.L. drafted the first version of the manuscript. All authors were involved in all stages of the study design and participated in preparing manuscript, whereas submission to the ethical committee was done by S.-W.H. and L.-C.L. C.-W.W. and Y.-W.C. were involved in statistical analysis and interpretation. T.V. and L.-C.L. critically reviewed the manuscript. All authors approved the final manuscript. Data were accessed by T.-H.H. and L.-C.L. throughout and after the study. All authors have read and agreed to the published version of the manuscript.

Funding: This research was funded by the Taipei Medical University–Shuang Ho Hospital (110TMU-SHH-14). The funding source had no role in the design, implementation, data analysis, interpretation or reporting of this study.

Institutional Review Board Statement: The study was conducted according to the guidelines of the Declaration of Helsinki, and approved by the Institutional Review Board of Taipei Medical University (N202011086).

Informed Consent Statement: Patient consent was waived due to de-identified retrospective study design.

Data Availability Statement: Data available on request due to restrictions, e.g., privacy or ethical.

Acknowledgments: The authors would like to thank You Yi-Shuan for her assistance with the evaluation methods used in the data analyses and technical consultation.

Conflicts of Interest: The authors declare no conflict of interest.

References

1. Obaid, H.; Connell, D. Cell therapy in tendon disorders: What is the current evidence? *Am. J. Sports Med.* **2010**, *38*, 2123–2132. [CrossRef] [PubMed]
2. Bass, E. Tendinopathy: Why the difference between tendinitis and tendinosis matters. *Int. J. Ther. Massage Bodyw.* **2012**, *5*, 14–17. [CrossRef]
3. Lewis, J.S. Rotator cuff tendinopathy. *Br. J. Sports Med.* **2009**, *43*, 236. [CrossRef] [PubMed]
4. Riley, G.P.; Harrall, R.L.; Constant, C.R.; Chard, M.D.; Cawston, T.E.; Hazleman, B.L. Tendon degeneration and chronic shoulder pain: Changes in the collagen composition of the human rotator cuff tendons in rotator cuff tendinitis. *Ann. Rheum. Dis.* **1994**, *53*, 359–366. [CrossRef]
5. Hashimoto, T.; Nobuhara, K.; Hamada, T. Pathologic evidence of degeneration as a primary cause of rotator cuff tear. *Clin. Orthop. Relat. Res.* **2003**, *415*, 111–120. [CrossRef] [PubMed]
6. Scott, A.; Backman, L.J.; Speed, C. Tendinopathy: Update on Pathophysiology. *J. Orthop. Sports Phys. Ther.* **2015**, *45*, 833–841. [CrossRef]
7. Neer, C.S., 2nd. Impingement lesions. *Clin. Orthop. Relat. Res.* **1983**, *173*, 70–77. [CrossRef]
8. Neer, C.S., 2nd. Anterior acromioplasty for the chronic impingement syndrome in the shoulder: A preliminary report. *J. Bone Jt. Surg.* **1972**, *54*, 41–50. [CrossRef]
9. Leroux, J.L.; Codine, P.; Thomas, E.; Pocholle, M.; Mailhe, D.; Blotman, F. Isokinetic evaluation of rotational strength in normal shoulders and shoulders with impingement syndrome. *Clin. Orthop. Relat. Res.* **1994**, *304*, 108–115. [CrossRef]
10. Seitz, A.L.; McClure, P.W.; Finucane, S.; Boardman, N.D., 3rd; Michener, L.A. Mechanisms of rotator cuff tendinopathy: Intrinsic, extrinsic, or both? *Clin. Biomech.* **2011**, *26*, 1–12. [CrossRef]
11. MacDermid, J.C.; Ramos, J.; Drosdowech, D.; Faber, K.; Patterson, S. The impact of rotator cuff pathology on isometric and isokinetic strength, function, and quality of life. *J. Shoulder Elb. Surg.* **2004**, *13*, 593–598. [CrossRef] [PubMed]
12. Tekeoglu, I.; Ediz, L.; Hiz, O.; Toprak, M.; Yazmalar, L.; Karaaslan, G. The relationship between shoulder impingement syndrome and sleep quality. *Eur. Rev. Med. Pharm. Sci.* **2013**, *17*, 370–374.
13. Østerås, H.; Arild Torstensen, T.; Arntzen, G.; Østerås, B.S. A comparison of work absence periods and the associated costs for two different modes of exercise therapies for patients with longstanding subacromial pain. *J. Med. Econ.* **2008**, *11*, 371–381. [CrossRef] [PubMed]
14. Vecchio, P.; Kavanagh, R.; Hazleman, B.L.; King, R.H. Shoulder pain in a community-based rheumatology clinic. *Br. J. Rheumatol.* **1995**, *34*, 440–442. [CrossRef] [PubMed]
15. Tempelhof, S.; Rupp, S.; Seil, R. Age-related prevalence of rotator cuff tears in asymptomatic shoulders. *J. Shoulder Elb. Surg.* **1999**, *8*, 296–299. [CrossRef]
16. Milgrom, C.; Schaffler, M.; Gilbert, S.; van Holsbeeck, M. Rotator-cuff changes in asymptomatic adults. The effect of age, hand dominance and gender. *J. Bone Jt. Surg.* **1995**, *77*, 296–298. [CrossRef]
17. Sambandam, S.N.; Khanna, V.; Gul, A.; Mounasamy, V. Rotator cuff tears: An evidence based approach. *World J. Orthop.* **2015**, *6*, 902–918. [CrossRef]
18. Redondo-Alonso, L.; Chamorro-Moriana, G.; Jiménez-Rejano, J.J.; López-Tarrida, P.; Ridao-Fernández, C. Relationship between chronic pathologies of the supraspinatus tendon and the long head of the biceps tendon: Systematic review. *BMC Musculoskelet. Disord.* **2014**, *15*, 377. [CrossRef]
19. Hsiao, M.S.; Cameron, K.L.; Tucker, C.J.; Benigni, M.; Blaine, T.A.; Owens, B.D. Shoulder impingement in the United States military. *J. Shoulder Elb. Surg.* **2015**, *24*, 1486–1492. [CrossRef]
20. Moor, B.K.; Bouaicha, S.; Rothenfluh, D.A.; Sukthankar, A.; Gerber, C. Is there an association between the individual anatomy of the scapula and the development of rotator cuff tears or osteoarthritis of the glenohumeral joint? A radiological study of the critical shoulder angle. *Bone Jt. J.* **2013**, *95-B*, 935–941. [CrossRef]

21. Moor, B.K.; Wieser, K.; Slankamenac, K.; Gerber, C.; Bouaicha, S. Relationship of individual scapular anatomy and degenerative rotator cuff tears. *J. Shoulder Elb. Surg.* **2014**, *23*, 536–541. [CrossRef] [PubMed]
22. Moor, B.; Röthlisberger, M.; Müller, D.; Zumstein, M.; Bouaicha, S.; Ehlinger, M.; Gerber, C. Age, trauma and the critical shoulder angle accurately predict supraspinatus tendon tears. *Surg. Res.* **2014**, *100*, 489–494. [CrossRef] [PubMed]
23. Li, H.; Chen, Y.; Chen, J.; Hua, Y.; Chen, S. Large Critical Shoulder Angle Has Higher Risk of Tendon Retear After Arthroscopic Rotator Cuff Repair. *Am. J. Sports Med.* **2018**, *46*, 1892–1900. [CrossRef]
24. Heuberer, P.R.; Plachel, F.; Willinger, L.; Moroder, P.; Laky, B.; Pauzenberger, L.; Lomoschitz, F.; Anderl, W. Critical shoulder angle combined with age predict five shoulder pathologies: A retrospective analysis of 1000 cases. *BMC Musculoskelet Disord.* **2017**, *18*, 259. [CrossRef] [PubMed]
25. Nyffeler, R.W.; Werner, C.M.; Sukthankar, A.; Schmid, M.R.; Gerber, C. Association of a large lateral extension of the acromion with rotator cuff tears. *J. Bone Jt. Surg.* **2006**, *88*, 800–805. [CrossRef]
26. Kim, J.R.; Ryu, K.J.; Hong, I.T.; Kim, B.K.; Kim, J.H. Can a high acromion index predict rotator cuff tears? *Int. Orthop.* **2012**, *36*, 1019–1024. [CrossRef]
27. Lee, M.; Chen, J.Y.; Liow, M.H.L.; Chong, H.C.; Chang, P.; Lie, D. Critical Shoulder Angle and Acromial Index Do Not Influence 24-Month Functional Outcome After Arthroscopic Rotator Cuff Repair. *Am. J. Sports Med.* **2017**, *45*, 2989–2994. [CrossRef]
28. Melean, P.; Lichtenberg, S.; Montoya, F.; Riedmann, S.; Magosch, P.; Habermeyer, P. The acromial index is not predictive for failed rotator cuff repair. *Int. Orthop.* **2013**, *37*, 2173–2179. [CrossRef]
29. Blonna, D.; Giani, A.; Bellato, E.; Mattei, L.; Calo, M.; Rossi, R.; Castoldi, F. Predominance of the critical shoulder angle in the pathogenesis of degenerative diseases of the shoulder. *J. Shoulder Elb. Surg.* **2016**, *25*, 1328–1336. [CrossRef]
30. Sankaranarayanan, S.; Saks, B.R.; Holtzman, A.J.; Tabeayo, E.; Cuomo, F.; Gruson, K.I. The critical shoulder angle (CSA) in glenohumeral osteoarthritis: Does observer experience affect measurement reliability on plain radiographs? *J. Orthop.* **2020**, *22*, 160–164. [CrossRef]
31. Khan, K.; Cook, J. The painful nonruptured tendon: Clinical aspects. *Clin. Sports Med.* **2003**, *22*, 711–725. [CrossRef]
32. Itoi, E.; Tabata, S. Incomplete rotator cuff tears. Results of operative treatment. *Clin. Orthop. Relat. Res.* **1992**, *284*, 128–135. [CrossRef]
33. Itoi, E.; Kido, T.; Sano, A.; Urayama, M.; Sato, K. Which is more useful, the "full can test" or the "empty can test," in detecting the torn supraspinatus tendon? *Am. J. Sports Med.* **1999**, *27*, 65–68. [CrossRef] [PubMed]
34. Ferri, M.; Finlay, K.; Popowich, T.; Stamp, G.; Schuringa, P.; Friedman, L. Sonography of full-thickness supraspinatus tears: Comparison of patient positioning technique with surgical correlation. *AJR. Am. J. Roentgenol.* **2005**, *184*, 180–184. [CrossRef] [PubMed]
35. Bianchi, S.M.C. *Ultrasound of the Musculoskeletal System, First*; Bianchi, S., Martinolo, C., Eds.; Springer: Berlin/Heidelberg, Germany, 2007; p. 190.
36. Roy, J.-S.; Braën, C.; Leblond, J.; Desmeules, F.; Dionne, C.E.; MacDermid, J.C.; Bureau, N.J.; Frémont, P. Diagnostic accuracy of ultrasonography, MRI and MR arthrography in the characterisation of rotator cuff disorders: A systematic review and meta-analysis. *Br. J. Sports Med.* **2015**, *49*, 1316–1328. [CrossRef] [PubMed]
37. Bjarnison, A.O.; Sørensen, T.J.; Kallemose, T.; Barfod, K.W. The critical shoulder angle is associated with osteoarthritis in the shoulder but not rotator cuff tears: A retrospective case-control study. *J. Shoulder Elb. Surg.* **2017**, *26*, 2097–2102. [CrossRef] [PubMed]
38. Seo, J.; Heo, K.; Kwon, S.; Yoo, J. Critical shoulder angle and greater tuberosity angle according to the partial thickness rotator cuff tear patterns. *Orthop. Traumatol. Surg. Res.* **2019**, *105*, 1543–1548. [CrossRef]
39. Lin, C.-L.; Chen, Y.-W.; Lin, L.-F.; Chen, C.-P.; Liou, T.-H.; Huang, S.-W. Accuracy of the Critical Shoulder Angle for Predicting Rotator Cuff Tears in Patients With Nontraumatic Shoulder Pain. *Orthop. J. Sports Med.* **2020**, *8*, 2325967120918995. [CrossRef]
40. Gerber, C.; Snedeker, J.G.; Baumgartner, D.; Viehöfer, A.F. Supraspinatus tendon load during abduction is dependent on the size of the critical shoulder angle: A biomechanical analysis. *J. Orthop. Res. Off. Publ. Orthop. Res. Soc.* **2014**, *32*, 952–957. [CrossRef]
41. Viehöfer, A.F.; Gerber, C.; Favre, P.; Bachmann, E.; Snedeker, J.G. A larger critical shoulder angle requires more rotator cuff activity to preserve joint stability. *J. Orthop. Res. Off. Publ. Orthop. Res. Soc.* **2016**, *34*, 961–968. [CrossRef]
42. Watanabe, A.; Ono, Q.; Nishigami, T.; Hirooka, T.; Machida, H. Association between the Critical Shoulder Angle and Rotator Cuff Tears in Japan. *Acta Med. Okayama* **2018**, *72*, 547–551. [CrossRef] [PubMed]
43. Pandey, V.; Vijayan, D.; Tapashetti, S.; Agarwal, L.; Kamath, K.; Acharya, K.; Maddukuri, S.; Willems, W.J. Does scapular morphology affect the integrity of the rotator cuff? *J. Shoulder Elb. Surg.* **2016**, *25*, 413–421. [CrossRef] [PubMed]
44. Zaid, M.B.; Young, N.M.; Pedoia, V.; Feeley, B.T.; Ma, C.B.; Lansdown, D.A. Anatomic shoulder parameters and their relationship to the presence of degenerative rotator cuff tears and glenohumeral osteoarthritis: A systematic review and meta-analysis. *J. Shoulder Elb. Surg.* **2019**, *28*, 2457–2466. [CrossRef]
45. Smith, D.L.; Campbell, S.M. Painful shoulder syndromes: Diagnosis and management. *J. Gen. Intern. Med.* **1992**, *7*, 328–339. [CrossRef] [PubMed]
46. Yamamoto, A.; Takagishi, K.; Osawa, T.; Yanagawa, T.; Nakajima, D.; Shitara, H.; Kobayashi, T. Prevalence and risk factors of a rotator cuff tear in the general population. *J. Shoulder Elb. Surg.* **2010**, *19*, 116–120. [CrossRef] [PubMed]

47. Balke, M.; Liem, D.; Greshake, O.; Hoeher, J.; Bouillon, B.; Banerjee, M. Differences in acromial morphology of shoulders in patients with degenerative and traumatic supraspinatus tendon tears. *Knee Surg. Sports Traumatol. Arthrosc.* **2016**, *24*, 2200–2205. [CrossRef] [PubMed]
48. Miyazaki, A.N.; Itoi, E.; Sano, H.; Fregoneze, M.; Santos, P.D.; da Silva, L.A.; Sella Gdo, V.; Martel, E.M.; Debom, L.G.; Andrade, M.L.; et al. Comparison between the acromion index and rotator cuff tears in the Brazilian and Japanese populations. *J. Shoulder Elb. Surg.* **2011**, *20*, 1082–1086. [CrossRef]
49. Balke, M.; Schmidt, C.; Dedy, N.; Banerjee, M.; Bouillon, B.; Liem, D. Correlation of acromial morphology with impingement syndrome and rotator cuff tears. *Acta Orthop.* **2013**, *84*, 178–183. [CrossRef]
50. Chalmers, P.N.; Beck, L.; Miller, M.; Kawakami, J.; Dukas, A.G.; Burks, R.T.; Greis, P.E.; Tashjian, R.Z. Acromial morphology is not associated with rotator cuff tearing or repair healing. *J. Shoulder Elb. Surg.* **2020**, *29*, 2229–2239. [CrossRef]
51. Andrade, R.; Correia, A.L.; Nunes, J.; Xará-Leite, F.; Calvo, E.; Espregueira-Mendes, J.; Sevivas, N. Is Bony Morphology and Morphometry Associated With Degenerative Full-Thickness Rotator Cuff Tears? A Systematic Review and Meta-analysis. *Arthrosc. J. Arthrosc. Relat. Surg.* **2019**, *35*, 3304–3315.e2. [CrossRef]

Interesting Images

Visualization of Dialysis-Related Amyloid Arthropathy on ^{18}F-FDG PET-CT Scan

Miju Cheon * and Jang Yoo

Department of Nuclear Medicine, Veterans Health Service Medical Center, Seoul 05368, Korea; jang8214.yoo@gmail.com
* Correspondence: diva1813@naver.com

Abstract: We report a case of dialysis-related amyloid arthropathy in a patient with end-stage renal disease. It presented in our patient as moderately increased FDG uptake in the amyloid deposition in the periarticular tissues and eroding into adjacent bones.

Keywords: dialysis-related amyloidosis; amyloid arthropathy; long-term dialysis; FDG; PET-CT

A 76-year-old male patient with end-stage renal disease, secondary to polycystic kidney disease, presented with worsening swelling and pain in both shoulders and hips. He had been on regular hemodialysis for 20 years. On examination, there was pain, swelling and restriction of movements of the shoulder, wrist and hip. ^{18}F-FDG PET-CT was performed to evaluate for renal mass observed during a regular follow-up for polycystic kidney disease. ^{18}F-FDG PET-CT was performed using a standard PET-CT scanner (Discovery Molecular Imaging Digital Ready, GE Healthcare, Waukesha, WI, USA). The patient had fasted for six hours before scanning, and two sequential PET and CT scans were acquired at 60 min after ^{18}F-FDG injection (175 MBq). The PET-CT demonstrated several hypermetabolic masses suggesting malignant lesions in both kidneys (Figure 1). There was also increased metabolic activity in thickened soft tissues surrounding hips (maximum SUV 5.52 on the left and 4.51 on the right), shoulders (Figure 2), left elbow and left wrist (Figure 3). A cystic collection along the right subscapularis and supraspinatus muscle was not hypermetabolic, but surrounded by a hypermetabolic rim. The associated non-contrast CT obtained in PET-CT imaging showed osseous erosions of both humeral and femoral heads.

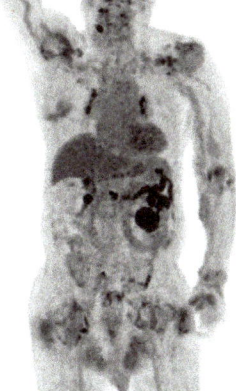

Figure 1. Maximum intensity projection of ^{18}F-FDG PET-CT demonstrated increased metabolic activity in the shoulders, left elbow, left wrist, left hand and hips.

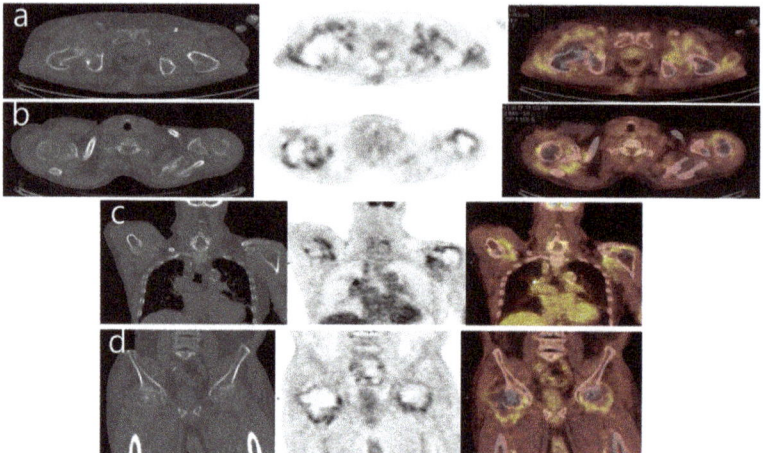

Figure 2. ^{18}F-FDG PET-CT axial (**a**,**b**) and coronal (**c**,**d**) images of both shoulders and hips demonstrate diffuse periarticular uptake. Non-contrast CT obtained in conjunction with PET-CT imaging showed osseous erosions involve both humeral and femoral heads.

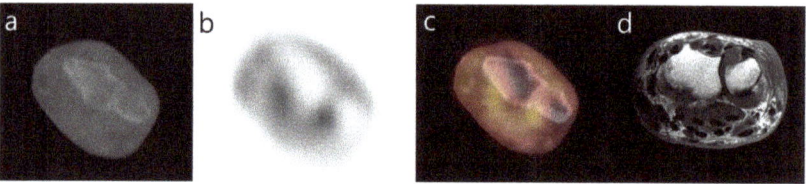

Figure 3. Axial ^{18}F-FDG PET-CT image (**a**–**c**) of the left wrist demonstrates periarticular uptake and associated osseous erosions. Axial T1-weighted MR image (**d**) reconfirms erosion and periarticular hypointense amyloid deposits.

Protein electrophoresis showed no monoclonal gammopathy. Serum kappa was 208.99 mg/L (normal 3.3–19.4 mg/L) and serum Lambda was 195.15 mg/L (5.71–26.3 mg/L) with a normal kappa-to-lambda ratio of 1.05 (normal 0.26–1.65). Serum β2-microglobulin was increased as 19.55 mg/L (normal 1.0–2.4 mg/L). Serum CRP and calcium were normal. Rheumatoid factor and anti-CCP antibodies were negative. No significant myocardial uptake was observed in the bone scan obtained after injection of ^{99m}Tc-hydroxymethylene diphosphonate (HDP), which was performed to exclude rheumatoid arthritis due to arthralgia (Figure 4). Eventually, the patient underwent joint aspiration, and cytology revealed the presence of amyloidal deposits. Those findings were compatible with dialysis-related amyloid arthropathy.

Amyloidosis is characterized by the extracellular deposition of protein and protein derivatives. Dialysis-related amyloidosis (DRA) is a well-recognized and serious complication in patients on long-term dialysis. The duration of dialysis appeared to be a predominant risk factor, because amyloidosis occurred in patients with dialysis duration above 15 years [1]. DRA is characterized by the amyloid deposition with β2-microglobulin in the osteoarticular structure and viscera. Amyloid deposition with β2-microglobulin has a high affinity for collagen and predominantly affects the osteoarticular system [2]. Frequent sites of involvement are the shoulders, wrists, hips, knees and the carpal tunnel. Because the clinical manifestations of amyloid arthropathy can be easily confused with other polyarticular forms of arthritis such as rheumatoid arthritis, we should consider this diagnosis, particularly in patients with multiple myeloma or other predisposing conditions.

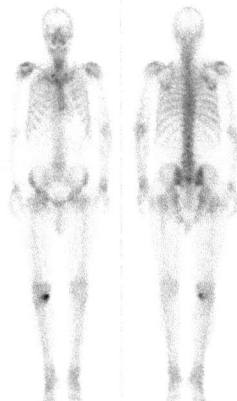

Figure 4. Bone scintigraphy with technetium-99m hydroxymethylene diphophonate (HDP) shows no cardiac accumulation.

We report a case where the ^{18}F-FDG PET-CT allows the identification of several DRA-associated lesions in the articular and periarticular soft tissues in a patient under long-term dialysis therapy. There were only a few reports dealing with ^{18}F-FDG PET-CT findings on DRA [3,4]. It suggests that ^{18}F-FDG PET-CT could be a non-invasive imaging modality showing the extent and distribution of osseous, articular and soft-tissue involvement in dialysis-related amyloid arthropathy.

Author Contributions: M.C.: involved in initial drafting of manuscript. J.Y.: involved in review of the images. All authors have read and agreed to the published version of the manuscript.

Funding: This research received no external funding.

Institutional Review Board Statement: The study was conducted according to the guidelines of the Declaration of Helsinki, and ethical review and approval were waived for the single case report.

Informed Consent Statement: Written informed consent has been obtained from the patient to publish this paper.

Data Availability Statement: The data that support the findings of this study are available from the corresponding author M.C., upon reasonable request.

Conflicts of Interest: The authors declare no conflict of interest.

References

1. van Ypersele de Strihou, C. Morphogenèse des dépôts d'amyloïde à beta 2m (A beta 2m) chez le patient en dialyse [Morphogenesis of beta 2m (A beta 2m) amyloid deposits in dialysis patients]. *Bull. Mem. Acad. R. Med. Belg.* **2000**, *155*, 273–278. [PubMed]
2. Sigaux, J.; Abdelkefi, I.; Bardin, T.; Laredo, J.D.; Ea, H.K.; UreñaTorres, P.; Cohen-Solal, M. Tendon thickening in dialysis-related joint arthritis is due to amyloid deposits at the surface of the tendon. *Jt. Bone Spine* **2019**, *86*, 233–238. [CrossRef] [PubMed]
3. Santagati, G.; Cataldo, E.; Columbano, V.; Chatrenet, A.; Penna, D.; Pelosi, E.; Hachemi, M.; Gendrot, L.; Nielsen, L.; Cinquantini, F.; et al. Positron Emission Tomography Can Support the Diagnosis of Dialysis-Related Amyloidosis. *J. Clin. Med.* **2019**, *19*, 1494. [CrossRef] [PubMed]
4. Piccoli, G.B.; Hachemi, M.; Molfino, I.; Coindre, J.P.; Boursot, C. Doxycycline treatment in dialysis related amyloidosis: Discrepancy between antalgic effect and inflammation, studied with FDG-positron emission tomography: A case report. *BMC Nephrol.* **2017**, *6*, 285. [CrossRef] [PubMed]

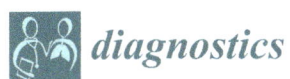

Article

Incidence of Spinal CSF Leakage on CT Myelography in Patients with Nontraumatic Intracranial Subdural Hematoma

Hyo Jin Kim [1,2], Joon Woo Lee [1,3,*], Eugene Lee [1], Yusuhn Kang [1] and Joong Mo Ahn [1]

[1] Department of Radiology, Seoul National University Bundang Hospital, 82 Gumi-ro 173 Beon-gil, Bundang-gu, Seongnam 13620, Korea; khjsm4@gmail.com (H.J.K.); eugene801027@gmail.com (E.L.); yskang0114@gmail.com (Y.K.); joongmoahn@gmail.com (J.M.A.)
[2] Department of Radiology, Seoul Metropolitan Government-Seoul National University Boramae Medical Center, Seoul National University College of Medicine, 20 Boramae-ro 5-gil, Dongjak-gu, Seoul 07061, Korea
[3] Department of Radiology, Seoul National University College of Medicine, Seoul 03080, Korea
* Correspondence: joonwoo2@gmail.com

Abstract: The aim of the present study was to demonstrate the incidence of spinal cerebrospinal fluid (CSF) leaks in patients with nontraumatic intracranial subdural hematoma (SDH) and determine clinical parameters favoring such leaks. This retrospective study was approved by the institutional review board. Patients diagnosed with nontraumatic intracranial SDH who underwent computed tomography (CT) myelography between January 2012 and March 2018 were selected. 60 patients (male: female, 39:21; age range, 20–82 years) were enrolled and divided into CSF leak-positive and CSF leak-negative groups according to CT myelography data. Clinical findings were statistically compared between the two groups. Spinal CSF leak was observed in 80% (48/60) of patients, and it was significantly associated with an age of <69 years ($p = 0.006$). However, patients aged ≥69 years also had a tendency to exhibit spontaneous intracranial hypotension (SIH)-induced nontraumatic intracranial SDH (60.87%; 14/23). Therefore, CT myelography is recommended to be performed for the evaluation of possible SIH in patients with nontraumatic intracranial SDH, particularly those aged <69 years. Patients aged ≥69 years are also good candidates for CT myelography because SIH tends to occur even in this age group.

Keywords: intracranial subdural hematoma; spontaneous intracranial hypotension; CT myelography; epidural blood patch

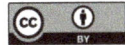

1. Introduction

Nontraumatic intracranial subdural hematoma (SDH) can be induced by a variety of causes. Hypertensive cortical artery rupture [1], middle meningeal artery aneurysm rupture [2], idiopathic bleeding, coagulopathy, oncological bleeding, and cocaine-induced bleeding have been reported as causative factors for acute SDH [3]. Causative factors for chronic SDH include stretching of bridging veins due to extensive brain atrophy, fragile neovasculatures associated with neomembrane formation after subdural hygroma or acute SDH [4]. For both acute and chronic SDH, conservative management (reversal of anticoagulation and prophylactic anticonvulsants) or surgical treatment (hematoma evacuation) is used depending on the patient's symptoms and extent of hematoma [4].

Spontaneous intracranial hypotension (SIH) can also result in nontraumatic SDH. SIH is a disorder characterized by decreased cerebrospinal fluid (CSF) volume and pressure, and it is caused by a persistent CSF leak through a dural defect along the neuraxis [5]. Spontaneous focal dural thinning and dehiscence are common causes of CSF leaks. Degenerative abnormalities of the spine, including disk protrusions and osteophytes, may also result in thecal sac tears. Although some authors also report CSF–venous fistula as one of the causes, this remains a topic of speculation [6]. A CSF leak can result in downward traction on the brain, causing headaches, subdural fluid collection, and possible brain herniation [5].

Occasionally, tearing of the bridging veins results in SDH [7]. In such cases, hematoma evacuation prior to repair of the CSF leak may be ineffective, and untreated downward traction can lead to further postoperative accumulation of SDH [8]. Therefore, for optimal treatment of some patients with SDH, clinicians should recognize the possibility of SIH as a cause of hematoma and search for CSF leaks requiring repair with procedures such as an epidural blood patch (EBP) [8]. When dealing with patients with SDH, the differential diagnosis of SIH should be emphasized, particularly in younger patients, patients without a history of head trauma, and patients with postural headaches [9]. Currently, computed tomography (CT) myelography is considered the gold standard for the initial evaluation of SIH [10–12] because it offers superior anatomic details [13].

Beck [14] conducted a prospective study and reported that spinal CSF leaks were present in 25.9% of nongeriatric patients ($\leq$60 years) with chronic SDH. However, to the best of our knowledge, there is no other structured study on the incidence of imaging-confirmed CSF leaks in patients with SDH. Since 2012, neurosurgeons at our institution request CT myelography to rule out SIH in patients with nontraumatic SDH without any explainable cause. If a CSF leak is detected on CT myelography, EBP is performed. Accordingly, we have observed a higher rate of CSF leaks than that reported in Beck's study. Therefore, we designed the present study to demonstrate the incidence of spinal CSF leaks and determine potential clinical parameters favoring such leaks in patients with nontraumatic SDH.

2. Materials and Methods

2.1. Patients

This retrospective study was approved by the institutional review board of our hospital, which waived the need for informed consent because of the retrospective study design. Neurosurgeons at our institution requested CT myelography to rule out SIH in patients with nontraumatic SDH without any explainable cause. Two research assistants went through the hospital's electronic medical records between January 2012 and March 2018 then retrieved the details of patients diagnosed with SDH and subjected to CT myelography. The following inclusion criteria were applied to the patients identified from the medical records: no history of trauma, absence of coagulopathy according to a coagulation panel and platelet count measurements, absence of intracranial mass lesions susceptible to spontaneous bleeding, no history of drug abuse, performance of follow-up brain imaging at three months after treatment for SDH, and age >18 years. Eventually, 60 patients (male:female, 39:21; mean age, 58.65 ± 15.52 years; range, 20–82 years) were included. According to the previously written reports of CT myelography, the patients were divided into CSF leak-positive and CSF leak-negative groups.

2.2. Retrospective Review of Electronic Medical Records and Imaging Findings

A radiologist who was blinded from CT myelography reports retrospectively reviewed the patients' demographic data, Glasgow coma scale scores, anticoagulant use, presence or absence of orthostatic headache at the first visit, laterality of SDH and the degree of midline shift in initial images, treatment the patients underwent, and follow-up findings in brain images taken within, and at three months [15,16] after treatment for SDH. The radiologist also recorded whether recurrence had developed on follow-up brain images. We defined 'recurrence' of SDH as a subsequent increase in hematoma volume in subdural space and compression of the brain surface after treatment by referring to the previous several studies [16,17].

2.3. Statistical Analysis

To determine variables that were significantly associated with CSF leaks, the medical records for CSF leak-positive and leak-negative groups were analyzed using chi-square tests/Fisher's exact tests for discrete variables and t-tests for continuous variables. A p-value of <0.05 was considered statistically significant.

2.4. Our Routine CT Myelography Procedure & Interpretation

In a fluoroscopy room, the patient is placed on a radiolucent table in the lateral decubitus position, with the right side up and knee flexed. Using a midline interlaminar approach between the third and fourth lumbar vertebrae under fluoroscopy guidance, a trained musculoskeletal radiologist inserts a 22-gauge spinal needle into the CSF space. Following the confirmation of CSF drainage via the spinal needle, 15 cc of contrast medium (OMNIPAQUE 300, Amersham Health, Princeton, NJ, USA) is slowly injected through the needle. When the contrast medium reached the spinal canal at the atlantooccipital level, the patients are transferred to the CT unit for whole-spine imaging, and the acquired data are presented in axial, sagittal, and coronal planes (Brilliance 64 CT scanner, Philips Healthcare, Best, Netherlands; helical; beam collimation, 64×0.625 mm; kVp, 120; mAs, 250; pitch, 0.798; rotation time, 0.5 s; thickness, 2 mm; increment, 1 mm).

Trained musculoskeletal radiologists immediately interpret the obtained images to confirm the presence of contrast media leakage (=CSF leak) exists. A positive CSF leak is defined as extrathecal CSF accumulation at any level. Meningeal diverticula are not considered as CSF leaks because single or multiple nerve root sleeve diverticula of various sizes and configurations can be seen as incidental findings [6].

2.5. Our Routine EBP Procedure

If CSF leaks are confirmed by CT myelography, targeted EBP with autologous blood is performed under fluoroscopic guidance. If there are multiple leaks, EBP is performed at the mid-level of the leaks in order to ensure the widest coverage. Generally, 10 cc of blood is used for each targeted level, and a total of up to 20 cc of blood is used.

3. Results

In total, 48 of the 60 (80%) patients exhibited CSF leaks on CT myelography. Differences in parameters between the leak-positive and leak-negative groups are shown in Table 1.

Table 1. Statistical Analysis of Parameters for Patients with Cerebrospinal Fluid Leaks and Those without Leaks among a Cohort of Patients with Nontraumatic Intracranial Subdural Hematoma.

	Leak (+) Total N = 48	Leak (−) Total N = 12	*p*-Value
Male sex, n (%)	31 (64.58)	8 (66.67)	1.000
Mean age ± standard deviation	56.85 ± 15.50	65.83 ± 13.93	0.165
Age < 69, n (%)	34 (70.83)	3 (25.00)	0.006
Wafarin, n (%)	0 (0.00)	1 (8.33)	0.200
Aspirin, n (%)	8 (16.67)	1 (8.33)	0.671
Clopidogrel, n (%)	3 (6.25)	0 (0.00)	1.000
Orthostatic headache, n (%)	12 (25.00)	1 (8.33)	0.628
Glasgow coma scale score of 15, n (%)	48 (100.00)	12 (100.00)	N/A
Unilateral subdural hematoma, n (%)	9 (18.75)	5 (41.67)	0.13
The degree of midline shift (mm ± standard deviation)	3.34 ± 3.47	3.82 ± 4.46	0.29

The proportions of patients aged <69 years ($p = 0.006$) were significantly higher in the leak-positive group than in the leak-negative group. However, patients aged ≥69 years also had a tendency to exhibit SIH-induced SDH (14/23; 60.87%).

Targeted EBP was performed for all 48 leak-positive patients, with 31 undergoing surgical removal of hematoma as well as EBP. From these 31 patients, three developed recurrence repeatedly after several surgeries but showed complete resolution following one or two EBP procedures; 10 patients developed recurrence after a single EBP procedure and necessitated repeated EBP from one to three times with surgical evacuation (eight patients needed one surgery and two patients required two surgeries) until there was no recurrence; 18 underwent surgery and EBP at about the same time (within 24 h), and among them, one had additional surgery due to recurrence; meanwhile, the other 17 did not have to undergo further invasive procedures (Figures 1 and 2A–E).

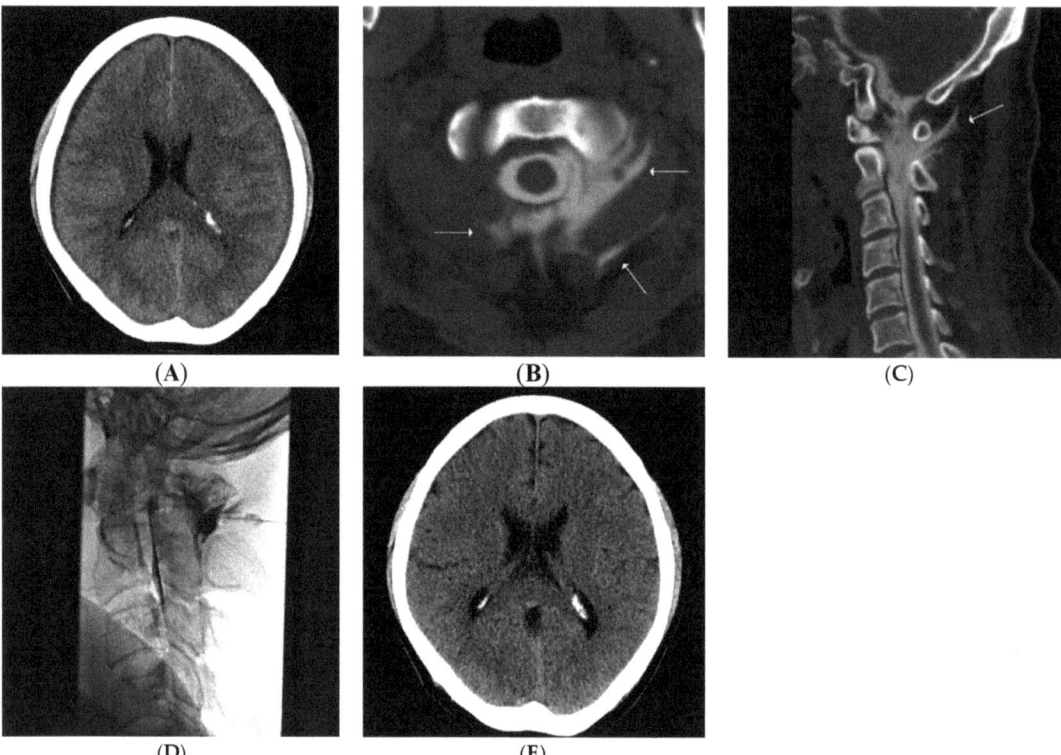

Figure 1. (A–E) Findings for a representative case involving a 53-year-old man with nontraumatic intracranial subdural hematoma (SDH). The patient presented with a chief complaint of headache not related to a specific posture. (A). Brain computed tomography (CT) image shows bilateral intracranial SDH. He was referred to us for CT myelography and epidural blood patch (EBP) the day after undergoing burr-hole trephination and hematoma removal. (B,C). Axial and sagittal CT myelography images show a large amount of cerebrospinal fluid leaks at the level of the C1/2 left extradural space (solid arrows). (D) EBP is performed at the C1/2 level. (E). Follow-up brain CT performed after 3 months shows no evidence of SDH.

Of the 17 patients who underwent EBP only, 14 developed no recurrence (Figure 3A–F) and three developed recurrence after a single EBP procedure; the latter three patients underwent a second EBP procedure and did not develop recurrence thereafter.

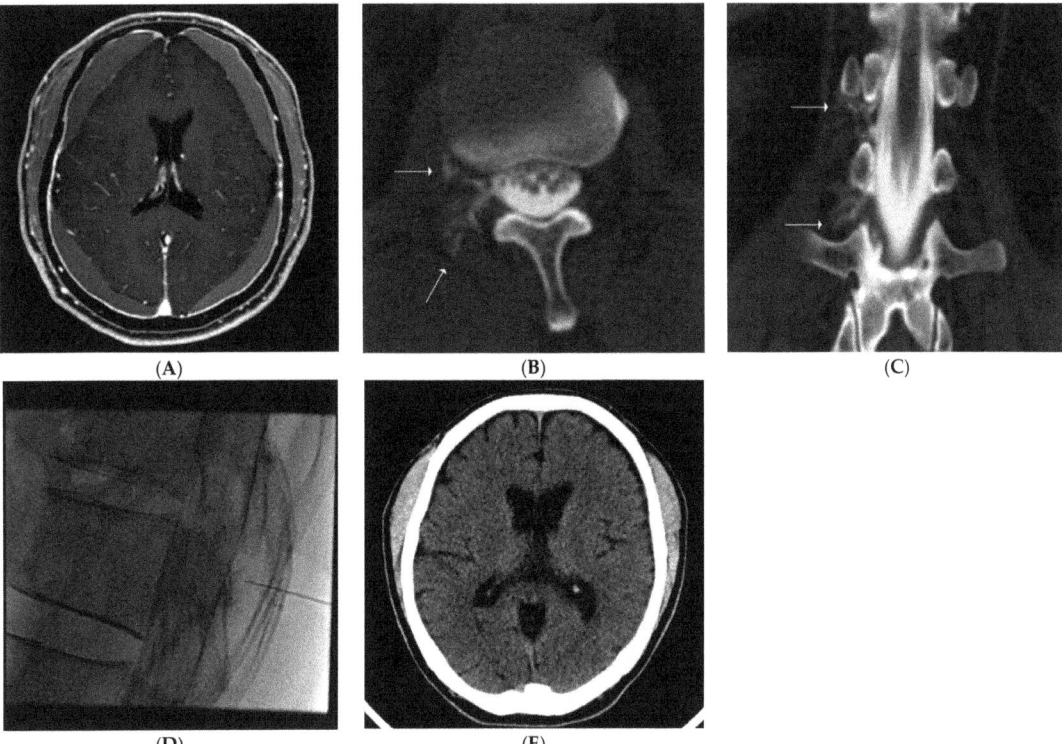

Figure 2. (**A–E**). Findings for a representative case involving a 70-year-old man with nontraumatic intracranial subdural hematoma (SDH). The patient presented with a chief complaint of headache not related to a specific posture. (**A**). Contrast-enhanced, fat-suppressed T1 weighted image shows bilateral nontraumatic SDH with pachymeningeal thickening and enhancement. (**B**,**C**). Axial and coronal computed tomography (CT) myelography images show cerebrospinal fluid leaks at the level of the T12/L1 and the L1/2 right extradural space (solid arrows). (**D**). An epidural blood patch is performed at the T12/L1 level. Intrathecal staining is present due to a previously injected contrast agent for CT myelography. (**E**). Follow-up brain CT performed after 3 months shows no evidence of SDH.

Of the 12 leak-negative patients, eight underwent surgical removal of hematoma, one underwent both surgical removal of hematoma and EBP, and one underwent EBP alone. The latter two patients underwent empirical nontargeted EBP at the discretion of neurosurgeons, although they showed negative CT myelography findings. The remaining two patients only received conservative management. All 12 leak-negative patients showed hematoma resolution with no recurrence after treatment.

A total of 40 patients required surgery for nontraumatic SDH. In the leak-positive group, a total of 31 patients underwent surgery; burr-hole trephination and hematoma removal in 25 patients, and craniotomy in 6 patients. In the leak-negative group, a total of 9 patients underwent surgery; burr-hole trephination and hematoma removal in 7 patients and craniotomy in 2 patients. The reoperation rate after EBP was 7.5%.

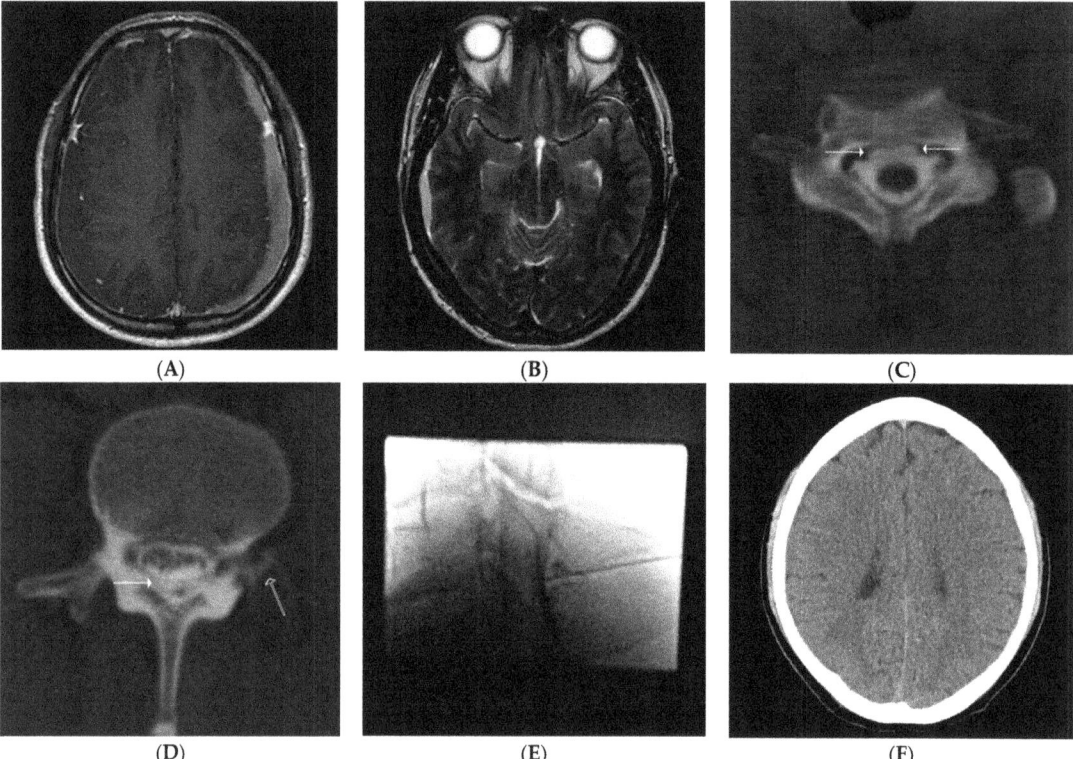

Figure 3. (**A**–**F**). Findings for a representative case involving a 41-year-old man with nontraumatic intracranial subdural hematoma (SDH). The patient presented with a chief complaint of headache not related to a specific posture. (**A**). Contrast-enhanced, fat-suppressed T1 weighted image shows bilateral nontraumatic SDH with pachymeningeal thickening and enhancement. (**B**). T2 weighted image at the initial presentation shows cisternal obliteration. (**C**,**D**). Computed tomography (CT) myelography performed to evaluate possible spontaneous intracranial hypotension shows cerebrospinal fluid leaks at the level of the C6/7 ventral epidural space (solid arrows, (**C**)), the L2/3 dorsal epidural space (a solid arrow, (**D**)), and the left extraforaminal space (a hollow arrow, (**D**)). (**E**). Subsequent epidural blood patch is performed at the C6/7 and L2/3 (not shown) levels. (**F**). Follow-up brain CT performed after 3 months shows no evidence of SDH.

4. Discussion

The present study revealed that the incidence of spinal CSF leaks was 80% in patients with nontraumatic SDH. An age of <69 years was significantly associated with the presence of CSF leaks, although patients aged ≥69 years also tended to exhibit SIH-induced SDH (60.87%). A total of 40 patients required surgery. The reoperation rate after EBP was 7.5%.

The standard management strategy for SDH generally involves decompression surgery or conservative care with close observation depending on the age of the hematoma, degree of the midline shift, clot thickness, and neurological status [4,18]. However, a different treatment strategy is necessary for the sealing of CSF leaks in patients with SIH-induced SDH [19–22]. Therefore, for optimal treatment in some patients with SDH, recognition of the possibility of SIH as a cause of SDH is important [8]. In a study of the incidence of imaging-confirmed CSF leaks in patients with SDH, Beck [14] found that spinal CSF leaks were present in 25.9% nongeriatric patients (≤60 years) with chronic SDH. In the present study, we detected leaks in 80% patients with nontraumatic SDH who underwent CT myelography to rule out suspected SIH. This rate is considerably higher than that reported by Beck. Additionally, SIH-induced SDH was also seen in older age groups than in the study by Beck. These suggest that clinicians need to broaden their scope of doubt regarding SIH and expand the indications for studies to detect CSF leaks, such as CT myelography, in patients with nontraumatic SDH.

It would be interesting to know why the leak-positive and leak-negative groups showed no significant difference with regard to the presence of orthostatic headache, one of the most famous clinical findings of SIH. One reason could be that orthostatic headache may be seen even in the presence of relatively small leaks that are not large enough to be detected on CT myelography. In such cases, magnetic resonance myelography with intrathecal gadolinium, which is considered an effective medium for the detection of low flow leaks, can be considered [6]. However, considering that all of our leak-negative patients who did not receive EBP showed no recurrence or aggravation of symptoms, we recommend that slow, intermittent, or small leaks that are not detectable on CT myelography may not always require identification or EBP.

The percentage of reoperation in patients with SDH varies depending on the literature. According to one study, the reoperation rate for chronic SDH is 9.4 to 19.5% [15]. In the current study, 40 patients underwent surgical removal of hematoma, and among them, three patients needed reoperation (7.5%) after EBP. This figure is lower than previously reported, and it suggests that timely EBP may allow a good outcome in patients with SIH-induced SDH.

This study has several limitations. First, although the leak-positive rate revealed by imaging studies was higher than that in the previous study, there could have been differences in the CT myelography protocol between the previous study and our study in terms of the radiation dose, slice thickness, pitch, and reconstruction interval. Because there was no exact match between the test conditions, the comparison between the two studies may have limited value. Second, this was a retrospective study, and the sample size was relatively small. Larger-scale, prospective studies may be needed to further clarify our findings.

5. Conclusions

In conclusion, the findings of the present study suggest that CT myelography is recommended to be performed for the evaluation of possible SIH in patients with nontraumatic SDH, particularly those aged <69 years. Patients aged ≥69 years are also good candidates for CT myelography because SIH tends to occur even in this age group.

Author Contributions: Conceptualization, J.W.L.; methodology, J.W.L. and H.J.K.; data acquisition, analysis, and interpretation, J.W.L., E.L. and H.J.K.; writing—original draft preparation, J.W.L. and H.J.K.; writing—review and editing, E.L., Y.K and J.M.A. All authors have read and agreed to the published version of the manuscript.

Funding: This research received no external funding.

Institutional Review Board Statement: The study was conducted according to the guidelines of the Declaration of Helsinki and approved by the Institutional Review Board of Seoul National University Bundang Hospital (B-1809-492-108, 30 August 2018).

Informed Consent Statement: Patient consent was waived because of the retrospective study design.

Data Availability Statement: The data presented in this study are available on request from the corresponding author. The data are not publicly available due to privacy.

Conflicts of Interest: The authors declare no conflict of interest.

References

1. Avis, S.P. Nontraumatic acute subdural hematoma: A case report and review of the literature. *Am. J. Forensic Med. Pathol.* **1993**, *14*, 130–134. [CrossRef] [PubMed]
2. Korosue, K.; Kondoh, T.; Ishikawa, Y.; Nagao, T.; Tamaki, N.; Matsumoto, S. Acute subdural hematoma associated with nontraumatic middle meningeal artery aneurysm: Case report. *Neurosurgery* **1988**, *22*, 411–413. [CrossRef] [PubMed]

3. Coombs, J.B.; Coombs, B.L.; Chin, E.J. Acute spontaneous subdural hematoma in a middle-aged adult: Case report and review of the literature. *J. Emerg. Med.* **2014**, *47*, e63–e68. [CrossRef] [PubMed]
4. Ducruet, A.F.; Grobelny, B.T.; Zacharia, B.; Hickman, Z.; DeRosa, P.L.; Anderson, K.; Sussman, E.; Carpenter, A.; Connolly, E.S. The surgical management of chronic subdural hematoma. *Neurosurg. Rev.* **2012**, *35*, 155–169. [CrossRef] [PubMed]
5. Davidson, B.; Nassiri, F.; Mansouri, A.; Badhiwala, J.H.; Witiw, C.D.; Shamji, M.F.; Peng, P.W.; Farb, R.I.; Bernstein, M. Spontaneous intracranial hypotension: A review and introduction of an algorithm for management. *World Neurosurg.* **2017**, *101*, 343–349. [CrossRef]
6. Kranz, P.; Luetmer, P.H.; Diehn, F.E.; Amrhein, T.J.; Tanpitukpongse, T.P.; Gray, L. Myelographic techniques for the detection of spinal CSF leaks in spontaneous intracranial hypotension. *Am. J. Roentgenol.* **2016**, *206*, 8–19. [CrossRef]
7. Ferrante, E.; Rubino, F.; Beretta, F.; Regna-Gladin, C.; Ferrante, M.M. Treatment and outcome of subdural hematoma in patients with spontaneous intracranial hypotension: A report of 35 cases. *Acta Neurol. Belg.* **2018**, *118*, 61–70. [CrossRef]
8. Inamasu, J.; Moriya, S.; Shibata, J.; Kumai, T.; Hirose, Y. Spontaneous intracranial hypotension manifesting as a unilateral subdural hematoma with a marked midline shift. *Case Rep. Neurol.* **2015**, *7*, 71–77. [CrossRef]
9. Wan, Y.; Xie, J.; Xie, D.; Xue, Z.; Wang, Y.; Yang, S. Clinical characteristics of 15 cases of chronic subdural hematomas due to spontaneous intracranial hypotension with spinal cerebrospinal fluid leak. *Acta Neurol. Belg.* **2016**, *116*, 509–512. [CrossRef]
10. Wendl, C.M.; Schambach, F.; Zimmer, C.; Foerschler, A. CT myelography for the planning and guidance of targeted epidural blood patches in patients with persistent spinal CSF leak. *Am. J. Neuroradiol.* **2012**, *24*, 1711–1714.
11. Mokri, B.; Piepgras, D.G.; Miller, G.M. Syndrome of orthostatic headaches and diffuse pachymeningeal gadolinium enhancement. *Mayo. Clin. Proc.* **2007**, *72*, 400–413. [CrossRef]
12. Schievink, W.I.; Deline, C.R. Headache secondary to intracranial hypotension. *Curr. Pain. Headache Rep.* **2014**, *18*, 457. [CrossRef] [PubMed]
13. Kranz, P.G.; Malinzak, M.D.; Amrhein, T.J.; Gray, L. Update on the diagnosis and treatment of spontaneous intracranial hypotension. *Curr. Pain Headache Rep.* **2017**, *21*, 37. [CrossRef]
14. Beck, J.; Gralla, J.; Fung, C.; Ulrich, C.T.; Schucht, P.; Fichtner, J.; Andereggen, L.; Gosau, M.; Hattingen, E.; Gutbrod, K.; et al. Spinal cerebrospinal fluid leak as the cause of chronic subdural hematomas in nongeriatric patients. *J. Neurosurg.* **2014**, *121*, 1380–1387. [CrossRef]
15. Motiei-Langroudi, R.; Stippler, M.; Shi, S.; Adeeb, N.; Gupta, R.; Griessenauer, C.J.; Papavassiliou, E.; Kasper, E.M.; Arle, J.; Alterman, R.L.; et al. Factors predicting reoperation of chronic subdural hematoma following primary surgical evacuation. CT-guided epidural blood patching of directly observed or potential leak sites for the targeted treatment of spontaneous intracranial hypotension. *J. Neurosurg.* **2017**, *129*, 1143–1150. [CrossRef] [PubMed]
16. Nakaguchi, H.; Tanishima, T.; Yoshimasu, N. Factors in the natural history of chronic subdural hematomas that influence their postoperative recurrence. *J. Neurosurg.* **2001**, *95*, 256–262. [CrossRef] [PubMed]
17. Torihashi, K.; Sadamasa, N.; Yoshida, K.; Narumi, O.; Chin, M.; Yamagata, S. Independent predictors for recurrence of chronic subdural hematoma: A review of 343 consecutive surgical cases. *Neurosurgery* **2008**, *63*, 1125–1129. [CrossRef] [PubMed]
18. Bullock, M.R.; Chesnut, R.; Ghajar, J.; Gordon, D.; Hartl, R.; Newell, D.W.; Servadei, F.; Walters, B.C.; Wilberger, J.E. Surgical management of acute subdural hematomas. *Neurosurgery* **2006**, *58*, S2-16–S2-24.
19. Nishizaki, T.; Ikeda, N.; Nakano, S.; Sakakura, T.; Fujii, N.; Okamura, T. Clinical status of patients with cerebrospinal fluid hypovolemia treated with an epidural blood patch. *Open J. Mod. Neurosurg.* **2015**, *5*, 107–112. [CrossRef]
20. Ferrante, E.; Olgiati, E.; Sangalli, V.; Rubino, F. Early pain relief from orthostatic headache and hearing changes in spontaneous intracranial hypotension after epidural blood patch. *Acta Neurol. Belg.* **2016**, *116*, 503–508. [CrossRef]
21. Staudt, M.D.; Pasternak, S.H.; Sharma, M.; Pandey, S.K.; Arango, M.F.; Pelz, D.M.; Lownie, S.P. Multilevel, ultra-large-volume epidural blood patch for the treatment of neurocognitive decline associated with spontaneous intracranial hypotension: Case report. *J. Neurosurg.* **2018**, *129*, 205–210. [CrossRef] [PubMed]
22. Wong, K.; Monroe, B.R. Successful treatment of postdural puncture headache using epidural fibrin glue patch after persistent failure of epidural blood patches. *Pain Pract.* **2017**, *17*, 956–960. [CrossRef] [PubMed]

MDPI
St. Alban-Anlage 66
4052 Basel
Switzerland
Tel. +41 61 683 77 34
Fax +41 61 302 89 18
www.mdpi.com

Diagnostics Editorial Office
E-mail: diagnostics@mdpi.com
www.mdpi.com/journal/diagnostics

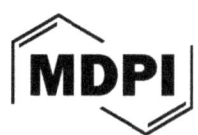

www.ingramcontent.com/pod-product-compliance
Lightning Source LLC
LaVergne TN
LVHW070451100526
838202LV00014B/1703